Ingomar-Werner Franz

Ergometry in Hypertensive Patients

Implications for Diagnosis and Treatment

Translated by Terry Telger

Foreword by P. Schölmerich

With 78 Figures and 63 Tables

Springer-Verlag
Berlin Heidelberg New York Tokyo

Prof. Dr. med. Ingomar-Werner Franz

Institut für Leistungsmedizin und Kardiologische Abteilung,
Klinikum Charlottenburg, Freie Universität Berlin,
Forckenbeckstraße 20, 1000 Berlin 33, BRD

Terry Telger
3429 Cloer Drive, Fort Worth
Texas 76109, USA

ISBN-13: 978-3-642-70374-4 e-ISBN-13: 978-3-642-70372-0
DOI: 10.1007/978-3-642-70372-0

Library of Congress Cataloging in Publication Data

Franz, I.-W. (Ingomar-Werner)
Ergometry in hypertensive patients. Translation of: Ergometrie bei Hochdruckkranken.
Bibliography: p. Includes index. 1. Hypertension-Diagnosis. 2. Exercise tests. 3. Heart function tests. 4. Treadmill exercise tests. I. Title. [DNLM: 1. Blood Pressure Determinationinstrumentation. 2. Exertion. 3. Heart Function Testsmethods. 4. Hypertension-diagnosis. 5. Hypertensiontherapy. WG 340 F837e]
RC685.H8F6313 1985 616.1'32'075 85-17313

Softcover reprint of the hardcover 1st edition 1986

Dedicated to

Gaby, Thorid

Göran, Ragna

and my mother

Foreword

Within the field of general medicine, the last two decades have seen the curative procedures increasingly supplemented by functions that can be summed up under the heading of "preventive health care." There is a close link between this development and the changing morbidity pattern. In highly developed countries the morbidity rate attributable to infectious diseases has been much reduced, while the various types of arteriosclerosis, some tumorous conditions, and so-called functional syndromes have attained massive incidence rates.

Systematic epidemiologic studies have yielded the concept of risk factors, i.e., certain exogenous and endogenous factors whose elimination, ideally, would make it possible to avoid the manifestation of an illness or to ensure it did not become manifest until later in life or in a milder form. The socioeconomic and sociomedical significance of these aspects is considerable, as can be seen from all the statistics on the reasons for incapacity and early retirement and on the relative contributions of different illnesses to total mortality.

Effective avoidance of illnesses by primary prophylaxis (elimination of the causes of disease) or early detection of the symptoms of disease (secondary prophylaxis) leading to early treatment would be a particularly significant step forward, since in the case of most of the conditions mentioned above only palliative forms of treatment are available, and none that have any curative effect.

Attempts to apply sound knowledge collected in epidemiologic studies in practical programs are certainly fraught with difficulties. These lie in the varying degrees of health consciousness, with social-class-specific gradations in the intensity of utilization of the prophylactic facilities available, especially while there are no symptoms to justify a visit to the doctor. The problems are also concerned with the cost-benefit ratio, however; if screening is not performed in a controlled manner it can lead to cost escalations that can hardly be supported, while a more favourabel cost-benefit ratio is possible when risk groups can be identified. Finally, however, there are still numerous difficulties in the assessment of the findings from the viewpoint of diagnosis and prognostic significance. This applies particularly to one of the most effective risk factors in the pathogenesis of arteriosclerosis, viz. arterial hypertension. Epidemiologic data suggest that at least 10% of the adult population is affected, and that only a quarter of those affected receive adequate treatment. The most common reason for this is that people are unaware of their hypertension. The evaluation of the values obtained on measurement of arterial pressure is also not a simple matter. Variations in the blood pressure at rest, different limit values separating normal from elevated pressure, and different recommendations for treatment on the basis of these undermine the confidence of both patient and the doctor.

This is the first point of departure of the present work, which allows a nicer differentiation of the areas of normal pressure, borderline hypertension, and definite hypertension by applying graduated levels of physical stress.

The varying reactions to physical stress in different patient groups give information that is useful in assessment of the prognosis and the same time cast new light on some aspects of therapy. It has been shown in the present study that conventional antihypertensive agents do not by any means lower the resting blood pressure and the blood pressure on exertion in the same way. Finally, ergometric stress can also be used as a model for the evaluation of stress-dependent metabolic processes and hormonal reactions. This allows a better understanding of some of the side effects of the therapeutic agents used so that they can be more easily avoided.

The sociomedical significance of the conclusions, drawn from the findings recorded in a large number of subjects, is high. In addition, the examination procedure is universally applicable, does not take up much time, and can also be justified from the cost angle.

The panel of judges appointed by the Hufeland Award Foundation sees this volume as an important contribution to prophylactic health care, and has proposed that it be recognized as the prizewinning work of 1981. The Board of Governors of the Hufeland Award Foundation has accepted this proposal, thereby continuing their tradition of over 20 years' standing of honoring newly recognized and scientifically sound truths that can be applied in practical ways in the sector of health care.

P. Schölmerich
Hufeland Award Foundation

Preface

Blood pressure, the central parameter in the diagnosis of arterial hypertension, is a highly variable quantity. It can fluctuate markedly with the time of day and with the momentary physical and emotional state of the individual. This raises two fundamental problems with regard to the clinical assessment of arterial hypertension. First, it is apparent that the detection and evaluation of blood pressure in the office setting can be an extremely difficult matter, and that the WHO criteria for classifying patients as hypertensive, borderline hypertensive and normotensive are largely arbitrary. This particularly applies to the diagnosis of borderline hypertension, juvenile labile hypertension, and age-linked blood pressure elevations.

Second, the resting blood pressure does not reflect the excessive blood pressure increases that may occur in response to everyday stresses. The nature of these elevations appears to be important in determining the severity of hypertensive complications. They have a bearing not only on the progression of cardiovascular complications, but also on the danger of acute myocardial events in hypertensive patients with occult or overt coronary heart disease, since an excessive stress-induced rise of blood pressure greatly increases the myocardial oxygen demand.

The evaluation of high blood pressure would be greatly facilitated by a standardized test procedure that would enable comparable and *reproducible* blood pressure determinations to be made. It would also be useful to have a standardized method for monitoring sympathetic activity so that the occurrence and magnitude of inordinate stress responses could be more accurately assessed.

One way of meeting these requirements is through standardized ergometric testing. Owing to its good reproducibility, ergometry is widely used to evaluate cardiocorporeal performance in sports and occupational medicine, as well as for detecting coronary heart disease in the hospital or office setting.

When one considers the good standardizability and convenience of ergometry on the one hand, and the formidable diagnostic problems involved in the evaluation of high blood pressure on the other, ergometry appears to be a rational technique for the diagnosis of hypertension. Because hypertension is so prevalent, such a method can be of practical value only if it relies on relatively simple equipment and is well tolerated by the patient. Moreover, a single examination should not be so cost-intensive that it would prohibit serial testing, nor so time-consuming that it would preclude routine outpatient examinations.

One of the main goals of this book, therefore, is to establish whether indirect blood pressure determinations made during and after standardized ergometric exercise can discriminate between an arbitrarily defined normal and pathologic resting blood pressure, and thus facilitate evaluation, and also whether ergometric data are of value in the early recognition of hypertensive disease, the assessment of its severity, and the selection of patients for drug therapy. In answering these questions, it will be necessary to address three main aspects:

1. Does ergometric testing facilitate the assessment of borderline hypertension?
2. Does ergometry facilitate the evaluation of marginally to mildly elevated blood pressures in the elderly?
3. Is the blood pressure response to ergometry of prognostic significance in arterial hypertension?

A positive answer to these three questions would be of major relevance to preventive medicine and public health, for it would facilitate the selection of patients for antihypertensive therapy, which in turn could prevent or at least delay the onset of serious sequelae. This assumes particular significance in the light of recent U.S. and Australian intervention studies which showed a significant reduction of mortality over a five-year period in mildly hypertensive patients who received antihypertensive treatment.

The importance of arterial hypertension as a risk factor and the severity of its vascular complications are determined not only by the level of the resting blood pressure, but also by the magnitude, frequency and duration of blood pressure elevations that are elicited by ordinary physical and emotional stresses. Given the frequency of these stress responses, a central goal of antihypertensive therapy must be to alter these responses in such a way as to relieve the burden on the cardiovascular system. Thus, antihypertensive agents must lower not only the resting blood pressure but also the transient elevations of blood pressure which accompany physical and emotional stresses – a goal that is not realized in all cases. In the second part of the book, therefore, the following questions are addressed:

1. Do different beta-blocking agents, administered in equivalent doses, influence the rise of blood pressure during ergometry to an equal degree, and do they differ in their duration of action?

2. Do diuretics, calcium antagonists and beta-blocking agents which lower the blood pressure at rest have similar effects on blood pressure elevations during ergometry?
3. Do diuretics and calcium antagonists enhance the antihypertensive effect of beta-blocking agents and may they be used in combination with them?
4. Is the combined use of diuretics and beta-blocking agents a rational treatment for hypertension in the elderly?
5. How is the increased myocardial oxygen consumption in hypertensive patients, and the associated risk of myocardial infarction as well as fatal hypoxia-induced arrhythmias, influenced by different modes of therapy?
6. Do endurance training and weight reduction have a salutary effect on hypertension, and what possibilities, positive or negative, are offered by sport?

The resolution of these questions is of major practical importance, for it would facilitate the treatment of arterial hypertension, improve the efficacy of treatment, and also affirm the need to consider the pressor effects of environmental stresses when developing a treatment strategy.

I.-W. Franz

Table of Contents

I. Methodology

1. Principles of Ergometry

Ergometric function tests ensure accurate measurements and comparable, reproducible results in the determination of cardiopulmonary performance parameters. They are useful in internal medicine and in occupational and sports medicine, for they provide the examiner with rapid, objective information through relatively simple means. But the conduct and interpretation of ergometric tests require a detailed knowledge of methodology and of how specific performance parameters may respond to exercise. Therefore we shall discuss briefly the methodologic and physiologic principles which underlie the ergometric technique. For a more detailed introduction the reader is referred to the book *Ergometry* by Mellerowicz [300].

1.1. Methodologie Principles

1.1.1. Physical Principles

Ergometry is unique among cardiopulmonary-corporeal function tests in that it accurately measures the energy expended by the body in kpm/s or in watts. This is done by means of a mechanically or electromagnetically braked device called an *ergometer.* The mechanically braked ergometer of Åstrand (Fig. 1) is widely used and will serve here as a model for demonstrating the basic principles of performance measurement. But how is *ergometric performance* measured?

Perfmanance is defined physically as the rate at which work is done or, more specifically, as the product of force and distance per unit of time. In exercise physiology the term *workload* is commonly used to describe this quantity. The *ergometric workload,* then, is the product of the *braking force* and the *braking distance* per unit of time.

The braking force is adjusted and measured differently on different ergometers. The measuring apparatus of the ergometer in Fig. 1 is designed in the form of a pendulum balance on which the frictional force is read directly in kiloponds (kp). The braking distance depends on the design of the ergometer and is a fixed quantity. In the Astrand bicycle ergometer, a point on the friction surface of the bicycle wheel covers a branking distance of 6 m with each complete revolution of the wheel.

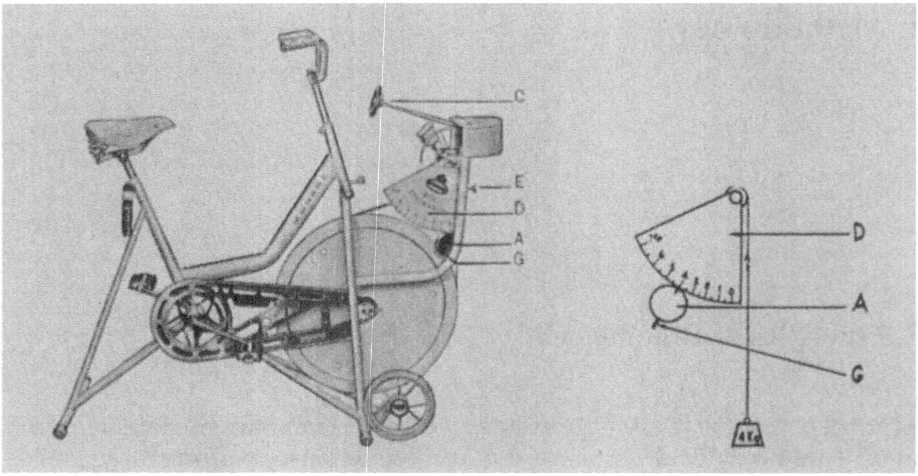

Fig. 1. The mechanically braked bicycle ergometer of Åstrand.

To illustrate how the ergometric workload is calculated, we shall take the case of a bicycle ergometer that is adjusted to a *braking force* of 1 kp. Then, with each complete rotation of the pedals, the subject will do work (force × distance) equal to 6 kpm. At a pedaling rate of 1 rpm, the workload would be equal to 6 kpm/min. At 50 rpm the workload would be 50 times 6, or 300 kpm/min (5 kpm/s). This is equivalent to approximately 50 watts (1 kpm/s = 9.81 W).

It is apparent that the ergometric workload can be increased in either of two ways: by increasing the braking force (e.g., from 1 to 2 kp), or by increasing the pedaling rate (e.g., from 50 to 60 rpm).

When conducting an ergometric test, then, it is important to understand that the results on a rate-dependent device are subject to considerable error if the subject deviates from a specified pedaling speed (e.g., 50 rpm).

Even on rate-independent devices, it is important to maintain a constant, standardized pedaling rate, because the biologic workload will vary at different rates even if the physical workload remains the same [274]. It is significant, then, whether exercise is done at a pedaling rate of 30 rpm or 70 rpm. This fact is too often neglected during cardiologic follow-up examinations or when assessing response to treatment.

Factors influencing the biologic workload on the bicycle ergometer are the *pedal crank length, pedal crank height* and *wheel mass,* and particularly the *exercise stages* and *workload increments* that are employed [300]. We shall take a closer look at these crucial factors on the basis of our own comparative tests of the Physical Work Capacity 170. The results of these tests are of particular interest, for they provide the methodologic groundwork for the exercise stages and increments used in evaluating the blood pressure response to ergometry.

1.1.2. Exercise Stages and Workload Increments

By analyzing the individual response of the heart rate to ergometric exercise, it is possible to evaluate the subject's aerobic capacity by referring the measured

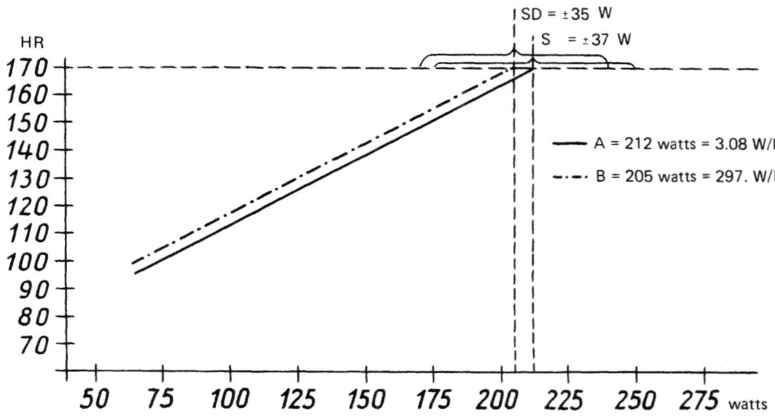

Fig. 2. PWC 170 determined with workload increments of 25 watts/2 min (protocol A) and 50 watts/6 min (protocol B).

heart rates to the corresponding workload in watts and comparing them with normal values in a control population.

Of the various ergometric test procedures that have been devised, the *Physical Work Capacity 170* (PWC 170) is one of the most useful [105, 306, 331].

The PWC 170 was introduced by Wahlund [439] and is measured by excercising the subject at three different stages, each lasting 6½ minutes and each separated from the previous stage by a workload increment of 50 watts. The heart rate during each stage is measured, and the PWC 170 is determined by plotting the heart rates on a graph and extrapolating the line to 170 (Fig. 2). The idea is to determine how many watts of energy the subject can or would expend at a heart rate of 170 beats/min.

The main disadvantage of this protocol is that the use of three consecutive, 6½-minute stages is too time-consuming for routine daily testing. This prompted us to conduct a study on 35 male subjects aged 20–30 years to determine whether PWC 170 tests using shorter exercise stages of varying duration and intensity would furnish consistent, reproducible results [105]. We administered the following three protocols to all subjects in varying sequence, with each test lasting a total of 6 min:

Protocol A.: Increment = 10 watts/1 min. For the first minute the workload in watts was approximately equal to the subject's body weight in kg. Thereafter the workload was increased by 10 watts/1 min.

Protocol B: Increment = 25 watts/2 min. The initial workload was 75 watts for all subjects and was increased by 25 watts/2 min.

Protocol C: Increment = 1 watt/kg body weight/3 min. The initial workload was 1 watt/kg body weight for 3 min. This was increased to 2 watts for the second 3-minute stage.

Using these methods, we obtained a PWC 170 of 170 watts in protocol A, 177 watts in protocol B, and 176 watts in protocol C. Thus, almost identical PWC 170 values were obtained in 6-minute tests using three different incremental workloads. This was true both for a relatively high PWC 170 of 261 watts (highest value determined) and for a low PWC 170 of only 108 watts (lowest value determined).

The heart rates attained during the 6th minute of the final stage averaged 140 beats/min in protocol A and 143 beats/min in protocol B, and so the PWC 170 was obtained by extrapolating to a rate of 170. It should be noted that the linearity of the plot from 140 to 170 beats/min has been well established, both by our own observations of subjects in protocol C and by the experimental findings of other authors [17, 30, 198, 306].

Thus, the PWC 170 as determined by our modified technique provides an objective measure of the subject's *cardicorporeal performance capacity.* The majority of authors [17, 299, 306, 331, 386] continue to use the more time-consuming protocols with stages 6 minute in duration. At this point it is reasonable to ask whether stages of only 1 or 2 minutes' duration provide less accurate PWC 170 values, since the heart rate may be unable to reach a steady state before the next stage is commenced. We therefore conducted another study designed to show whether the PWC 170 obtained in 6-minute stages, and thus under known steady-state conditions, differs from that obtained in 2-minute stages and, if so, to what degree. The following two protocols were compared in 30 male subjects aged 18-38 years [105]:

Protocol A: Two-minute stages with increments of 25 watts/2 min.

Protocol B: Six-minute stages with increments of 50 watts/6 min.

The PWC 170 determined in protocol A was 212 watts or 3.08 watts/kg body weight; that determined in protocol B was 205 watts or 2.97 watts/kg body weight (Fig. 2). The difference of 7 watts, or 0.11 watts/kg body weight, is not significant. It is particularly noteworthy that the *stabilization time of the heart rate* was only two minutes in protocol A, and so there was sufficient time to attain a steady state in healthy individuals [105]. It may be concluded, then, that the PWC 170 measured with increments of 25 watts/2 min provides an objective and reproducible measure of cardiopulmonary-corporeal performance. This is further indicated by the highly significant ($p < 0.001$) correlation between the PWC 170 determined with increments of 25 watts/2 min and with maximal oxygen consumption [142]. This result is not surprising when one considers that the stabilization time of the exercise heart rate (time to steady state) is not solely dependent on the duration of the exercise stage, but also depends on the initial workload (not too high) and especially on the size of the workload increment between stages. Thus, increments in excess of 10 and 25 watts require stabilization times exceeding 1 and 2 minutes, respectively.

These results, show that with a proper choice of workload increments, even short test stages can yield results that are just as reliable and reproducible as the results obtained with 6-minute stages. We believe that increments of 10 watt/1 min or 25 watts/2 min are the most favorable for ergometry owing to the substantial time saving that is achieved. Increments of 10 watts/1 min are advised for higher-risk patients.

1.1.3. Standards for Ergometric Testing

Based on earlier recommended standards, recent research, continuing experience, and a poll taken at the Fourth International Seminar for Ergometry in Berlin in 1981, the following standards have been recommended by the Association for the Study of Ergometry of the International Council of Sports and Physical Education (ICSPE) of UNESCO [299, 300]:

1. *Standard ergometers* that are in compliance with 1956 ICSPE specifications (circular flywheel, weight 100 kg, uniform diameter, inertial moment 5.55 kgm^2, with equal flywheel and crank velocities. Devices with different flywheel weights and velocities may be used if an equivalent kinetic energy is developed. Crank length or double crank length 33.3 cm).
2. *Pedaling rate* of 50 ($\pm$10) rpm (for submaximal exercise) or 60–100 rpm (for maximal exercise) (> -2 SD of HR_{max}).
3. *Exercise stages* of specified intensity and duration. The following may be employed:
   a) Stages of 10 watts/1 min or 25 watts/2 min for subjects with a limited exercise capacity and for children and adolescents (start with 25, 30 or 50 watts).
   b) Stages of 25 watts/2 min for subjects (male and female) considered to have an average exercise capacity (start with 50 or 75 watts).
   c) Stages of 25 watts/2 min or 50 watts/3 min for subjects considered to have a large exercise capacity (start with 100 or 150 watts).
   d) All subjects should be exercised at a minimum of three stages.
   e) An energy expenditure of 1 watt/1 kg body weight for 3 or 6 minutes is a convenient standard workload.
   f) When determining maximal ergometric parameters, stages of 25 watts/1 min or 50 watts/2 min should be used. Stages of 10 watts/1 min may be indicated for subjects or patients with limited exercise tolerance. The total test duration should be at least 6 and not more than 12 minutes.
   g) On occasion it may be necessary to depart from these general rules if the condition of the subject or purpose of the test warrants it. The reason for the departure should be noted on the test record.
4. *Environmental conditions and test preparations* as specified by the ICSPE [300] must be adhered to.
   a) The diet should be changed as little as possible before the day of the test. A light carbohydrate meal (two slices of bread with butter or jam, and a bland drink such as water, fruit juice or milk) may be consumed up to three hours before the test.
   b) The subject should avoid undue physical and psychologic stresses on the day before the test. On the day of the test he should avoid even minor stresses, as they might alter ergometric performance.
   c) The details of the procedure should be explained to the subject. All extraneous stimuli should be avoided, including noise, conversation, drafts, window views of traffic, etc.
   d) The subject should rest in a sitting or preferably a recument position for at least 10 minutes before the test.

e) The *ambient temperature* should be between 18 and 22 °C and should not exceed the range of 16–24 °C. Relative humidity should be 30–60%. Ergometric tests should not be done on hot, humid days if possible, or the results should be interpreted accordingly.
f) To facilitate thermoregulation, only short pants should be worn during the test.
g) All drugs, including coffee, tee and tobacco, should be avoided on the day of the test, and longer-acting drugs should be discontinued several days beforehand. Necessary drugs that were not discontinued should be noted on the record.
h) The time of day of the test should be indicated. Repeat comparative tests should be done at the same time of day if possible, because work capacity varies during the course of the day.
i) Any unusual circumstances should be noted on the test record.

5. Attention should be given to quality criteria such as calibration, objectivity, reproducibility, sensitivity and specificity. These have not yet been standardized on an international basis.

1.2. Physiology and Pathophysiology of Ergometry

Besides strict adherence to standard conditions, the interpretation of ergometric results requires an accurate knowledge of how certain physiologic parameters respond to ergometry [135, 300]. For example, it has been well established experimentally that the heart rate, systolic blood pressure and oxygen consumption increase linearly with the ergometric workload [15, 16, 17, 300]. This linearity forms the basis for *ergometric performance measurements,* in which measured perfomance parameters such as heart rate and oxygen uptake are referred to the physical workload, in watts, that is attained during exercise. Knowledge of the mean values and standard deviations in a normal population has made it possible to develop ergometric protocols that are widely used for the evaluation of cardiocorporeal performance. By the same token, knowledge of the normal blood pressure to response to ergometry should make it possible to develop a standard ergometric protocol for blood pressure evaluations that would be of major clinical value.

This seems all the more plausible when one considers that the *arterial blood pressure* at any given time is based on the interaction between the cardiac output (stroke volume times heart rate), the elasticity coefficient É, and the total peripheral resistance. The *systolic* blood pressure is determined essentially by the cardiac output, while the *diastolic* blood pressure depends chiefly on the *peripheral vascular resistance.* Thus, the level of the blood pressure may be influenced both by hemodynamic factors and by changes in the arterial wall.

1.2.1. Hemodynamic Changes

Because physical exertion increases the cardiac output, a rise of the systolic blood pressure is a natural consequence of ergometric testing. However, this pressure rise is appreciably greater in hypertensives than in normotensives at the same workload, and it is lower in trained than in untrained individuals [113]. This disparity relates mainly to differences in heart rate, total peripheral resistance and cardiac function for a given intensity of exercise.

1.2.2. Arterial Wall Changes

With advancing age the aorta becomes less efficient in its function as an *expansion chamber.* In extreme cases this allows the full pressure of the stroke volume to act directly on the wall of the aorta with each opening of the aortic valve and may cause the systolic pressure of elderly patients to be elevated both at rest and during ergometry.

Of greater importance, however, are changes in the *arterioles* involving a *thickening of the media* [102]. These changes are responsible for the increased peripheral resistance seen in arterial hypertension and result in an elevated diastolic pressure. Even during ergometry, the peripheral vascular resistance is the principal determinant of diastolic pressure. Exercise in normal persons triggers

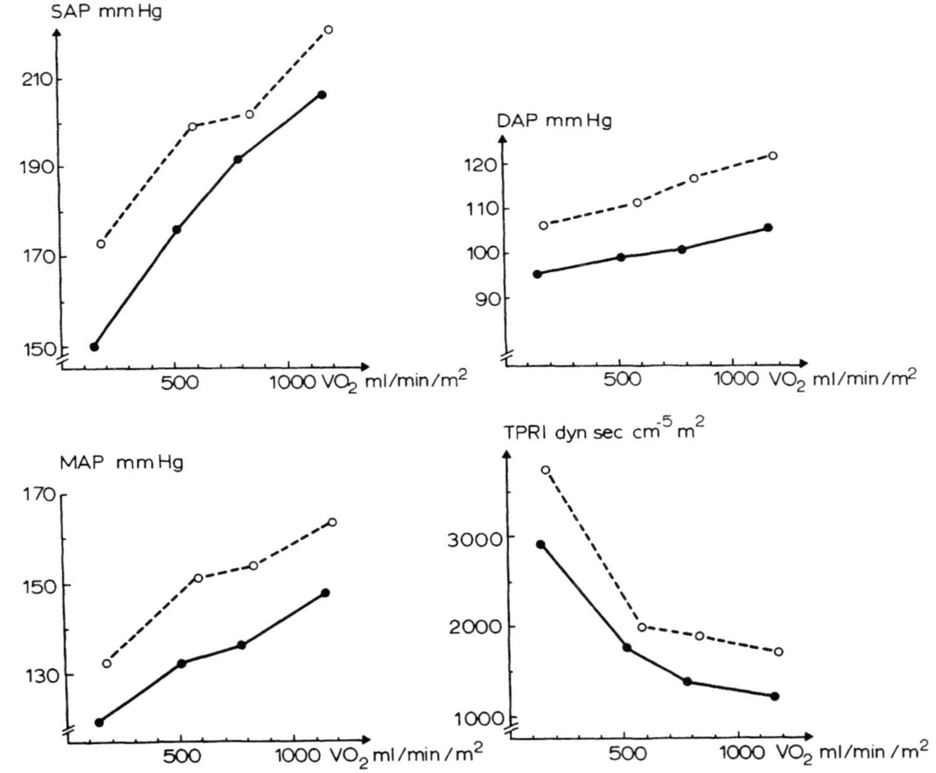

Fig. 3. Hemodynamic changes at rest and during ergometry after 10 years (- - -) in untreated hypertensives. There are marked increases in the systolic blood pressure (SAP), diastolic blood pressure (DAP), mean arterial pressure (MAP), and especially in the total peripheral resistance index (TPRI) (after Lund-Johannsen [274].

a metabolic vasodilatation which significantly lowers the total peripheral resistance [215, 216, 277, 278], thereby minimizing the rise of diastolic pressure which accompanies the high cardiac output. Hypertensives, on the other hand, experience a significant rise of diastolic pressure during ergometry, because the capacity of vasodilatation to lower the the peripheral resistance is restricted in varying degrees depending on the serverity of the hypertension. Thus, the response of the diastolic blood pressure to ergometry is an important criterion for discriminating between normotension and hypertension (Fig. 3).

2. Blood Pressure Measurement during Ergometry

2.1. Study Population

During the period from February, 1976, to July, 1980, a total of 829 male and female subjects were tested. Data regarding age, height and body weight for the separate test groups are presented together with the results, as are the criteria for participation in the various studies.

For each subject a thorough history was taken and a clinical examination was performed prior to testing. Patients with acute and chronic illnesses (except for arterial hypertension) and patients taking medications were excluded from further evaluation. We also excluded persons who were considered to be athletically trained on the basis of questioning and ergometry, or in whom accurate ergometric testing and blood pressure determinations were not possible.

The great majority of hypertensives in the study had not received prior drug treatment for their high blood pressure. Previously treated hypertensives were admitted only if they had not received treatment for at least eight weeks prior to the study.

2.2. Test Methodology

2.2.1. The Ergometer

All tests were done on the mechanically braked ERG 301 bicycle ergometer of the firm Robert Bosch Ltd., Berlin. The pedal crank length and wheel weight of this ergometer are in full compliance with international ergometric standards [300]. The device is also equipped with a calibrating mechanism which allows the calibration to be checked and adjusted easily and quickly. Unfortunately this feature is still lacking in many ergometers and should be a fundamental requirement for accurate scientific ergometric studies [192]. The braking force is fully adjustable and permits even small load increments (e.g., 5 or 10 watts) to be made with high accuracy. This is also facilitated by an expanded scale on the device which indicates the exact workload in watts over a range from 0 to 100 W. A 0-300 W scale may be used if higher loads are desired.

The ergometer is used in conjunction with a special reclining chair which enables the distance to the pedals to be adjusted for any subject height in accordance with recommended standards [300]. The seat of the chair is horizontal, while the back rest is inclined about 45° to serve as a support for the upper body and arms. The pedals are mounted below the seat to permit full downward extension of the legs as on an upright ergometer. Thus, the semiupright position offers a rational compromise between the advantages of supine and upright ergometry. The calm and relaxed position of the upper body and arms facilitates blood pressure measurements and permits high-quality ECG tracings to be obtained. At the same time, this posture avoids the leg elevation and consequent unphysiologic increase in venous return which accompany supine ergometry. From the subject's standpoint, the pedaling motion is better tolerated both objectively and subjectively in the semiupright position than in recumbency [17].

2.2.2. Exercise Stages and Workload Increments

Normal blood pressure values during and after exercise were obtained by exercising the normotensive subjects on the ergometer in the semiupright position. The initial workload was 30 watts for the females and 50 watts for the males, progressing to 80 and 100 watts, respectively, in increments of 10 watts/min. In all cases care was taken that a constant pedaling rate of 50 rpm was maintained.

We also tested the hypertensive patients over a range of 50–100 watts. We selected this range because we felt it corresponded well to ordinary levels of exertion [402, 456]. Because even exercise of this intensity can elicit marked blood pressure elevations [21, 109, 113, 258, 259, 272, 416, 456], the vascular risk of arterial hypertension is accurately characterized by this range.

The decision to avoid higher or even maximal workloads is also based on methodologic considerations. On the one hand, as will be shown, false-low diastolic blood pressure readings become more prevalent as the workload increases. Furthermore, the systolic blood pressure, which is essentially a function of cardiac output, becomes difficult to evaluate at maximal exercise levels, because even robust, normotensive athletes may attain systolic pressures of 250 mm Hg or more on account of their large maximum cardiac outputs.

The use of increments of 10 watts/1 min not only yields more accurate and reproducible results than stages of longer duration (see Chap. II, 1.1.2.) but also offers a substantial time saving, which is essential if tests are to be conducted routinely.

Moreover, the use of small increments and brief stages permits the immediate detection and even avoidance of inordinate blood pressure increases. This is particularly desirable for elderly and high-risk patients who may have overt coronary insufficiency, for example. Of course, the examiner may elect to employ different stages and increments (e.g., 25 watts/2 min with blood pressure readings at 50, 75 and 100 watts) if the nature of the inquiry warrants it. This applies particularly to evaluations of the blood pressure response of athletically trained hypertensives who do not raise their heart rate sufficiently at 100 watts. When the workload is increased to a heart rate of approximately 125 beats/min (reached by untrained subjects at 100 watts), a marked elevation of the systolic and diastolic blood pressures can then be demonstrated in these patients.

2.3. Heart Rate Measurement

The heart rate was monitored by taking an ECG during the final 10 seconds of each 1-minute stage. The ECG was recorded on the six-channel Cardioscript C 6000 recorder of the firm Schwarzer, Munich. The paper feed was checked at regular intervals to avoid errors.

Heart action was monitored continuously with a two-channel storage oscilloscope (Memory Twenscobe MTS 102, Simonsen and Weel). Together with the ECG, this made it possible to exclude or detect rhythm abnormalities and coronary disease, and to terminate the test prematurely if indicated [110].

2.4. Blood Pressure Measurement

Given the prevalence of high blood pressure, a method for the diagnosis of arterial hypertension can be of practical value only if it is applicable on a broad, general basis and does not require overly complicated equipment. The direct, intravascular measurement of arterial blood pressure using telemetry, as advocated by Bachmann [19-21], Floras [101], Krönig [253-259], Littler [272, 273], Rost [361, 362], Taylor [416] and others, permits accurate and above all continous blood pressure monitoring in hypertensive patients and has contributed much to our present understanding of arterial hypertension. Unfortunately, measurements of this type are not practical for hospital and office use on a widespread basis.

We therefore dispensed with direct arterial blood pressure measurements in favor of the classic *auscultation method* of Riva-Rocci, Korotkov and Recklinghausen using a calibrated *mercury manometer* [251, 344, 356] so that we could evaluate the accuracy and practicality of the technique.

The recommendations of the Commission of the German Society for Circulatory Research and the German League for Hypertension Prevention and Control [80] regarding the indirect determination of blood pressure were strictly followed. Only accurate and conscientious adherence to recommended standards can guarantee blood pressure readings of sufficiently high accuracy, comparability and reproducibility. This applies most especially to the proper selection of the *cuff* and its correct placement on the arm. Care also is taken to place the membrane stethoscope at the correct *auscultation site* over the brachial artery and to apply minimal pressure so that a false-low diastolic reading is not obtained.

Blood pressure readings were taken at 1-minute intervals during the last 20 seconds of each minute, both during ergometry and for 5 minutes during the recovery period. The point where the Korotkoff sounds were first audible (Korotkoff phase I) was designated as the *systolic blood pressure,* and the point at which the sounds were abruptly muffled was considered to be the *diastolic blood pressure* (Korotkoff phase IV). The blood pressure was read in increments of 2 mm Hg, though it is known that respiratory movements and vibrations transmitted to the mercury column by the pulse wave necessarily introduce a degree of error. To minimize the error, the mercury column of the manometer should be in a vertical position, and the examiner's eye should be level with the meniscus.

As stated earlier, ergometric testing in a *semiupright posture* is highly advantageous for blood pressure measurements owing to the relaxed position of the arm. When ergometry is done in an upright sitting position, it is necessary to have the patient release the handlebar to eliminate noise transmission and relax the arm muscles. The esaminer stands in front of the patient, places his left arm under the patient's right forearm and elbow for support, and raises the forearm approximately to the level of the heart. The examiner's left hand fixes the stethoscope over the brachial artery on the medial surface of the elbow. It is also helpful to clamp the patient's right hand gently between the left elbow and body to immobilize the arm and relax it. The examiner should confirm that the arm is relaxed before proceeding with the measurement.

Invasive studies by Bevegard and Holmgren [37] on the effect of posture on circulatory function during ergometry showed no significant difference between blood pressure readings in the upright and semiupright positions. On comparing *upright* and *supine ergometry,* the authors found no differences in systolic and diastolic blood pressure responses despite a significant disparity in cardiac stroke volume. This result has been confirmed by Poliner et al. [332]. In addition, the normal values reported by other authors, some of which were obtained in the sitting position (cf. Chap. III.2.4.), point to a close similarity of readings in the semiupright and upright postures.

2.5. Comparison of Direct and Indirect Blood Pressure Measurements

Numerous comparative studies have been published on the value of direct and indirect measurements during ergometry. There is general agreement that indirect measurements yield systolic blood pressure readings which do not differ significantly from direct intravascular measurements [9, 10, 227, 237, 290, 291, 313]. Thus, indirect blood pressure determinations are by no means inferior to direct measurements, and they furnish reliable and reproducible results.

By contrast, Matthes et al. [291] and Rost [362] report that direct and indirect measurements of the diastolic pressure correlate well only at very mild ergometric workloads (Fig. 4). A similar observation is made by Anschütz [10]. As the workload is increased, statistically significant differences appear in the indirect blood pressure readings, which become spuriously low. Thus, tests conducted by Rost at a 110-watt load indicated an indirect blood pressure of 189/85 mm Hg, which was consistent with the 185/87 reading obtained intravascularly. At 190 watts, however, the diastolic reading obtained by auscultation was 10 mm Hg too low.

A survey of the literature indicates that diastolic blood pressures measured indirectly during exercise are always spuriously low [10, 227, 237, 291, 313]. In

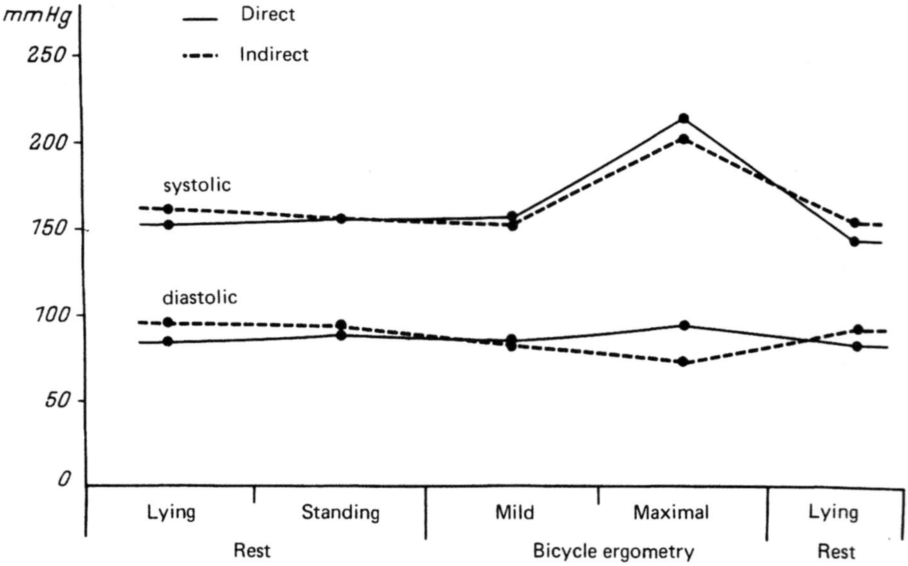

Fig. 4. Comparative schematic representation of direct and indirect blood pressure determinations (after Matthes et al. [291]).

practical terms, this means that a diastolic reading of, say, 120 mm Hg definitely represents an elevation of the diastolic pressure, though it cannot be said with certainty whether the actual pressure is 125 or even 130 mm Hg [10].

Based on their comparison of direct and indirect blood pressure determinations, Matthes and coworkers state the following:

> Comparing these results and considering what is involved technically in indirect blood pressure measurements by the Riva-Rocci-Korotkov method versus direct measurements using telemetry, we believe that the latter should be reserved for very special inquiries.
>
> For routine hospital and office blood pressure determinations and for ordinary exercise testing, indirect blood pressure determinations by the Riva-Rocci-Korotkov method provide results of sufficient accuracy when the foregoing criteria are observed.

The studies presented here show convincingly that the indirect measurement of diastolic blood pressure during ergometry is of major value for both scientific and practical inquiries. This is evidenced in part by the high correlation that was found between diastolic pressures measured during ergometry and those measured in the 3rd and 5th minute of the recovery period, when measurements are no longer encumbered by problems of methodology (s. Chap. II.2.6.). This correlation was observed in normotensives and hypertensives alike (Fig. 5). It was found that patients with high diastolic pressures during ergometry also showed markedly elevated pressures in the recovery period after the heart rate had declined, making it possible to estimate the blood pressure level in the 3rd and 5th minute postexercise from the level of the exercise blood pressures, and vice-versa. Thus, measurement of the postexercise blood pressure is an important aid to clinical diagnosis and should always be included in the ergometric

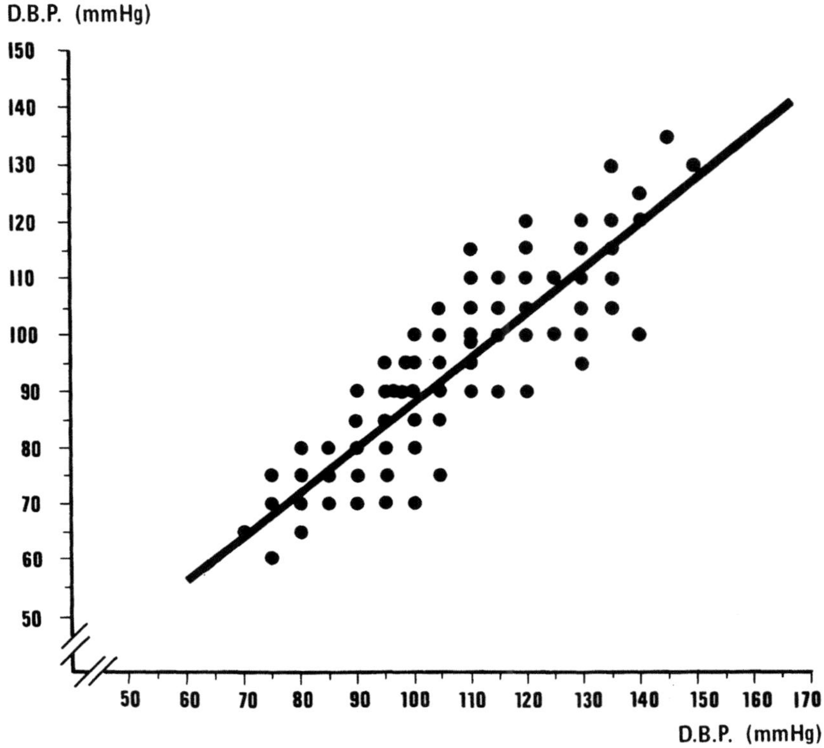

Fig. 5. Correlation (y=0.776 × +11.5; r=0.86; p 0.001) between the diastolic blood pressure at 100 watts (× axis) and the diastolic blood pressure in the 3rd minute of recovery in 156 males (47 normotensives, 52 borderline hypertensives, 57 hypertensives).

examination. It also provides a check of the diastolic blood pressure measured during exercise and therefore aids in its correct evaluation. This can be particularly useful in tests of antihypertensive drug efficacy (s. Chap. III).

As further evidence for the value of indirect diastolic pressure determinations during ergometry, we note that the different groups of hypertensives could be accurately differentiated with regard to age and severity on the basis of their diastolic as well as systolic blood pressures when the indirect method was employed (s. Chap. II.3.). It is noteworthy that the diastolic pressure variations in the different groups showed similar trends and magnitudes both during ergometry and in the recovery period.

We may also point to the good agreement between the diastolic blood pressures reported here and the pressures measured by other authors using invasive techniques (s. Chap. 3.4. and 5.1.).

On rare occasions the examiner may still be able to hear the Korotkoff sounds when the cuff is completely deflated. This "peristence phenomenon" is partly a result of low wall tension but is due mainly to an excessive blood flow velocity, which further increases with the heart rate during exercise [10]. Thus, the phenomenon tends to occur at higher levels of exercise and is most common in juveniles with hyperkinetic heart syndrome who have an exessive heart rate and peripheral vasodilatation. For example, an accurate diastolic blood pressure reading in phase IV could not be obtained during ergometry in 7 out of 49 exercise-negative borderline hypertensives (s. Chap. II.4.1.). In such cases the diastolic pressure must be evaluated on the basis of readings taken during the recovery period following a decline of the heart rate. This could be done without difficulty in all exercise-negative borderline hypertensives. Of the 409 hypertensives tested, none showed a persistence of Korotkoff sounds, which is understandable in view of the high peripheral resistance and consequent restriction of vasodilatation. Thus, if the persistence phenomenon occurs during submaximal exercise at 50-100 watts such that a diastolic pressure cannot be determined, it is highly doubtful that arterial hypertension is present.

2.6. Environmental Specifications and Test Preparations

Ergometric performance can be affected by various factors. This is why the Standardization Committee for Ergometry of the ICSPE established environmental specifications and preparations for ergometric testing at the Second International Ergometry Seminar in Berlin in 1967 ([300], s. Chap. I.1.1.3.).

It was not difficult to satisfy these conditions when establishing normal exercise and postexercise blood pressure values, because all subjects had been thoroughly instructed beforehand. Supervision was not possible, of course, aside from questions asked on the day of the test. All conditions could not be fully satisfied in the hypertensive patients, but any major violations noted at interview caused the patient to be excluded from the study.

II. Ergometry as an Aid to Diagnosis

1. Statement of Problem

As a risk factor, arterial hypertension poses a significant challenge to preventive and curative medicine. When we consider the fact that of the estimated 6.3 million hypertensive persons in the Federal Republic of Germany, 40% are undiagnosed and only about 25% are receiving proper treatment [166, 167, 200, 225, 319, 355, 440, 449], we can appreciate how far we are from adequately coping with hypertension and its major sequelae [74, 205, 211, 269, 295, 359]. Approximately 50% of all deaths before age 65 in the Federal Republic of Germany are due to the effects of high blood pressure [449], and 40% of early disability retirements are occasioned by cardiovascular disease, for which hypertension is the principal risk factor [411].

Numerous epidemiologic studies have demonstrated a direct link between high blood pressure and morbidity and mortality from cardiovascular disease [205, 295, 413, 430–433]. The results of the U.S. Hypertension Detection and Follow-up Program study, published in late 1979, clearly show that even mild blood pressure elevations can have major pathologic significance [205, 206].

The Australian Therapeutic Trial in Mild Hypertension also showed that treatment with antihypertensive drugs could significantly reduce cardiovascular mortality and morbidity in mildly hypertensive patients compared with patients treated with placebos [286]. A similar result was obtained by Trafford and coworkers in their study of 961 patients in England [422].

In the Framingham Study, 75% of patients with cardiac failure were found to have hypertension [225]. As the level of the blood pressure increases, moreover, so does the incidence of coronary heart disease [224, 359, 299, 413] and myocardial infarction [421]. Hypertensives also suffer cerebral infarctions more frequently than the normotensive population [316, 449].

These facts prompted Sturm and Schuster to write in the journal *Deutsche Medizinische Wochenschrift* in 1977 [411], "Given the poor prognosis of untreated hypertension and the excellent results of modern antihypertensive therapy, it is extremely dangerous to neglect the proper evaluation, treatment and supervision of the hypertensive individual." Thus, a solution to the hypertension problem is of vital importance from the standpoint of preventive medicine and public health [95, 96, 166, 167, 199, 200, 392, 399, 449]. This can be accomplished only through the early detection of hypertension and above all through the correct evaluation of outpatient blood pressure determinations. Here we face a complex problem, however, because blood pressure, the central parameter in the diagnosis of arterial hypertension, is subject to a high degree of variability. The dilemma for the evaluating physician is that he has no true value for the resting blood pressure that is both comparable and reproducible. In most cases the readings are taken under conditions of apparent physical rest, upon which are superimposed effects relating to emotion, circadian rhythms and prior physical exertion. Consequently, the result is not reproducible. But reproducibility is an essential requirement for all diagnoses in medicine, particularly in view of the WHO recommendation that such readings be utilized to classify patients as normotensive, hypertensive and borderline hypertensive.

Various authors [21, 258, 259, 272, 416] have used direct, continuous blood pressure monitoring over a period of many hours to show that hypertensive patients frequently become normotensive under conditions of rest, especially at night. As early as 1921, Fahrenkamp [97] reported that blood pressure readings taken three times daily showed variations of up to 70 mm Hg in the systolic blood pressures of hypertensive persons. Diehl [82], in 1929, confirmed that the diurnal blood pressure variations were so great that the morning blood pressure may well be normal while the evening pressure is elevated. Kain and coworkers [221] reported in 1964 on direct blood pressure measurement performed in 62 hypertensive patients over a 12-hour period on 2 to 3 consecutive days. They found that the systolic blood pressures varied over a range of 50 mm Hg (135 to 185 mm Hg), and the distolic pressures over a range of 33.3 mm Hg (79.6 to 111.9 mm Hg). Mancia et al. [288], monitored blood pressures intra-arterially for 24 hours in 48 hypertensives and showed that a trial indirect blood pressure measurement by a physician during that time elicited a maximal blood pressure increase of 21 mm Hg systolic and 15 mm Hg diastolic. A similar increase was observed when a second reading was taken at a different time.

This extreme *variability of the blood pressure* has been confirmed by other authors [13, 43, 259, 416] in direct and indirect measurements. Thus, a striking diversity of blood pressure readings may be obtained, depending on the time of day and the subject's momentary physical and emotional [259, 381, 416, 435] state.

In 1959 the World Health Organization established criteria for the classification of blood pressures as normotensive, borderline hypertensive, and hypertensive. In this classification blood pressures below 140 mm Hg systolic, 90 mm Hg diastolic are considered to be normal; pressures from 140 mm Hg systolic, 90 diastolic to 160 mm Hg systolic, 95 diastolic are borderline; and pressure above 160 mm Hg systolic, 95 diastolic are hypertensive.

Considering the extreme variability in the blood pressure of normotensive persons and especially of hypertensives, it is understandable that this group classification of blood pressures has proved to be of limited value in practical evaluations. Thus, Moeller and Heyden reported in 1959 [307] that only 3.9% of 432 patients with labiel hypertension still had elevated blood pressures after 6 days in the hospital. The difficulties of group classification into normotension, borderline hypertension and hypertension are particularly well illustrated in a study described by Schulte et al. [379, 381]. Based on casual blood pressure readings taken on hospital admission, 20% of patients were classified as normo-

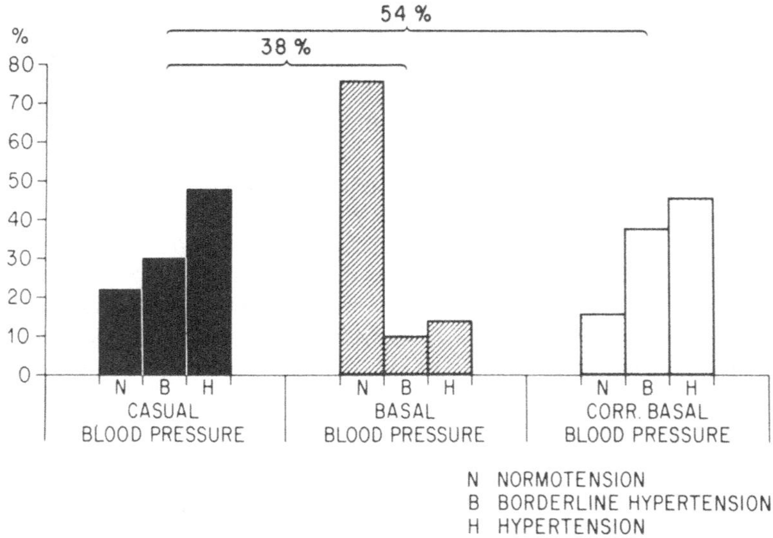

Fig. 6. Percentage distribution of normotension, borderline hypertension and hypertension in 50 males based on the casual blood pressure (left), basal blood pressure (center), and basal blood pressure corrected for the casual blood pressure by a linear regression technique (right). The braces at the top indicate the percentage agreement with the classification by casual blood pressure (after Schulte [379])

tensive, 30% as borderline hypertensive, and 50% as hypertensive (Fig. 6). When repeat readings were taken in the laboratory under conditions of strict rest, 75% had normal blood pressures, 10% had marginal elevations, and 15% were hypertensive. Moreover, only 38% of the patients were assigned to the same group as on admission.

The marked instability of blood pressures in the borderline range became apparent during the course of the Australian intervention study. In the control group treated with a placebo, the mean blood pressure was found to decrease from 158/102 mm Hg to 144/91 mm Hg over the 3-year period of the study. It should be noted, however, that only 50% of these patients displayed a marked fall of blood pressure; 32% stayed in the range from 95 to 109 mm Hg, and 12% even experienced an increase. The marked reduction of blood pressure in nearly 50% of the patients with mild hypertension illustrates how difficult it can be to select patients for treatment on the basis of the resting blood pressure, as Littler et al. [272] have pointed out.

In a strict sense, then, it must be concluded that blood pressure readings can be compared with one another only if they are obtained under external conditions that are equivalent in terms of physical and psychologic stress. This is extremely difficult in most clinical settings, however, which prompted Smirk, in 1944, to describe the determination of the "basal blood pressure" [394] as a reproducible reference value for the blood pressure level. The basal blood pressure is then lowest of multiple readings taken in the early morning on an empty stomach under resting conditions, it being assumed that this value is constant and reproducible from one day to the next. Besides the serious drawback that hospitalization is required for the determination, it was shown by Kilpatrick [231] in 1948 that the "basal" pressure measured in this way actually can vary by up to 35 mm Hg systolic and 25 mm Hg diastolic in hypertensive individuals and is clearly subject to superimposed emotional effects.

Neither is there any evidence that the "relaxation blood pressure" of Meesmann [296, 297], defined as the lowest recumbent blood pressure reading following five minutes' active orthostasis, is of any greater diagnostic value than multiple casual blood pressure determinations [250]. Through continous 24-hour telemetric blood pressure monitoring, Krönig showed that the casual blood pressure taken after 2–3 minutes' rest in a sitting or recumbent position corresponded most closely to the blood pressure levels occurring throughout the day [250].

The problems of blood pressure determination and evaluation described here illustrate the extreme difficulty of diagnosing high blood pressure, particularly the marginal or occasional elevations which are characteristic of borderline hypertension, juvenile labile hypertension, and mild hypertension in the elderly. The situation is further complicated by the need to take multiple blood pressure readings, which may raise problems of patient cooperation [166]. At the same time, the examining physician is frequently plagued with doubt as to the pathologic significance of marginally to mildly elevated blood pressures and the necessity of initiating antihypertensive treatment. In asymptomatic individuals and especially in juveniles, there is a tendency to ascribe mild blood pressure elevations to transitory "excitement" [181, 182] and neglect the need for further evaluation [166]. Also, as mentioned earlier, it is common even for hypertensive persons to have occasional periods of normotension [259, 416] that may be misleading to the examiner. Even when the blood pressure is markedly elevated but is still at the WHO Stage 1 level, the physician may be hesitant to initiate treatment due to uncertainties of assessment and interpretation [364].

At the first meeting of the German League for Hypertension Prevention and Control, Wollheim [450] presented a paper which stressed the "urgent need for clinically objectifiable features which would enable a positive characterization of essential hypertension." In this regard he pointed to a 1936 study by Hines [187] in which a "cold pressor test" was used to differentiate hypertensive from normotensive individuals. The 127 hypertensives responded to the test with a mean blood pressure rise of 47.2 mm Hg systolic, 34.3 diastolic, as opposed to opposed to a rise of only 11.4 mm Hg systolic, 10.6 diastolic in the normotensive subjects.

Schulte et al. [379, 382] claimed that a reliable diagnostic and prognostic evaluation of high blood pressure could be most readily achieved through the use of a standardized stressor. The authors used mental arithmetic for this purpose, but the objection may be raised that such a test is very difficult to standardize and compare on an interindividual basis. Moreover, the authors observed the occurrence of *adaptation phenomena* in subjects who were given the stress test a second time, resulting in poor reproducibility and marked overlaps between normotensive and hypertensives [318].

Isometric exercise also has been suggested and utilized for the purpose of stress testing. A number of studies have shown that the static muscle contraction of isometric exercise produces a very sharp rise of diastolic blood pressure, and thus of total peripheral resistance, in both normotensive and hypertensive individuals [294, 320, 455, 456]. This typical response could be demonstrated by means of a very simple isometric test, such as the lifting of a specified weight. Unfortunately, the studies of Zerzawy [455] as well as our own experience seem to indicate that even a standardized isometric test procedure would be of little value in the diagnosis of hypertension. This is due mainly to the poor specificity of the test, i.e., the fact that both normotensives and hypertensives respond to isometric exercise with marked diastolic blood pressure increases, often with a high degree of overlap. This contrasts sharply with the dynamic ergometric test, in which normotensives and hypertensives have opposite hemodynamic patterns in terms of diastolic blood pressure response. Another problem with isometric testing is that of standardization. For example, the circulatory response to static exercise depends largely on the state of training of the muscles being used, which is not the case in dynamic exercise.

Eckberg [91] tried unsuccessfully to use baroreflex sensitivity as a method of discriminating between normal and elevated blood pressures.

Krönig [259], summarizing the results of his long-term telemetric studies, stressed the crucial importance of exercise testing in mild hypertension as follows: "It may be concluded that hypertensive patients at WHO Stage I usually have normal blood pressures at rest, and that hypertension, being an aberration of response, is demonstrable only during exercise, at which time physical and emotional factors may play equally important roles."

It has already been stated that, owing to the extreme variability of the blood pressure and its dependence on physical and emotional state, blood pressure readings can be compared with one another only if they are obtained under equivalent external conditions. On way of producing these conditions is through standardized ergometric testing. Ergometry has found worldwide applications for the evaluation of cardiocorporeal performance capacity in sports and occupational medicine, and for the detection of ischemic heart disease in the hospital and physician's office, precisely by virtue of its good reproducibility. It has been shown that at workloads greater than 1 watt/kg body weight, the heart rate increases linearly with the increase in workload and is free of superimposed effects [306], yielding a result that is not altered by emotional influences. A similar result has been demonstrated for the systolic and diastolic blood pressure (see Chap. II.3.1.).

Besides good standardizability, an examination method should use relatively simple equipment and should be well tolerated by the patient if it is to gain wide acceptance. In addition, a single examination must not be so cost-intensive that frequent testing becomes impractical.

The ergometric test consists of six minutes of exercise and five minutes of recovery (or less in many cases) and thus is brief enough to permit routine outpatient testing on a broad basis. Additional time is saved by a reduced need for frequent follow-up examinations, which could make it much easier to cope with the hypertension problem in practical terms.

When one considers the good standardizability and practicality of this method on the one hand, and the formidible diagnostic problems involved in hypertension evaluation on the other, it would appear that ergometric testing represents an ideal solution. A major goal of the present investigations, therefore, was to address the question of whether blood pressure readings taken indirectly during and after standardized ergometry can demonstrate the dividing line between an arbitrarily defined normal and pathologic resting blood pressure and thus facilitate evaluation, and whether ergometry can provide a new, measurable clinical parameter that is of value in the early detection of hypertensive disease, the assessment of its severity, and the identification of patients who would benefit from drug therapy.

2. Blood Pressure and Heart Rate Responses of Normal Individuals

Because knowledge of normal values forms the basis for all diagnostic stress testing, we investigated the blood pressures of healthy, normotensive subjects of varying age and gender before, during and after ergometric exercise [123, 129].

2.1. Blood Pressure Responses of Men 20-50 Years of Age

2.1.1. Study Population

A total of 231 men of varying occupations were recruited from the staffs of three large Berlin companies and their affiliates. The men responded voluntarily to posted notices which offered the opportunity for a preventive cardiac examination and also specified the conditions for participation in the study and the criteria for exclusion.

Table 1. Age, height, weight, PWC_{170}/kg b.w. and mean testing time (means ± SD) for the study population as a whole of 173 healthy normotensive males aged 20 to 50 years and for the seperate age groups

	AGE (years)	HEIGHT (cm)	WEIGHT (kg)	PCW_{170}/kg b.w. (watts)	Mean testing time (hours)
All subjects Age group 20-50 yrs. n=173	35.3±7.5	178.2±6.6	74.9±7.7	2.32±0.4	13.02 p.m. ±2.7
Age group 20-29 yrs. n=49	26.1±2.1	178.7±8.3	73.0±7.7	2.33±0.4	13.78 p.m. ±3.3
Age group 30-39 yrs. n=71	35.5±2.7	178.8±5.5	75.7±7.7	2.37±0.43	12.68 p.m. ±2.3
Age group 40-49 yrs. n=53	44.4±2.5	176.6±6.2	75.0±8.3	2.27±0.34	12.49 p.m. ±2.4

Of the 231 volunteers, a total of 173 healthy, normotensive subjects were evaluated. The remaining 58 had to be excluded – 53 due to elevated blood pressures at rest and during ergometry, and 5 due to pathologic ECG changes involving ST segment depression or ventricular premature contractions during ergometry.

The anthropometric data, age and PWC 170 of the healthy subjects are presented in Table 1. The mean age distribution was clustered about the middle of each of the three age ranges. This means that the age groups could be compared with one another, and that representative values could be derived for each. In addition, height and weight data were very similar within the groups, with body weight tending to increase with age [249].

The cardiocorporeal performance capacity of the different groups was evaluated in terms of the PWC 170 or PWC 170/kg body weight. These determinations showed that aerobic capacity did not differ significantly within the age groups and, overall, was on an untrained level.

To keep conditions as uniform as possible, all tests were conducted on Saturdays between the hours of 9:30 a.m. and 4:30 p.m. The mean testing time was calculated in order to eliminate circadian effects. Again, no significant difference was found within the groups.

Table 2. Systolic blood pressures (means ± SD) at rest and during and after ergometry in healthy normotensive males aged 20 to 50 years (*p < 0.05)

Systolic b.p. (mmHg)				
Rest	All subjects n = 173	Age group 20–29 yrs n = 49	Age group 30–39 yrs n = 71	Age group 40–49 yrs n = 53
Casual b.p.	131.4 ± 11.4	135.4 ± 13.4	129.1 ± 9.5	131.7 ± 11.6
After 10 min recumbency	125.7 ± 8.1	128.4 ± 7.6	124.6 ± 8.6	124.5 ± 8
After 1 min standing	127.3 ± 9.7	129.7 ± 8.8	126.7 ± 10.1	126.0 ± 10.3
Before work	134.3 ± 9.7	137.1 ± 8.5	134.1 ± 10.1	132.7 ± 10.4
Ergometric work (watts)				
50	154.5 ± 12.3	156.8 ± 10.2	154.0 ± 13	153.4 ± 13.2
60	163.3 ± 11.8	163.3 ± 10.2	160.0 ± 12.6	161.5 ± 12.4
70	167.7 ± 12.1	169.8 ± 10.2	166.1 ± 12.3	167.8 ± 13.5
80	174.5 ± 13.3	176.6 ± 11.2	172.3 ± 13.2	175.7 ± 15.4
90	180.8 ± 13.5	182.5 ± 12.6	178.9 ± 13.0	181.8 ± 15.2
100	187.7 ± 14.1	188.4 ± 13.8	186.1 ± 13.5	189.1 ± 15.7
Recovery period				
1st	165.8 ± 13.6	168.3 ± 12.9	164.6 ± 13.6	165.0 ± 13.4
2nd	150.8 ± 11.1	153.8 ± 11.7	149.9 ± 10.9	149.1 ± 10.2*
3rd	142.9 ± 9.9	146.2 ± 10.1	141.8 ± 10.0	141.1 ± 8.5*
4th	137.8 ± 9.6	141.2 ± 9.5	137.3 ± 10.1	135.4 ± 8.5*
5th	134.0 ± 8.7	137.5 ± 8.5	133.5 ± 8.8	131.1 ± 8.2*

Table 3. Diastolic blood pressures (means ± SD) at rest and during and after work in healthy normotensive males aged 20 to 50 years (*p < 0.05; **p < 0.01; ***p < 0.001)

Diastolic b.p. (mmHg)				
Rest	All subjects n = 173	Age group 20–29 yrs n = 49	Age group 30–39 yrs n = 71	Age group 40–49 yrs n = 53
Casual b.p.	79.8 ± 6.8	79.2 ± 6.7	78.8 ± 6.1	81.7 ± 7.4
After 10 min recumbancy	78.8 ± 6.2	77.6 ± 6.9	78.5 ± 5.9	81.0 ± 5.7*
After 1 min standing	86.5 ± 6	85.2 ± 5.5	86.1 ± 5.9	88.2 ± 6.1*
Before work	84.5 ± 6	82.8 ± 7.7	85.0 ± 5.4	85.6 ± 4.9
Ergometric work (watts)				
50	86.2 ± 6.5	83.6 ± 8.2	85.8 ± 5.2	89.2 ± 4.8***
60	87.1 ± 7.1	84.0 ± 8.6	86.5 ± 5.5	90.6 ± 5.6***
70	88.1 ± 7.3	85.1 ± 8.5	87.8 ± 6.2	91.7 ± 6***
80	89.5 ± 7.7	86.2 ± 8.4	89.1 ± 6.5	93.4 ± 6.4***
90	90.7 ± 8.2	87.1 ± 9.1	90.5 ± 7.1*	95.2 ± 6.3***
100	91.9 ± 8.8	87.6 ± 9.5	92.0 ± 7.6**	96.8 ± 6.9***
Recovery period (min)				
1st	81.6 ± 7.3	78.8 ± 8.7	81.1 ± 6.4	84.6 ± 5.9**
2nd	80.1 ± 7	77.3 ± 7.7	80.0 ± 6.4*	82.9 ± 5.7*
3rd	79.4 ± 7.3	75.8 ± 7.6	79.5 ± 6.5*	82.9 ± 6.1**
4th	79.7 ± 7	76.4 ± 7.5	79.6 ± 6.7*	83.1 ± 5.9**
5th	80.3 ± 6.8	76.6 ± 6.8	80.5 ± 6.2*	83.8 ± 5.6**

2.1.2. Resting Blood Pressure

As shown in Tables 2 and 3, a total of four blood pressure readings were taken prior to ergometry. A casual reading was taken in the sitting position during the clinical examination, a second reading was taken after 10 minutes' recumbency, and a third after 1 minute of standing immediately following the recumbency. A fourth reading was taken after the subject had mounted the ergometer, the ECG leads had been placed and the blood pressure cuff applied.

Under all four resting conditions, no statistically significant increase of systolic blood pressure was found within the age groups. However, the diastolic blood pressure after 10 minutes' recumbency and 1 minute of standing showed a significant ($p < 0.05$) age dependence when the 30–40 age group was compared with the 40–50 group, and the 20–30 group was compared with the 40–50 group.

Overall, the subjects experienced a minimal systolic pressure increase of 1.6 mm Hg and a diastolic increase of 6.5 mm Hg when changing from the recumbent to the standing position ($p < 0.001$). Both the systolic and diastolic ($p < 0.001$) pressures recorded prior to ergometry were higher than the casual blood pressures and the pressures taken after 10 minutes' recumbency.

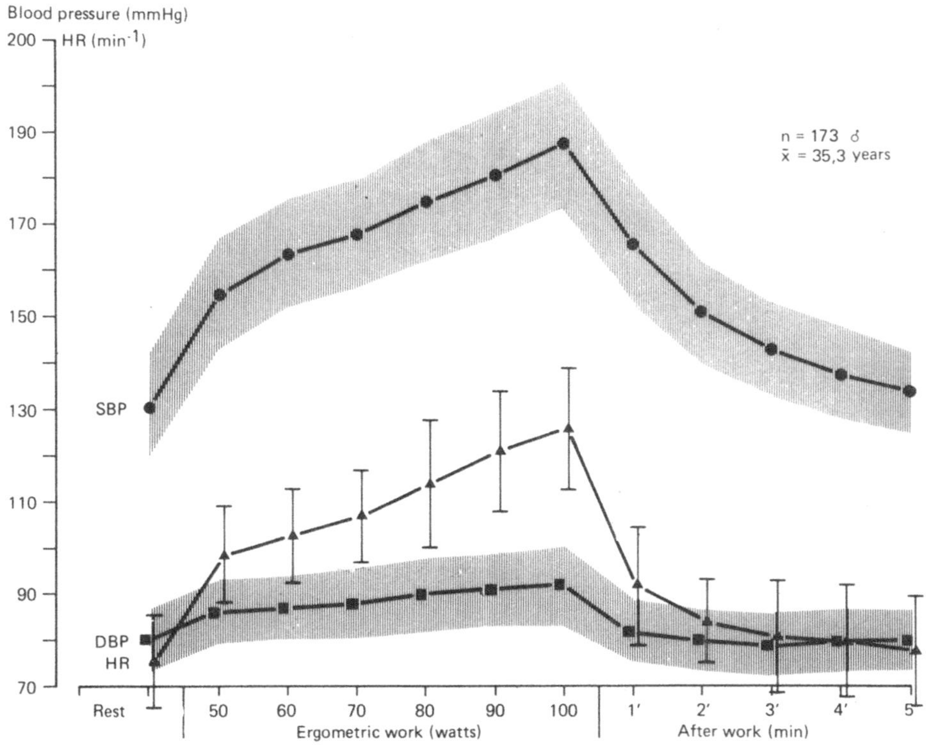

Fig. 7. Blood pressure and heart rate responses of normotensive males 20–50 years of age. The shaded areas denote the standard deviation. (SBP = systolic blood pressure; DBP = diastolic blood pressure; HR = heart rate).

2.1.3. Blood Pressure during Ergometry

Starting from a systolic blood pressure of 154.5 mm Hg at 50 watts, all subjects experienced a steady rise of blood pressure averaging 6.6 mm Hg/10 watts and attained a maximum of 187.7 mm Hg at 100 watts (Fig. 7). Broken down by age group, the data show no significant differences in terms of mean values and blood pressure increments per 10 watts (Table 2, Fig. 8).

In all subjects the mean diastolic blood pressure rose steadily from 86.2 mm Hg at 50 watts to a maximum of 91.9 mm Hg at 100 watts, increasing at a rate of 1.1 mm Hg/10 watts. Unlike the systolic blood pressure, the diastolic pressure showed a significant age dependence, as it did during rest. Thus, a significant difference was observed between the 20–30 and 30–40 groups ($p < 0.05$), the 30–40 and 40–50 groups, and 20–30 and 40–50 groups ($p < 0.001$) (Table 3, Fig. 8).

2.1.4. Blood Pressure during Recovery

As expected, the fall of systolic blood pressure was greatest at the end of the first minute of recovery and became progressively smaller each minute thereafter. By the 4th minute the mean systolic pressure had fallen to 137.8 mm Hg and

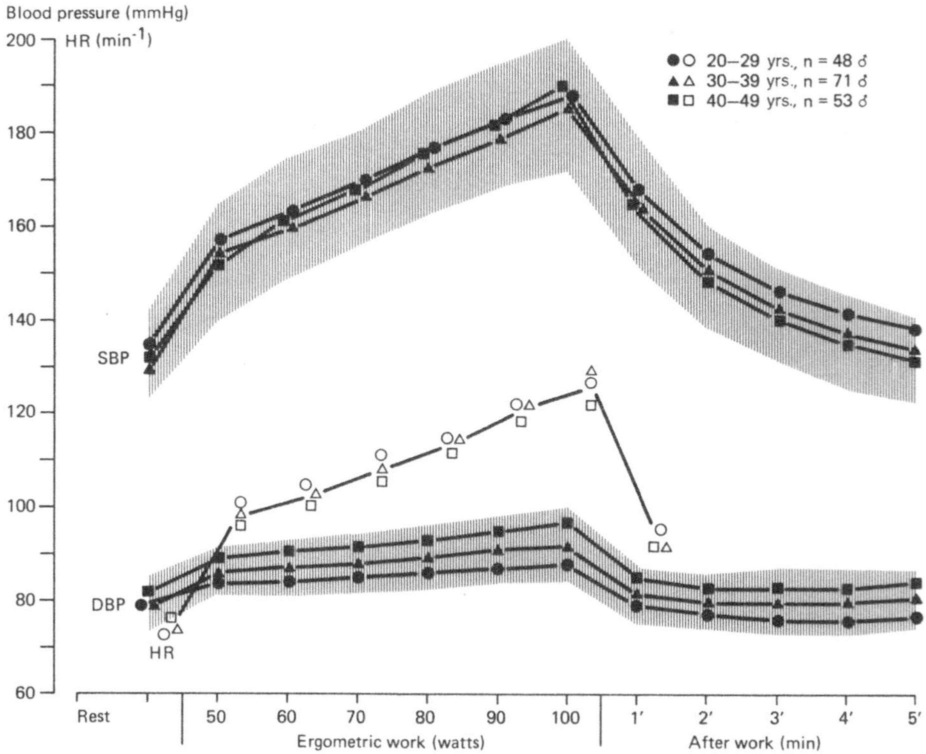

Fig. 8. Blood pressure and heart rate responses of normotensive males 20-50 years of age, broken down by age range (20-30, 30-40, 40-50).

thus was below the upper limit for the normotensive range (140 mm Hg). Systolic recovery pressures were lowest in the 40-50 age group, with a statistically significant difference (except for the 1st minute) occurring between the 20-30 and 40-50 groups ($p < 0.05$).

The fall of diastolic blood pressure also was greatest during the first minute of recovery, falling below the immediate pre-exercise level. No further significant pressure drop occurred during the remainder of the recovery period. A comparison by age group again showed an age-dependent increase of diastolic blood pressures, with the 40-50 group showing significantly higher pressures than the 30-40 group ($p < 0.01$) and the 20-30 group ($p < 0.001$) throughout the recovery period. A comparison of the 20-30 and 30-40 groups showed a statistically significant difference ($p < 0.05$) from the 2nd to the 5th minute of recovery.

2.1.5. Heart Rate before, during and after Ergometry

The mean values for the resting heart rate corresponded to the physiologic range of variation and showed no significant age-related effects (Table 4). This also applied to the rise of the heart rate after orthostasis, which was 12.2 beats/

Table 4. Heart rates (means ± SD) at rest and during and after work in healthy normotensive males aged 20 to 50 years

Heart rate (bts/min)				
Rest	All subjects n = 175	Age group 20–29 yrs n = 49	Age group 30–39 yrs n = 71	Age group 40–49 yrs n = 53
Casual b.p.	74.4 ± 10.1	75.3 ± 9.5	74.4 ± 11.3	75.6 ± 9.4
After 10 min recumbancy	67.6 ± 9.5	65.1 ± 9.4	66.0 ± 9.4	69.0 ± 10.2
After 1 min standing	79.8 ± 10.2	83.5 ± 9.4	78.8 ± 11.5	79.3 ± 9.4
Before work	67.6 ± 10.8	69.2 ± 8.4	66.4 ± 12.5	67.3 ± 9.6
Ergometric work (watts)				
50	98.1 ± 11.4	100.8 ± 9.8	97.8 ± 13.1	95.8 ± 10.0
60	102.9 ± 10.6	104.5 ± 10.9	103.4 ± 11.1	100.6 ± 9.7
70	108.3 ± 11.3	110.9 ± 11.7	108.0 ± 11	105.9 ± 11
80	113.9 ± 13.8	115.3 ± 12.4	114.9 ± 16.2	111.4 ± 11.8
90	120.5 ± 13.1	121.8 ± 12.4	122.1 ± 12.6	117.5 ± 12.8
100	126.3 ± 13.4	127.2 ± 13.8	128.9 ± 13.1	122.2 ± 13.2
Recovery period (min)				
1st	92.0 ± 13.4	95.5 ± 14.2	91.1 ± 13.0	91.3 ± 13.2
2nd	83.5 ± 13.2	85.2 ± 14.3	82.8 ± 13	82.8 ± 12.4
3rd	80.9 ± 12.4	82.9 ± 13.6	79.8 ± 11.7	81.2 ± 12.6
4th	79.3 ± 12.1	80.8 ± 12.5	78.1 ± 11.9	79.9 ± 12.2
5th	78.2 ± 11.6	79.4 ± 11.7	78.1 ± 12.1	78.0 ± 11.4

min for the population as a whole and thus corresponded to the heart rate increment reported by Thulesius [420].

During ergometry the heart rate rose steadily by an average of 5.6 beats/min/10 watts for all subjects, starting at 98.1/min at 50 watts and increasing to 126.3/min at 100 watts. Thus, the response of the heart rate was similar to that of the systolic blood pressure. The subjects in their 50's tended to have lower heart rates during ergometry.

During the postexercise recovery period the decrease in heart rate was most pronounced in the first minute, analogous to the blood pressure response. By the end of the fifth minute the heart rate was still above the initial pre-exercise level.

2.2. Blood Pressure and Heart Rate Responses of Men 55–80 Years of Age

2.2.1. Study Population

The subjects consisted of 50 healthy, normotensive men ranging from 55 to 80 years of age (average 64.4 years, height 177.1 ± 8.3 cm, weight 79.4 ± 8.7 kg) who had presented for a routine preventive cardiac examination. Blood pressures were taken before, during and after ergometry.

Table 5. Systolic (S.B.P.), diastolic (D.B.P.) blood pressures and heart rates (H.R.) (means ± SD) before, during and after work in 50 healthy normotensive males aged 55 to 80 years

n = 50		Rest	Ergometric work (watts)						Recovery period (min)				
		supine	50	60	70	80	90	100	1st	2nd	3rd	4th	5th
Mean age	S.B.P.	140.1	165.9	173.5	178.3	184.2	191.1	196.3	173.4	159.1	150.4	144	140.1
64.4 yrs	(mmHg)	15.3	16.8	18.4	19.5	19.5	20.2	19.5	23	21.3	18.9	18.6	19.3
	D.B.P.	83.1	91.1	93.2	93.8	94.6	95.4	96.1	83.9	82.3	81.7	82.2	82.5
	(mmHg)	8.1	8.9	8.1	9.2	8.7	8.6	8.2	10.2	8.6	9.4	9.4	8.4
	H.R	63.9	89.1	93.3	96.6	101.1	106.3	110.3	84.6	77.2	73.7	72.3	72.1
	$(min.^{-1})$	9	4.9	11.5	13.1	16.0	16.0	16.8	14.3	14.5	12.9	11.3	11.6

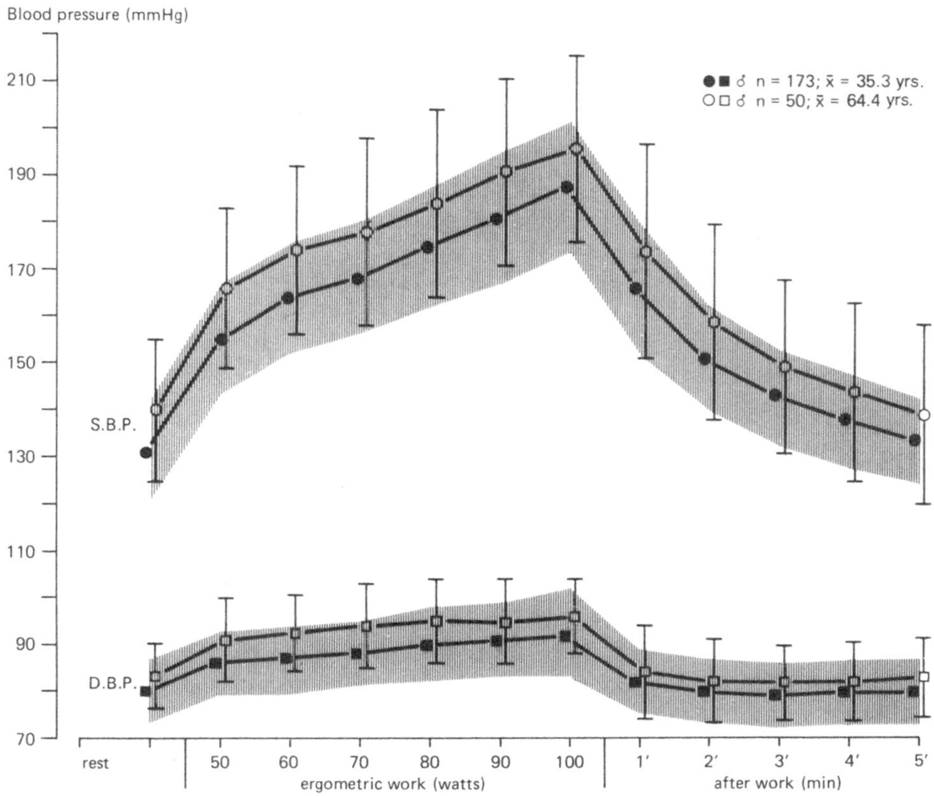

Fig. 9. Comparative representation of the blood pressure responses of older (average 64.4 years) and younger (average 35.5 years) normotensive males. The shaded areas denote standard deviation in the younger subjects.

2.2.2. Resting Blood Pressure

The mean casual blood pressure in these subjects was 140/83 mm and thus significantly higher ($p < 0.5$) than the 132/82 mm Hg recorded in the 40–49 age group (Table 5, Fig. 8, 9).

2.2.3. Blood Pressure during Ergometry

The systolic blood pressure rose continuously from 165.9 mm Hg at 50 watts to 196.3 mm Hg at 100 watts at a rate of 6.1 mm Hg/10 watts. This was significantly higher ($p < 0.05$) than in the 40–50 age group (Fig. 9).

The diastolic blood pressure also rose steadily at 1 mm Hg/10 watts in the range from 50 to 100 watts, and thus at a rate comparable to the normal population of younger men. The diastolic readings did not differ significantly from the readings in the 40–50 group, but they did differ significantly from the 20–30 group ($p < 0.01$) and 30–40 group ($p < 0.05$).

2.2.4. Blood Pressure during Recovery

The greatest fall of systolic blood pressure occurred during the first minute of recovery. Throughout the recovery period the systolic blood pressure was significantly higher ($p < 0.05$) than in the 40–50 age group but returned to the high-normal range (140 mm Hg) in the 5th minute of recovery. The diastolic pressure did not differ significantly from that of the subjects 20 years younger.

2.2.5. Heart Rate before, during and after Ergometry

The heart rates were significantly lower ($p < 0.01$–$p < 0.001$) before, during and after ergometry than in the 40–50 age group.

2.3. Blood Pressure and Heart Rate Responses of Women 20–50 Years of Age

2.3.1. Study Population

Normal blood pressure values for women were established in the same way as for the men, and identical test conditions were employed. A total of 170 women aged 20 to 50 years were recruited from the same firms as the men, and of these, 150 were evaluated. Fifteen women had to excluded because of blood pressure elevations, and five others were eliminated because of abnormal ECG findings involving ST segment depression or ventricular premature beats during ergometry.

Table 6 shows the mean values and standard deviations for age, height, weight, mean testing time, and PWC 170/kg body weight for the study population as a whole and for the separate age groups. As in the males, these parameters could be readily compared within the different groups, and thus between the sexes as well.

Table 6. Age, height, weight, PWC_{170}/kg b. w. and mean testing time (means ± SD) for the study population as a whole and for the separate age groups in 50 healthy normotensive females aged 20 to 50 years

	Age (yrs)	Height (cm)	Weight (kg)	PWC_{170}/kg b.w. (watts)	Mean testing time (hours)
All subjects Age group 20–50 yrs n = 150	34.7 ± 8.2	165.1 ± 5.1	60.5 ± 6.7	2.0 ± 0.38	12.9 p.m. ± 3.0
Age group 20–29 yrs n = 50	25.3 ± 2.9	165.2 ± 5.2	58.0 ± 6.2	2.01 ± 0.39	14.3 p.m. ± 3.1
Age group 30–39 yrs n = 50	34.7 ± 3.1	165.2 ± 5.3	61.0 ± 7.5	1.96 ± 0.37	12.4 p.m. ± 2.8
Age group 40–49 yrs n = 50	44.1 ± 2.7	164.7 ± 5.1	62.6 ± 5.7	2.04 ± 0.4	12.2 p.m. ± 2.7

Table 7. Systolic blood pressures (means ± SD) at rest and during and after work in 150 healthy normotensive females aged 20 to 50 years

Systolic b.p. (mmHg)				
Rest	All subjects n = 150	Age group 20-29 yrs n = 50	Age group 30-39 yrs n = 50	Age group 40-49 yrs n = 50
Casual b.p.	125.5 ± 10.4	122.6 ± 9.4	125.6 ± 10.8	127.9 ± 10.4
After 10 min recumbancy	120.4 ± 8.7	119.2 ± 9.3	121.4 ± 8.4	120.5 ± 8.4
After 1 min standing	121.1 ± 9.6	119.8 ± 9.8	122.8 ± 9.7	120.9 ± 9.4
Before work	128.8 ± 11.1	127.5 ± 10.8	128.2 ± 10.2	130.7 ± 12.3
Ergometric work (watts)				
30	146.0 ± 14.0	144.0 ± 13.1	146.9 ± 15.3	146.8 ± 13.8
40	152.1 ± 14	150.7 ± 12.9	151.6 ± 15.2	153.9 ± 13.9
50	156.7 ± 14.6	156.6 ± 13.7	155.2 ± 15.6	158.3 ± 14.7
60	164.3 ± 14.3	163.2 ± 14.6	163.6 ± 14.5	166.2 ± 13.8
70	172.3 ± 15	170.0 ± 15.8	171.2 ± 14.9	175.7 ± 13.9
80	178.8 ± 14.7	174.0 ± 15.3	178.1 ± 13.5	183.7 ± 13.8
Recovery period (min)				
1st	158.2 ± 13.3	157.1 ± 14	156.6 ± 14.1	160.8 ± 11.5
2nd	143.2 ± 11	142.8 ± 12.1	141.9 ± 11.2	144.8 ± 9.4
3rd	134.0 ± 9.7	133.9 ± 10.6	133.4 ± 10.3	134.6 ± 8.4
4th	129.2 ± 9.4	129.1 ± 10.4	128.5 ± 9.7	130.0 ± 8.2
5th	125.9 ± 9.4	125.3 ± 10	125.6 ± 10.4	126.9 ± 7.9

2.3.2. Resting Blood Pressure

The resting systolic blood pressures measured at four different times showed no statistically significant differences within the three female age groups (Table 7). This also applied to the diastolic blood pressure (Table 8), with the exception of casual readings obtained on arrival, which showed a statistically significant age dependence when the 20-30 and 30-40 groups ($p < 0.05$) and the 20-30 and 40-50 groups ($p < 0.01$) were compared. The highest resting systolic and diastolic pressures were measured immediately prior to ergometry ($p < 0.001$).

For the subjects as a whole, the change from recumbency to standing produced only a minimal, 0.7-mm Hg rise of the systolic blood pressure. However, this was associated with a significant ($p < 0.001$) 4.9-mm Hg rise of the diastolic pressure.

2.3.3. Blood Pressure during Ergometry

The mean systolic blood pressure of the subjects (Fig. 10) rose steadily at a rate of 6.6 mm Hg/10 watts, increasing from 146 mm Hg at 30 watts to 178.8 mm Hg at 80 watts. These values showed a marked tendency to increase with age, espe-

Table 8. Diastolic blood pressures (means ± SD) at rest and during and after work in 150 healthy normotensive females aged 20 to 50 years

Diastolic b.p. (mmHg)				
Rest	All subjects n = 150	Age group 20–29 yrs n = 50	Age group 30–39 yrs n = 50	Age group 40–49 yrs n = 50
Casual b.p.	76.7 ± 9.1	73.0 ± 8.5	77.5 ± 9.9	79.3 ± 8.1
After 10 min recumbency	76.7 ± 7.5	74.9 ± 8	77.6 ± 7	77.6 ± 7.4
After 1 min standing	81.6 ± 7.8	80.5 ± 8.4	81.7 ± 8	82.5 ± 6.8
Before work	82.1 ± 7.5	80.5 ± 7.6	82.3 ± 7.6	83.5 ± 7.3
Ergometric work (watts)				
30	83.9 ± 7.2	81.1 ± 6.2	84.5 ± 7.6	86.2 ± 7.1
			***	
40	85.5 ± 8.4	83.1 ± 7.7	85.4 ± 8.4	87.9 ± 8.6
			**	
50	87.1 ± 8.3	84.7 ± 8.0	87.1 ± 8.0	89.4 ± 8.4
			**	
60	88.7 ± 8.6	86.1 ± 8.5	89.2 ± 8.2	90.7 ± 8.6
			*	
70	90.1 ± 8.9	87.5 ± 9.1	90.9 ± 8.5	91.9 ± 8.6
			*	
80	91.0 ± 8.5	88.4 ± 8.8	92.1 ± 8.3	93.8 ± 7.8
			**	
Recovery period (min)				
1st	78.6 ± 8.8	77.2 ± 8.8	77.8 ± 9	80.7 ± 8.3
			*	
2nd	75.2 ± 8.1	73.7 ± 7.6	74.4 ± 8.5	77.4 ± 7.8
			*	
3rd	73.9 ± 7.6	72.7 ± 7.3	73.0 ± 7.9	76.0 ± 7.2
			*	
4th	74.3 ± 7.5	72.9 ± 6.8	73.6 ± 7.8	76.3 ± 7.6
			*	
5th	74.8 ± 7.4	73.6 ± 6.7	74.4 ± 7.9	76.3 ± 7.4

cially on comparison of the 30–40 and 40–50 age groups, but no statistically significant differences could be shown (Table 7, Fig. 11).

The mean diastolic blood pressure (Fig. 10) rose continuously from 83.9 mm Hg at 30 watts to 91.5 mm Hg at 80 watts, increasing at a rate of 1.5 mm Hg/10 watts. Comparison of the age groups showed a statistically significant difference ($p < 0.05$) between the 20–30 and 30–40 groups at workloads of 30 and 80 watts, and between the 20–30 and 40–50 groups at all workloads ($p < 0.01$–$p < 0.001$) Table 8, Fig. 11).

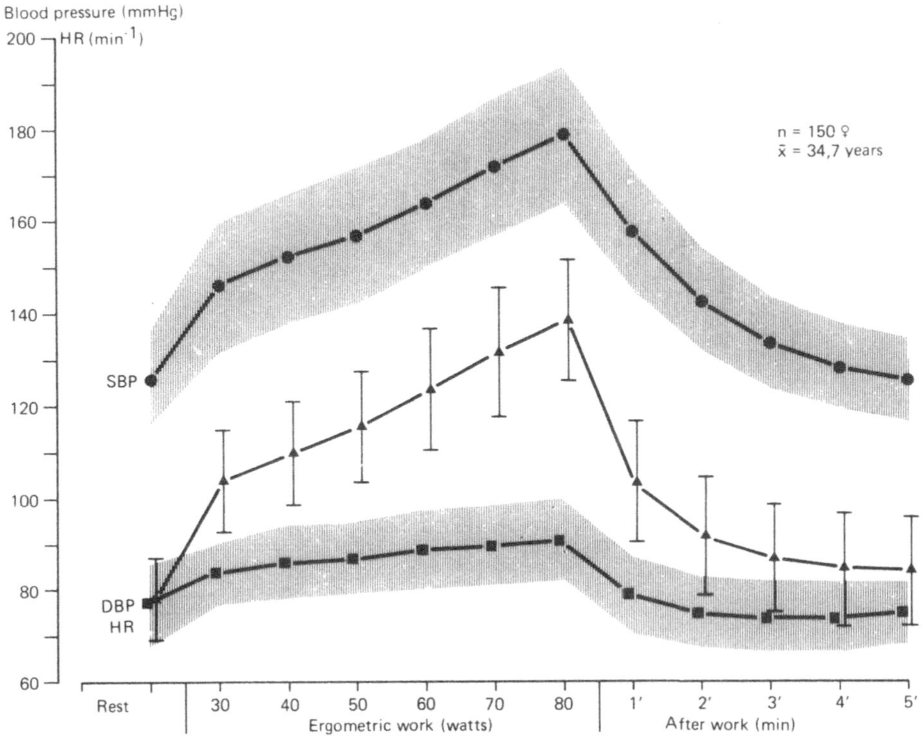

Fig. 10. Blood pressure and heart rate responses of normotensive females 20-50 years of age.

2.3.4. Blood Pressure during Recovery

As in the male subjects, the greatest systolic blood pressure fall occurred during the first minute of recovery. During the 3rd minute the mean systolic pressure fell well below the borderline range. In minute 5 it reached 134 mm Hg, which also was below the pre-exercise systolic reading.

By the end of minute 1 the mean diastolic blood pressure had already fallen to 78.6 mm Hg, at which time it was below the reading prior to ergometry ($p < 0.05$). In minute 4 the diastolic blood pressure reached 74 mm Hg, which was significantly ($p < 0.05$) below the reading after 10 minutes' recumbency. As during exercise, the 40-50 age group had the highest absolute diastolic blood pressures during recovery, though a statistically significant difference was found only between the 20-30 and 40-50 age groups for the first 4 minutes of recovery (Fig. 11, Table 8).

2.3.5. Heart Rate before, during and after Ergometry

We found the resting heart rate to be unaffected by age (Table 9). The 10.6 beats/min rise of the heart rate during orthostasis was consistent with normal values reported by Thulesius [420]. During ergometry the mean heart rate

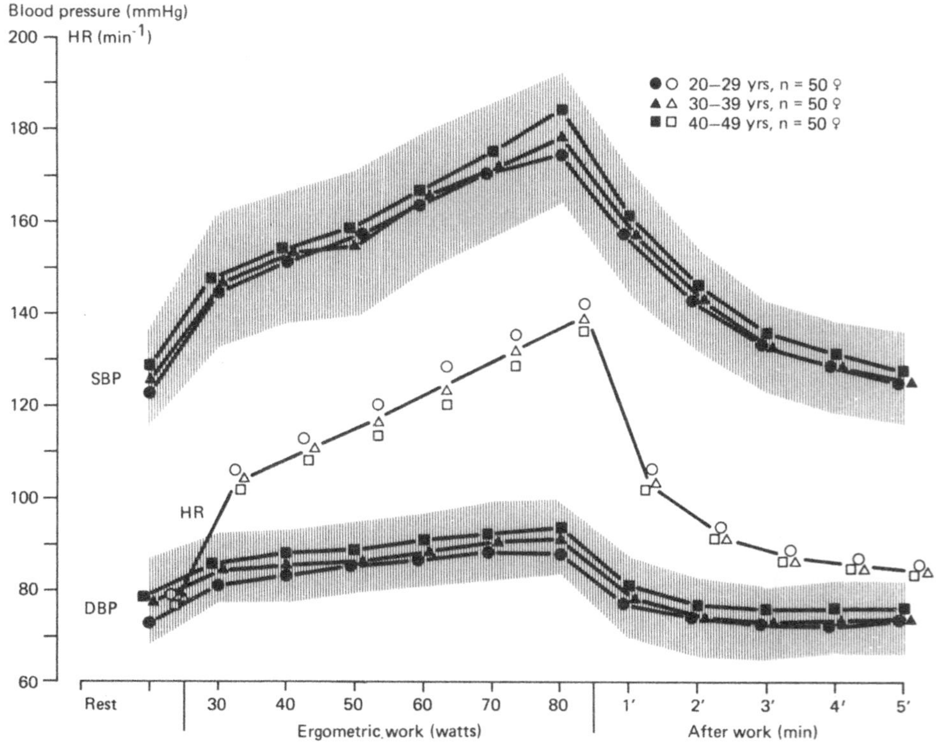

Fig. 11. Blood pressure and heart rate responses of normotensive females aged 20–50 years, broken down by age range (20–30, 30–40, 40–50)

Table 9. Heart rates (means ± SD) at rest and during and after work in 150 healthy normotensive females aged 20 to 50 years

Heart rate (bts/min)				
Rest	All subjects n = 150	Age group 20–29 yrs n = 50	Age group 30–39 yrs n = 50	Age group 40–49 yrs n = 50
Casual b.p.	78.1 ± 8.8	79.0 ± 9.1	78.5 ± 9.8	77.1 ± 7.7
After 10 min recumbancy	71.5 ± 8.7	71.6 ± 9.4	72.4 ± 7.5	70.4 ± 9.0
After 1 min standing	82.1 ± 10.9	83.7 ± 13	82.4 ± 9.9	80.0 ± 9.3
Before work	71.2 ± 9.6	72.0 ± 10.4	71.7 ± 8.4	69.7 ± 9.8
Ergometric work (watts)				
30	104.0 ± 11.4	105.7 ± 11.7	104.6 ± 11.4	101.7 ± 10.8
40	110.2 ± 11.4	112.2 ± 11.1	110.7 ± 12	107.6 ± 10.9
50	116.4 ± 11.9	119.7 ± 12	116.3 ± 11.8	113.0 ± 11.2
60	123.6 ± 12.9	127.7 ± 12.7	123.4 ± 13	119.9 ± 11.9
70	131.8 ± 14.1	135.4 ± 14.2	131.6 ± 14.3	128.4 ± 13.1
80	138.8 ± 12.9	142.2 ± 12.4	138.0 ± 12.4	136.4 ± 13.5

Table 9 continued.

Rest	All subjects n=150	Age group 20–29 yrs n=50	Age group 30–39 yrs n=50	Age group 40–49 yrs n=50
Recovery period (min)				
1st	103.7±13.2	106.3±13.7	103.0±14.1	101.8±11.3
2nd	91.8±12.7	92.6±14.2	91.5±12.4	91.2±11.5
3rd	87.3±11.9	88.3±13.4	87.2±11.3	86.3±11.1
4th	85.4±11.1	86.1±12.7	84.8±10.1	85.3±10.5
5th	84.1±12	84.8±13	84.1±10.9	83.5±12.2

rose at a rate of 7 beats/10 watts, increasing from 104 at 30 watts to 138.8 at 80 watts and paralleling the rise of the systolic blood pressure. No differences were apparent within age groups, although values tended to diminish with age, as in the males (Table 9).

The greatest fall of heart rate occurred at the end of the first minute of recovery. After five minutes the heart rate had not yet returned to the initial pre-exercise level.

2.4. Comparative Assessment of the Blood Pressure Responses of Normotensive Men and Women

The 20- to 50-year-old men in our study developed a blood pressure of 188±14 over 92±9 mm Hg at a workload of 100 watts. These values are in good agreement with the normal range of 170–210/85–100 mm Hg reported by Kirchhoff [233] at the same workload. Al-Eshaiker and Mellerowicz [2] found a mean blood pressure of 180/105 mm Hg at 100 watts in 50 men aged 20–30 who pedaled a cycle ergometer in the supine position. Unfortunately, the workload increment of 25 watts/1 min used in that study was inadequate for the subjects tested. Halhuber [168] reports a mean blood pressure of 200/95 mm Hg for cycling in the sitting position at a 100-watt load. Hollmann [195] reported a markedly lower blood pressure at 100 watts, but it must be considered that his subjects underwent regular endurance training.

Renner et al. [349] found a mean systolic blood pressure of 176 (range of 196–154) mm Hg in 219 18-year-old males who were exercised at 100 watts on an upright cycle ergometer. Åstrand [16] measured a blood pressure of 180±24/92±11 mm Hg in 80 healthy men (average age 54 years) who were exercised on an upright cycle to a heart rate of 100±5 beats/min. These values are intermediate between the blood pressures determined at comparable heart rates in the two oldest groups tested in our study (average age 44.4 and 64.4 years) and thus are also consistent with our results.

If we compare the normotensive blood pressures determined here with the direct intravascular measurements of other authors, we again find a good agreement of results. A normal population tested by Körnig [259] had a mean resting blood pressure of 118.9/69.9 mm Hg, which rose to 163 ± 22.9/82.1 ± 11.6 mm Hg during exercise at 75 watts. The normotensive population in our study had a mean pressure of 167.7 ± 12/88.1 ± 7.3 mm Hg at a 70-watt load. The systolic pressure increase of 42 mm Hg between recumbency and 75-watt exercise in our study agrees well with the 44.1 mm Hg increase reported by Krönig. Rost and Hollmann [361] used direct intra-arterial measurements to monitor the blood pressure responses of young, untrained subjects to ergometry and found a mean blood pressure of 170 mm Hg systolic, 87.5 diastolic at 100 watts. For comparison, the authors also tested 10 older, untrained men with an average age of 60.1 years and found a mean blood pressure of approximately 217/98 mm Hg. These findings confirm the age dependence of blood pressure response that is demonstrated in our study.

Like the males, the population of normotensive females responded to ergometry with a continuous rise of systolic and diastolic blood pressure. The diastolic response showed a significant age dependence. Allowing for the difference in age and resting blood pressure, it may be said that the normal age-dependent values determined here agree well with those obtained by Åstrand [16] in 103 normotensive women (average age 54 years) during upright cycle ergometry.

On comparing the 20- to 50-year-old women and men, we found significantly lower ($p < 0.001$) systolic and diastolic blood pressures in the women both at rest and in the recovery period. On the other hand, no statistically significant differences were noted between males and females at the same level of exercise for the study population as a whole. When the sexes were compared within the three age ranges, however, a significant age effect became apparent. Thus, women in the 40–50 age range had significantly ($p < 0.01$) higher systolic blood pressures at a given level of exercise than did men of the same age.

2.5. Practical Utilization of Normal Values

On the whole, the systolic and diastolic blood pressures of our male and female populations were comparable at the same workloads. At 80 watts, for example, the women had a blood pressure of 179 ± 15/92 ± 9 mm Hg, compared to 175 ± 13/90 ± 8 mm Hg for the men. When we examine the corresponding heart rates, however, we find that a striking difference emerges. While the men had a heart rate of 114 ± 14/min at 80 watts, for example, the women attained a rate of 139 ± 13/min – a 22% higher value. This discrepancy is not surprising when one considers that 80 watts respresents a workload of 1.32 watts/kg body weight for the women, compared to only 1.07 watts/kg body weight for the men. The relative ergometric workload, in other words, was 23% greater for the women than the men. Thus, a *sex comparison* is biologically valid only if it is based upon relatively equal levels of exertion, i. e., equal heart rates or equal relative workloads. For example, if we compare the blood pressure response of the females at 50 watts (HR = 116/min) with that of the males at 80 watts (HR = 114/min), we find that at approximately equal heart rates, and thus at equal relative workloads, the female subjects develop lower systolic and dia-

Table 10. Systolic (S. B. P.), diastolic (D. B. P.) blood pressures and heart rates (H. R.) (means ± SD) during ergometric work in 172 males and 150 females aged 20 to 50 years (+n = 50)

n = 323	Males (n = 172) 20 to 50 years, mean 35.3 yrs			Females (n = 150) 20 to 50 years, mean 34.7 yrs		
Ergometric work	H. R. (bts/min)	S. B. P. (mmHg)	D. B. P. (mmHg)	S. B. P. (mmHg)	D. B. P. (mmHg)	H. R. (bts/min)
50 watts	98.1 11.4	154.5 12.3	86.2 6.5	156.7 14.6	87.1 8.3	116.4 11.9
60 watts	102.9 10.6	161.3 11.8	87.1 7.1	164.3 14.3	88.7 8.6	123.6 12.9
70 watts	108.3 11.3	167.7 12.1	88.1 7.3	172.3 15	90.1 8.9	131.8 14.1
80 watts	113.9 13.8	174.5 13.3	89.5 7.7	178.8 14.7	91.5 8.5	138.8 12.9
90 watts	120.5 13.1	180.8 13.5	90.7 8.2	184.3+ 14.3	91.2+ 8.3	142.6+ 12.3
100 watts	126.3 13.4	187.7 14.1	91.9 8.8	185.5+ 7.3	93.2+ 7.3	144.6+ 10.4

stolic blood pressures than the males. This is consistent with the pattern observed before and after ergometry (s. Table 10, Fig. 12).

For the practical utilization of normal blood pressure values in ergometry, then, one should not just refer the upper limit of normotension in 20- to 50-year-olds of 200/100 mm Hg (mean + 1 SD) to a workload of 100 watts. It is important to relate the normotensive limit to the subject's *heart rate response* to ensure that equivalent relative workloads apply. This means that an upper normal limit of 200/100 mm Hg is valid for a heart rate of 126 ± 13/min in untrained men and for a rate of 145 ± 10/min in untrained women. In all cases the upper normal is considered to be the mean value plus one standard deviation.

Correction of the blood pressure for the heart rate response is of major practical importance in two respects. First, it is significant whether the body weight of a subject (male or female) exercised at 100 watts is 50 or 80 kg, because this materially affects the relative workload that is imposed.

Second, it is important to consider that referring the blood pressure to a constant workload of, say, 100 watts can introduce a substantial technical error. As recent investigations have shown [192], the workload actually imposed on the subject may differ from the workload in watts that is indicated on the ergometer dial. This can occur on all devices but is especially common on older, uncalibrated models. By evaluating the blood pressure in terms of a specified level of the heart rate, it is possible to avoid these errors.

On calibrated ergometers, comparison of the blood pressure responses to relatively equal workloads of, say, 1 watt/kg body weight also provides a reliable and reproducible parameter. The female subjects, with a mean body weight of 60.5 kg, develop a blood pressure of 164 ± 14/89 ± 9 mm Hg at 1 watt/kg body weight (i.e., approx. 60 watts) and a heart rate of 124 ± 13/min. The corre-

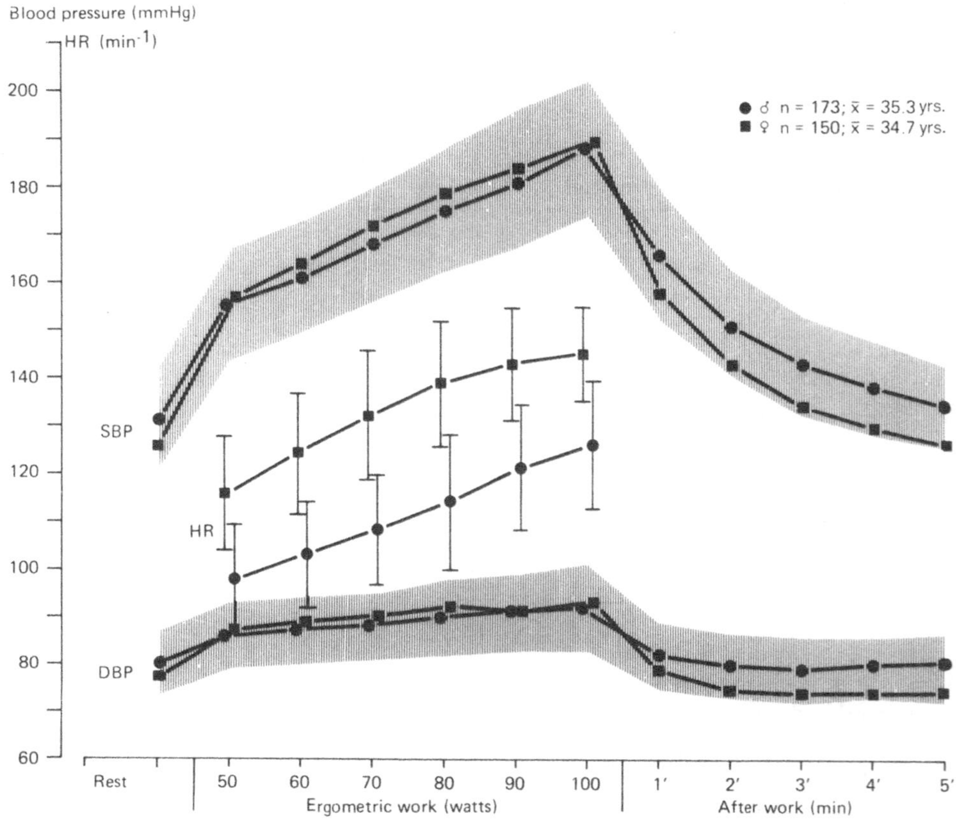

Fig. 12. Comparative representation of the blood pressure and heart rate responses of normotensive males and females 20–50 years of age

sponding value at 1 watt/kg in the male subjects, who have a mean body weight of 74.9 kg, is 171 ± 13/89 8 mm Hg with a heart rate of 111 ± 13/min.

As will be shown (see Chap. II.3.2.), blood pressure responses during the recovery period provide a highly specific means of differentiating normotension from hypertension. In the normotensive individual, the blood pressure reaches or falls below the resting upper normotensive limit of 140/90 mm Hg within five minutes after exercise is terminated.

The "upper normal" values discussed here for blood pressures during and after ergometry refer to the mean value plus one standard deviation of the total population of 20- to 50-year-old men and women and should be applied uniformly to all three age ranges for ordinary blood pressure evaluations. Even though the diastolic blood pressure varies with age, this approach nevertheless is justified because it facilitates the practice of ergometric testing and does not diminish its diagnostic value. This is confirmed by the good agreement with normal values reported by other authors [2, 15, 154, 168, 233].

The normal blood pressure values stated here were obtained through bicycle ergometry in the semiupright position. Based on invasive studies by Bevegård et al. [37] on the effect of posture on circulatory function during exercise, it may be concluded that the blood pressure response to ergometry is virtually the same in the semiupright, upright and supine positions.

On comparing upright and supine ergometry, the authors found no appreciable difference in systolic and diastolic blood pressures despite the significant difference in cardiac stroke volumes. This result was confirmed by Poliner et al. [332].

For 55- to 60-year-old men (see Chap. III.2.2.) it is necessary to employ higher blood pressure limits during and after ergometry. For this segment a blood pressure of 200/105 mm Hg is considered to be the upper limit of normal for a 70-watt load (HR = 97 ± 13/min), and 215/105 mm Hg is considered normal for a 100-watt load (HR = 110 ± 17/min). Referred to a relatively equal standard workload of 1 watt/kg body weight for a mean body weight of 79.4 kg (= approx. 80 watts), this results in a vlaue of 184 ± 20/95 ± 9 mm Hg for the normal blood pressure at a corresponding heart rate of 101 ± 16/min. At the end of the 5th minute of recovery, the diastolic blood pressure should be below 90 mm Hg and the systolic pressure below 150 mm Hg.

2.6. Correlative Assessment of Diastolic Blood Pressures before, during and after Ergometry

We analyzed our results for normotensive men and women to see whether a correlation existed between the resting diastolic blood pressure after 10 minutes' recumbency or 1 minute of standing and the diastolic pressures recorded during exercise. The correlation coefficients are shown in Table 11. It was found that the diastolic blood pressure after 10 minutes' recumbency and after 1 minute of standing correlated significantly with the diastolic pressures recorded at 30–80 watts for women and at 50–100 watts for men. In both sexes the correlation was stronger at lower workloads.

Table 11. The correlation coefficients between diastolic (D.B.P.) blood pressure after 1 min in the standing position or after 10 min recumbency and measured during ergometric work (50 to 100 watts for males and 30 to 80 watts for females) in normotensive subjects aged 20 to 50 years ($r = 0.56$ to 0.45; $p < 0.001$)

D.B.P. at work	Correlation coefficients between resting diastolic b.p. and during exercise			
	Males n = 173	Females n = 150	Males n = 173	Females n = 150
	D.B.P. Standing		D.B.P. Supine	
50, 30 watts	0.56	0.56	0.59	0.58
60, 40 watts	0.51	0.60	0.51	0.60
70, 50 watts	0.49	0.59	0.47	0.58
80, 60 watts	0.46	0.55	0.42	0.53
90, 70 watts	0.46	0.52	0.40	0.48
100, 80 watts	0.40	0.47	0.36	0.46

We also checked to see how the diastolic blood pressure at 80 watts for women and 100 watts for men correlated with the diastolic pressure during the 3rd minute of the recovery period. Again, we found a significant correlation ($p < 0.01$) with an r of 0.52 for men and 0.65 for women.

The significant correlations between diastolic blood pressures before, during and after ergometry also underscore the practical soundness of indirect blood pressure determinations in the range from 50 to 100 watts.

3. Blood Pressure and Heart Rate Responses of Hypertensive Patients

3.1. Reproducibility of Blood Pressure and Heart Rate Responses during and after Ergometry

As we have said, blood pressure readings can be validly compared with one another only if they are obtained under equivalent external conditions. Thus, a standardized test procedure is needed which will guarantee comparable and above all reproducible blood pressure readings and thereby facilitate the evaluation of hypertension.

In the emotional stress test, obvious signs of adaptation were apparent when the test was administered a second time [318]; hence the results of the test were not resproducible. Reproducibility, however, is an essential criterion for any diagnostic method.

We therefore investigated whether similar *adaptation phenomena* were operative in blood pressure and heart rate responses during and after standardized ergometry, and also whether these responses were subject to diurnal variations.

3.1.1. Hypertensives

Twenty male hypertensives with an average age of 25.8 years whose blood pressures were mildly elevated (WHO Stage 1) were tested. Their blood pressure responses during and after ergometry were tested 3 times on a work-free Saturday between the hours of 8:00 a.m. and 10:00 a.m., 10:00 a.m. and 12:00 noon, and 4:00 p.m. and 6:00 p.m. under otherwise identical conditions.

It was found that both the systolic and diastolic blood pressures measured under standardized rest conditions were lower in the second and third tests than in the initial test. Due to the large individual scatter of readings, however, a statistically significant difference could not be demonstrated (Table 12).

On comparing the systolic blood pressures during ergometry at the three testing times, we find that the readings obtained in the 2nd and 3rd tests at the first two exercise stages of 50 and 60 watts tend to be markedly lower than in the initial test. In fact, a statistically significant difference ($p < 0.05$) was demonstrated between the 1st and 2nd tests at 60 watts. As the workload increased, however, all three readings showed excellent agreement. At 100 watts, for example, the 1st, 2nd and 3rd readings were 203 ± 12 mm Hg, 200 ± 12 mm Hg and $203 \pm$

Table 12. Systolic (S. B. P.), diastolic (D. B. P.) blood pressures and heart rates (H. R.) (means ± SD) at rest and during and after work in 20 males with mild hypertension who were tested 3 times on a work-free saturday between the hours of 8:00 a. m. and 10:00 a. m., 10:00 a. m. and 12:00 noon, and 4:00 p. m. and 6:00 p. m. (*$p < 0.05$)

n = 20		Rest	Ergometric work (watts)						Recovery period (min)				
		Supine	50	60	70	80	90	100	1.	2.	3.	4.	5.
S. B. P. (mmHg)	8:00 and 10:00 a. m.	155.2 13	173.9 9.6	180.3 11.3	186.1 12.4	191.5 13	198.1 11.4	203.4 11.7	175 11.5	163.8 10.8	159.3 12.5	156.7 11.6	156.4 12.3
	10:00 a. m. and 12:00 noon	149.7 10.8	165.9 11.6	169.8 13.5*	177.5 10.7	183.5 9.8	191.9 9.3	200.3 12	170.2 13.7	158.7 12.3	151.8 11.5	150.5 12.1	147.3 10.4
	16:00 and 18:00 p. m.	150.5 17.5	165.2 12.1	176.6 12.6	181.4 10.8	188.9 12.5	196.5 9.8	203.2 9.8	174.4 10.8	162.2 11	156.4 11.2	153.8 12.4	150.9 13.1
D. B. P. (mmHg)	8:00 and 10:00 a. m.	105.2 9.4	110.6 12.5	111.4 12.9	112.2 12.9	113.4 13.2	114.6 14.4	116.4 13.2	107.5 10.4	105.3 11.1	104.5 11	102.9 11.3	104.0 12.2
	10:00 a. m. and 12:00 noon	104.2 8.2	106 11.3	106.9 11	107.9 11.7	111.2 11.9	111.8 11.9	114.2 12.8	105.1 10	103.3 10.7	102.2 10.3	102 10.5	102.1 10.4
	16:00 and 18:00 p. m.	101.2 12.1	106.3 13.7	106.5 13.5	107.9 14	109.7 14.4	111 13.9	113 13.5	102.1 12	100 11.1	99.5 11.6	99.2 12.1	99 11.9
H. R. (bts/min)	8:00 and 10:00 a. m.	63.9 9.4	90 8.8	93.3 8.7	98.4 9.8	103.4 9.1	107.7 10.9	111.6 10.7	78.2 12.4	71.8 10.9	69.2 12	68 11	67.4 10.9
	10:00 a. m. and 12:00 noon	62.1 7.1	90.9 9.4	91.7 9.0	96.2 9.7	101.7 9.3	105.9 10.6	110.4 10.5	74.6 11.9	71.5 11.1	66.8 10.4	67.6 9.2	66.8 10.2
	16:00 and 18:00 p. m.	68 11.1	91.9 8.4	97.2 8.6	98.7 9.4	105.4 7.9	110 8.4	114.3 9.4	76.9 9.7	73.4 10.4	71.4 9.9	72.8 10	72.4 11.8

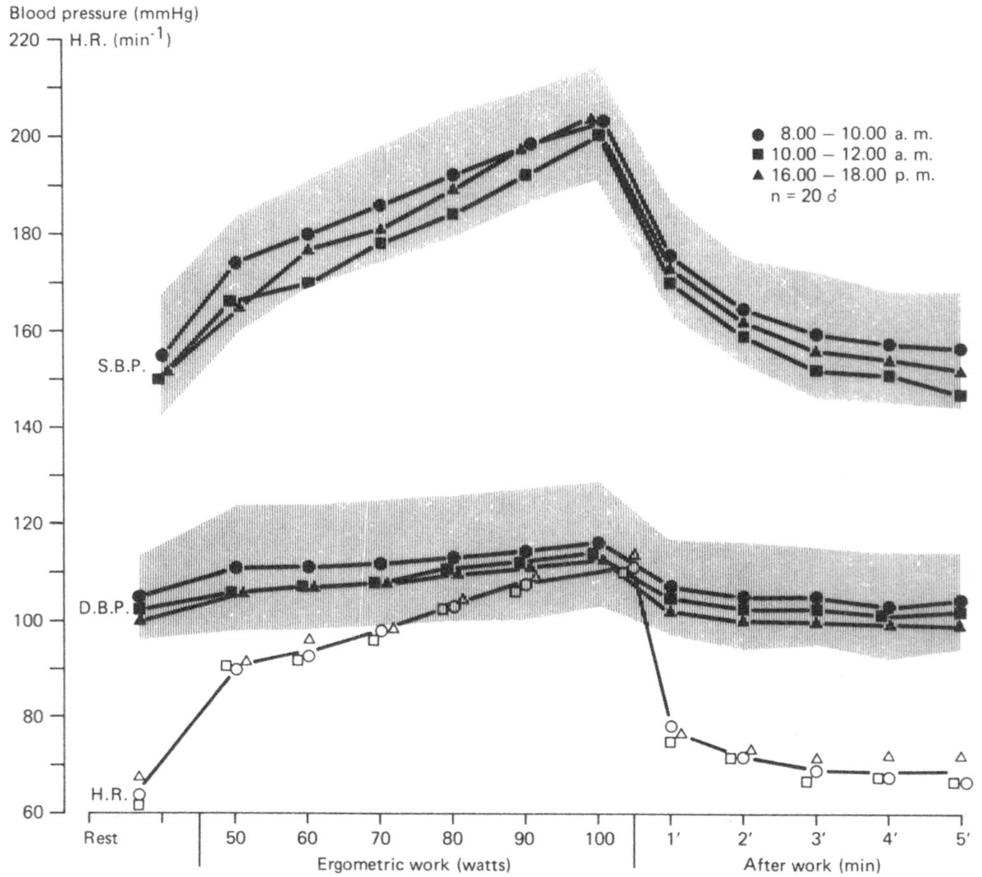

Fig. 13. Reproducibility of blood pressures readings in 20 male hypertensives and 13 borderline hypertensives taken at different times of day (8:00-10:00 a.m., 10:00 a.m. and 12:00-noon, 4:00-6:00 p.m.). The shaded area indicates the standard deviation of the initial reading

9 mm Hg, respectively. During the recovery period as well, similar systolic pressure readings were obtained on all three occasions, e.g., 175 ± 12 mm Hg, 170 ± 14 mm Hg and 174 ± 11 mm Hg at the end of the 1st minute (Table 12, Fig. 13).

Equally good agreement was found in the diastolic blood pressures measured before, during and after ergometry. As with the systolic pressures, the readings showed excellent agreement as the workload progressed, and diastolic pressures tended to be somewhat lower in the second and third tests.

The heart rates, too, showed no significant variation from one test to the next. Heart rates tended to be lower during exercise in the 2nd test between 10:00 a.m. and 12:00 noon, and higher during exercise in the evening test.

3.1.2. Borderline Hypertensives

Borderline hypertensives tend to have greater blood pressure fluctuations on repeat determinations [259]. We wished to learn whether this variability was also operative during and after ergometry. For our tests we selected eight borderline hypertensives who had exhibited marginal, labile blood pressure elevations during multiple readings at rest, and we subjected these patients to ergometric testing at three different times of day. All tests were done on work-free Saturdays, and the patients were advised to observe all conditions and restrictions pertaining to ergometric stress testing. The 1st test was performed between 8:00 a.m. and 10:00 a.m.; the 2nd was begun exactly 2 hours and the 3rd exactly 8 hours after the start of the 1st test.

Prior to ergometry the resting blood pressure was measured under 3 different conditions: after 10 minutes' recumbency, after 1 minute of standing, and immediately before the start of exercise. The systolic blood pressures after 10 minutes' recumbency became progressively lower during the course of the 3 tests; the afternoon reading of 133.4 mm Hg was well within the normotensive range and differed significantly ($p < 0.05$) from the first morning reading of 148.6 mm Hg (Table 13). The orthostatic systolic pressure also fell by about 10 mm Hg during the course of testing, although the difference was not statistically significant. The same pattern was seen in the systolic blood pressure prior to ergometry, with the 144.6 mm Hg afternoon reading differing significantly ($p < 0.05$) from the 152 mm Hg reading obtained in the first morning test. The diastolic blood pressures displayed a similar declining trend during the course of the examinations. Thus, the 95.7 mm Hg diastolic pressure measured in the afternoon immediately before exercise was significantly ($p < 0.05$) lower than the 105.7 mm Hg and 102.9 mm Hg readings taken in the first and second morning tests, respectively.

Interestingly, when we compare the systolic and diastolic pressures measured immediately before ergometry with the readings taken after 10 minutes' recumbency, we find that the latter are markedly higher. Presumably they represent a psychologic stress response. It is noteworthy that the increase of diastolic blood pressure relative to the orthostatic value became progressively smaller in the 2nd and 3rd tests, signifying a degree of adaptation on the part of the subjects.

Despite the marked variability of the blood pressure under resting conditions, the systolic and diastolic pressure levels showed no significant inter-test differences at higher workloads between 70 and 100 watts (Fig. 14). At the initial stages of 50 and 60 watts, the systolic blood pressure was in some cases significantly ($p < 0.05$) higher in the 1st measurement than in the 2nd and 3rd. At 100 watts, however, the 3 readings of 200 ± 7 mm Hg, 197 ± 11 mm Hg and 199 ± 7 mm Hg showed excellent agreement. Similar agreement was found among readings taken after the 1st minute of recovery: 171 ± 11 mm Hg, 167 ± 12 mm Hg and 170 ± 8 mm Hg.

The diastolic blood pressure at 100 watts was 111 ± 10 mm Hg in the 1st measurement, 108 ± 10 mm Hg in the 2nd, and 107 ± 8 mm Hg in the 3rd. The maximum mean difference of 4 mm Hg diastolic between the 1st and 3rd measure-

Table 13. Systolic (S. B. P.) and diastolic (D. B. P.) blood pressures and heart rates (H. R.) (means ± SD) at rest and during and after work in 8 male borderline hypertensives who were tested 3 times on a work-free saturday (*p < 0.05. **p < 0.01)

n = 8		Rest			Ergometric work (watts)						Recovery period (min)		
		Supine	Standing	Before work	50	60	70	80	90	100	1.	3.	5.
S. B. P (mmHg)	8:00 and 10:00 a.m.	148.6 12.7	142.9 17.0	152 7.1	171 9.7	177.6 7.7	180.3 6.7	187.6 8.1	193.1 6.5	200.3 6.6	170.8 11.3	154.5 7.6	151.5 7.6
	10:00 a.m. and 12:00 noon	141.1 8.7	141.4 6.9	145.1 5.0*	160.8 8.1*	164.6 10.8*	173.5 8.5	179.5 9.0	187.9 11.2	197.1 11.6	167.3 12.3	147.8 5.7	143.8 8.9
	16:00 p.m. and 18:00 p.m.	133.4 7.5*	132.6 5.1	144.6 8.7*	159.8 6.1*	170.8 6.3	176.6 4.8	185.3 8.8	192.5 7.3	199.0 6.6	170.3 7.7	150.8 6.6	145.1 8.6
D. B. P. (mmHg)	8:00 and 10:00 a.m.	98.3 6.5	96.6 5.6	105.7 5.5	105.6 10.1	106.9 11.1	107.1 10.6	107.4 10.4	109.3 11.2	111.5 10.1	105.8 9.5	99.8 6.7	101 9.0
	10:00 a.m. and 12:00 noon	97.1 9.5	98.0 6.9	102.9 6.4	102.3 10.8	101.3 7.6	102.1 9.8	106.3 10.2	106.0 9.9	108.1 10.1	100.8 6.4	98 7.9	98.4 7.9
	16:00 p.m. and 18:00 p.m.	91.4 6.9	93.4 5.5	95.7 4.2**	100.1 8.0	101.1 9.1	102.3 10.1	103.3 9.4	104.8 9.4	106.8 9.7	96.5 5.3*	95.5 6.7	95.3 6.8
H. R. (bts/min)	8:00 and 10:00 a.m.	62.4 8.4	69.6 11.0	70.5 15.1	90.0 8.8	93.3 8.7	98.4 9.8	103.4 9.1	107.7 10.9	111.6 10.7	78.2 12.4	69.2 12.0	67.4 10.9
	10:00 a.m. and 12:00 noon	56 5.5*	63.6 10.2	59.6 7.8	90.9 9.4	91.7 9.0	96.2 9.7	101.7 9.3	105.9 10.6	110.4 10.5	74.6 11.9	66.8 10.4	66.8 10.2
	16:00 p.m. and 18:00 p.m.	65.6 6.9	79.0 14*	65.9 11.6	91.9 8.4	97.2 8.6	98.7 9.4	105.4 7.9	110.0 8.4	114.3 9.4	76.9 9.7	71.4 9.9	72.4 11.8

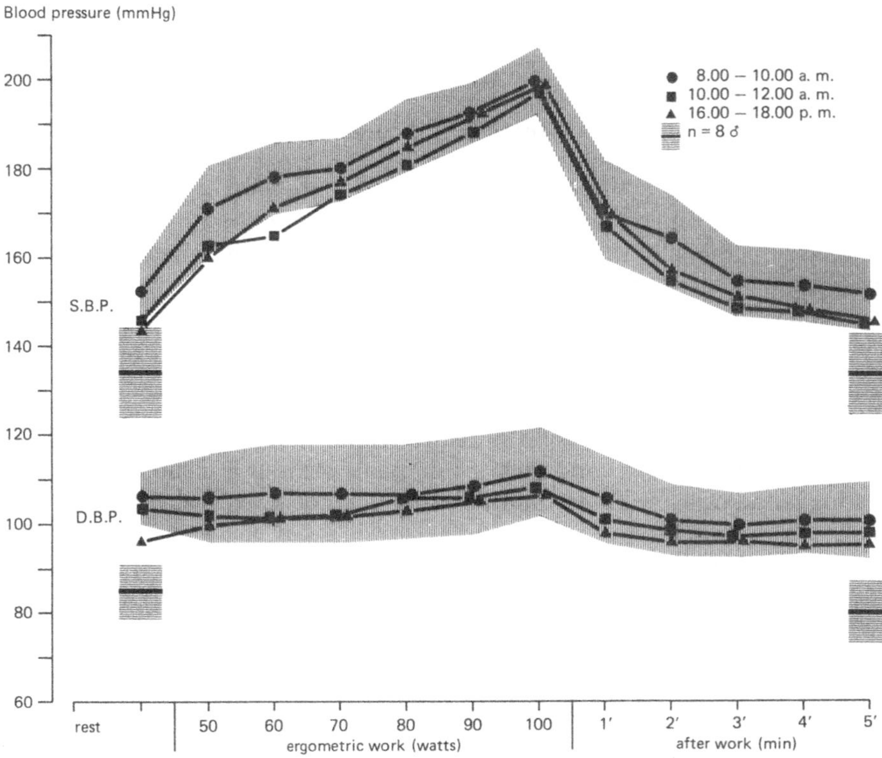

Fig. 14. Reproducibility of blood pressures readings in 20 male hypertensives and 13 borderline hypertensives taken at different times of day (8:00-10:00 a.m., 10:00-noon, 4:00-6:00 p.m.). The shaded areas indicate the standard deviation of the initial reading

ments is far smaller than the maximum mean difference of 10 mm Hg observed prior to ergometry.

As in the Stage 1 hypertensives, the heart rates of the borderline hypertensives during and after ergometry showed no significant differences from one test to the next.

The high reproducibility of blood pressure responses to ergometry has been confirmed by other authors [262, 264]. Lassvik, [264] for example, calculated a variance factor of 3 ± 2% for the maximum systolic blood pressure in ergometrc tests done on a single day, and a factor of 5 ± 4% for day-to-day variability.

Results on the reproducibility of blood pressures during and after ergometry permit the following conclusions to be drawn:

1. Repeat blood pressure determinations at workloads below 1 watt/kg body weight may reveal a decline of systolic blood pressures as a manifestation of an adaptation phenomenon.
2. The declining systolic pressures are attributable to the lower initial blood pressure level prior to ergometry, which in turn is determined by the altered emotional state of the patient.

3. At higher workloads of 80–100 watts we find excellent reproducibility of blood pressures and heart rates in agreement with invasive measurements by Drexler and Löllgen [86].
4. We observe no diurnal blood pressure fluctuations, a finding consistent with the telemetric data of Körnig for WHO Stage 1 hypertensives [259].
5. Even patients with labile and borderline hypertension, who had variable blood pressures under various "standardized" rest conditions, showed excellent reproducibility of their systolic and diastolic pressures when exercised at loads from 80 to 100 watts.
6. Accordingly, hypertensive individuals can invariably be recognized as such on the basis of their blood pressure responses during and after ergometry - a differentiation that cannot always be made on the basis of resting measurements.
7. Determination of of the blood pressure response during standardized ergometry at 50–100 watts and up to 5 minutes thereafter is clearly superior to resting blood pressure determinations in its diagnostic accuracy and specificity.
8. Ergometric testing is also useful in that it reduces the need for frequent follow-up visits, which could aid greatly in coping with the hypertension problem on a practical level.

3.2. Comparison of Hypertensive Males Varying in Age and Severity of Blood Pressure Elevation

In the sections that follow we shall examine on a comparative basis the blood pressure and heart rate responses of hypertensive patients varying in age, gender and hypertension severity during and after ergometric exercise. Besides describing relevant pathophysiologic processes, we shall make a particular effort to draw diagnostic and prognostic implications.

3.2.1. Patients

We tested a total of 281 hypertensive males ranging in age from 18 to 74 who had presented for a routine preventive cardiac examination. To aid in evaluating the results, we first divided the patients into two groups by age, with patients younger than 50 comprising group 1, and patients 50 or older comprising group 2. We then further divided each of these groups into two subgroups (A and B) according to the level of the casual blood pressure. Patients whose blood pressures were lower than 170/105 mmHg were assigned to groups 1A and 2A; patients with blood pressures higher than 170/105 mmHg were assigned to groups 1B and 2B (Table 14). The purpose of this arbitrary grouping was to enable comparisons by age and by severity of arterial hypertension.

Data regarding age, height, weight and patient numbers are given in Table 14. The groups were distributed such that there was an approximate 20-year age difference between the older groups (2A, 2B) and younger groups (1A, 2A), providing a good basis for age comparison. We also had a good basis for com-

Table 14. Age, height, weight and patient numbers (means ± SD) of 330 younger and older male and female hypertensives with different severities of hypertension

n = 330	Males Group 1 A S.B.P. < 170 mmHg D.B.P. < 105 mmHg	Males Group 2A S.B.P. < 170 mmHg D.B.P. < 105 mmHg	Males Group 1B S.B.P. > 170 mmHg D.B.P. > 105 mmHg	Males Group 2B S.B.P. > 170 mmHg D.B.P. > 105 mmHg	Females Group 1	Females Group 2
Age (years)	37 ± 8 (18-50)	59.7 ± 6.8 (51-78)	40.1 ± 6.3 (17-50)	60.9 ± 6.3 (51-73)	39.9 ± 6 (30-50)	60.4 ± 5.6 (51-67)
Height (cm)	178 7.9	176 6.2	175.9 7.2	173.6 6.5	164 5.5	158.2 7.4
Body weight	81.1 8.6	80.3 7.5	80.5 8.6	79.9 11.8	76.4 16.7	66.7 8.7
Number of patients	132	35	72	42	30	19

paring the severity of hypertension within a particular age group, because roughly the same age distribution was present in both the younger and older groups (average of 37 and 40.1 years in groups 1A and 1B, respectively, and 59.7 and 60.9 years in groups 2A and 2B).

The percentage deviation from normal weight (height in cm minus 100) was 3.9% for group 1A, 6% for group 1B, 5.7% for group 2A, and 8.6% for group 2B, so that the two groups with higher resting blood pressures also had a relatively greater degree of overweight.

We did not consider it reasonable to classify the hypertensive patients according th WHO stages, because the population included only Stage 1 and 2 hypertensives, the majority of whom belonged to Stage 1.

3.2.2. Age Comparison of Hypertensives with Blood Pressures below 170/105 mmHg

First we shall examine the patients' blood pressure and heart rate responses as a function of age for the milder forms of hypertension (Table 15, Fig. 15). The group of younger hypertensives with mild pressure elevations (group 1A) had significantly ($p < 0.001$) higher systolic blood pressures both during and after ergometry than the normotensive population of the same age. Looking at the older hypertensives (group 2A), we find that while their resting diastolic blood pressures were comparable to the diastolic pressures in group 1A, their systolic blood pressures were significantly higher ($p < 0.001$) before, during and after ergometry. It is noteworthy that the systolic blood pressures in both groups at the end of the fifth minute of recovery were still well above the pre-exercise level.

The diastolic blood pressure of groups 1A and 2A rose continuously during ergometry and remained elevated in the recovery period compared to the normal population ($p < 0.001$). While the initial, resting diastolic pressure readings were almost identical in the younger and older groups, the diastolic pressures of

Table 15. Systolic (S. B. P.) and diastolic (D. B. P.) blood pressures and heart rates (H. R.) response (means ± SD) as a function of age for the milder forms of hypertension (group 1A and group 2A; *p < 0.05. **p < 0.01. ***p < 0.001)

n = 167		Rest	Ergometric work (watts)						Recovery period (min)				
		Supine	50	60	70	80	90	100	1.	2.	3.	4.	5.
S. B. P. (mmHg)	Group 1A n = 132 37 yrs	151.6 10.7	181.7 18.6	188.3 18.3	195.1 19	200.8 20.6	204.3 20.8	213 22.4	186.6 18.8	173.2 17.2	166.2 14.9	160.6 17	158.1 14
	Group 2A n = 35 59.7 yrs	159.2 11.5***	189.8 21.6*	200.9 20.3***	207.7 20.4***	212.5 20.7***	219 20.9***	223.8 19***	198.8 16***	184.6 15.6***	174.8 15.3***	170.5 15.3***	168 15.3***
D. B. P. (mmHg)	Group 1A n = 132 37 yrs	98 5.5	108.2 9.5	110.3 9.3	111.8 9.3	113.1 10.3	114.1 11	115.8 11.1	104.2 8.5	103 7.8	102.8 8.3	102.8 8.6	103.5 8.5
	Group 2A n = 35 59.7 yrs	97.7 4.5	109.5 10.8	112.8 10.5	114 11.2	115.3 11.1	116 12.1	118.9 11.7	103.9 11.9	102.4 11.7	101.5 11.1	101.2 10.2	100.8 9
H. R. (bts/min)	Group 1A n = 132 37 yrs	70.8 12.9	97.8 12.6	102.5 13.4	107.2 14.5	111.8 15.2	116.3 15.2	121.2 16.8	90.1 17.8	82.9 16.8	79.2 14.5	79.4 15	78.3 15
	Group 2A n = 35 59.7 yrs	70.1 12.4	97.1 13.9	102.4 14.4	106.7 15.6	112.2 16.7	115.2 16.6	120.1 17.5	93.8 16.2	85.5 17.1	82.6 15.9	76.6 15.2	79.9 15.1

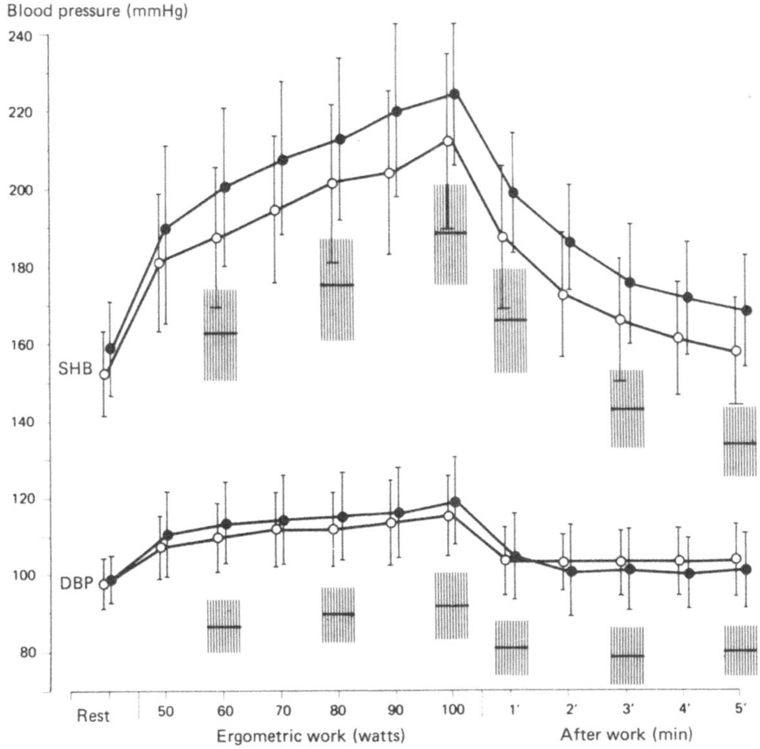

Fig. 15. Blood pressure responses of younger (group 1 A) and older (group 2 A) hypertensive patients with mild blood pressure elevations at rest. The shaded area indicates the normal blood pressure response

the older group were higher than those of the younger group at all stages of exercise, though statistical significance was not confirmed. Like the systolic blood pressure, the diastolic pressure did not reach or fall below the pre-exercise levels after five minutes of recovery.

The heart rate responses of both groups were virtually identical before, during and after ergometry.

3.2.3. Age Comparison in Hypertensives with Blood Pressures above 170/105 mmHg

A comparison of the hypertensive patients in groups 1B and 2B, who had resting blood pressures above 170/105 mmHg (Table 16, Fig. 16), demonstrated a higher systolic blood pressure in the older hypertensives (group 2B) at all workloads and during recovery, although no significant difference was apparent before exercise. The difference during exercise and recovery was statistically significant ($p < 0.05$–$p < 0.01$) only at 80 and 100 watts and in the 1st and 3rd minutes of recovery. Thus, the older hypertensives had greater blood pressure increases in both absolute and relative terms. This is also indicated by a comparison of group 1B with the older population in Chap. II.3.2.

Table 16. Systolic (S. B. P.) and diastolic (D. B. P.) blood pressures and heart rates (H. R.) response (means ± SD) as a function of age of the hypertensive patients in groups 1 and 2B (resting blood pressures above 170/105 mmHg) at rest and during and after work (*p < 0.05; **p < 0.01)

n = 114		Rest	Ergometric work (watts)						Recovery period (min)				
		Supine	50	60	70	80	90	100	1.	2.	3.	4.	5.
S. B. P. (mmHg)	Group 1B n = 72 40.1 yrs	172.5 14.3	195.1 20.1	205 20.6	210.2 20.5	213.9 20.8	219.8 22.1	224.9 21.7	194.8 20.5	183.6 17.8	176.9 17.2	175.5 19	173.4 18.1
	Group 2B n = 42 60.9 yrs	176.3 16.3	199.5 17.8	210.3 19.4	217 18.4	226 19.4**	230 19.1*	234.2 20.1*	208.5 23.7**	192.5 22.3*	185.5 20.5*	182.2 17.8	178.8 19.5
D. B. P. (mmHg)	Group 1B n = 72 40.1 yrs	113.7 7.2	119.7 9.2	121.7 10.5	122.2 10	124 10.8	124 10.5	126.3 11.4	113.7 11.2	112.8 10.7	112.7 10.4	113.6 10.9	113.8 11.3
	Group 2B n = 42 60.9 yrs	110.2 7.7*	121.3 11	123.1 13.2	123.5 13.3	124.9 13.9	126.6 13.4	128.2 13.3	114.6 14.7	113 12.8	111 11.7	112 12.7	113 13.1
H. R. (bts/min)	Group 1B n = 72 40.1 yrs	70.7 13.9	98.4 14.9	104.2 15.8	108.3 16.8	112.5 16.9	117.2 17.7	120.8 11.4	90.1 21	85.8 19.3	83.7 18.9	82.1 17.3	81.4 16
	Group 2B n = 42 60.9 yrs	72.8 10.5	96 12.2	101 11.2	105.3 11.2	110 11.4	114.5 12.7	118.1 14	90.6 12.8	84.2 13	81.1 12.1	80.6 11.5	79.7 10.9

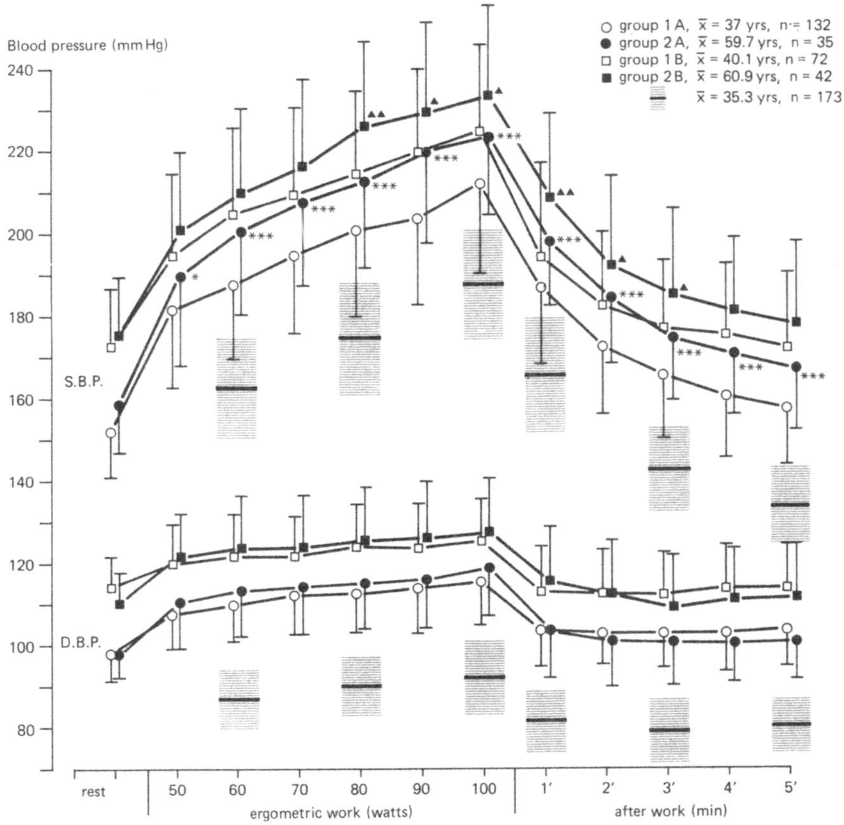

Fig. 16. Blood pressure responses of groups 1 A, 2 A, 1 B and 2 B of younger and older patients with different severities of hypertension

A similar pattern was evident in the diastolic blood pressure, which was higher in the older group at all stages of exercise despite a significantly ($p<0.05$) lower resting value. The difference during exercise was not statistically significant, however.

When we examined the systolic and diastolic blood pressures of both groups at the end of the fifth minute of recovery, we again found that these pressures had not yet returned to the pre-exercise levels.

The heart rates in the older group were lower at all stages of exercise, though the difference was not significant statistically.

3.2.4. Hypertensives of Equal Age but with Different Severities of Blood Pressure Elevation

The younger hypertensives of groups 1A and 1B showed a significant difference ($p<0.001$) in their resting blood pressures: 152/98 mmHg in the former vs. 173/114 mmHg in the latter. The difference remained at this level of significance throughout the range of 50 to 100 watts (e.g., 213/116 vs. 225/126 mmHg at 100 watts) and during the entire recovery period (Tables 15 and 16, Fig. 16).

The older hypertensives of groups 2A and 2B also had significantly different ($p < 0.001$) resting blood pressures: 159/98 mmHg vs. 176/110 mm Hg. During exercise the systolic blood pressures in group 2B were significantly higher ($p < 0.05$–$p < 0.01$) than in group 2A (e.g., 234 vs. 224 mmHg at 100 watts). A similar elevation of the systolic pressure was confirmed statistically ($p < 0.05$–$p < 0.01$) during all parts of the recovery period except for minute 2. The diastolic pressure in group 2B also attained a significantly higher level ($p < 0.01$–$p < 0.001$) during ergometry (e.g., 128 vs. 119 mmHg at 100 watts) and during recovery ($p < 0.001$) compared with group 2A.

Regardless of age, therefore, it is reasonable to expect that hypertensives with higher mean blood pressures at rest will also have higher mean blood pressures during exercise. We emphasize "mean pressure" because some individuals with low resting blood pressures may experience alarming blood pressure increases during exercise, causing the vascular risk in these patients to be grossly underestimated on the basis of readings obtained at rest. This problem is of clinical importance and will be explored further on the basis of case examples (II.3.4.5). Other patients, meanwhile, may show an opposite response: a relatively high resting blood pressure which increases little with exercise. This pattern is particularly characteristic of hypertension in the elderly (Chap. II.6.).

3.3. Comparison of Hypertensive Females of Varying Ages

3.3.1. Patients

We tested a total of 49 female outpatients who had presented for routine cardiac examinations. Given the limited number of participants in the study, we subdivided the patients into only two groups, with women under 50 assigned to group 1 and women over 50 assigned to group 2. The mean values and standard deviations for age, height and weight are shown in Table 14.

3.3.2. Blood Pressure and Heart Rate Responses

The younger women of group 1 (average age 39.9 years) and the older women of group 2 (average age 60.4 years) had resting systolic blood pressures of 157 and 162 mmHg, respectively, and thus showed no statistically significant difference (Table 17, Fig. 17).

During ergometry, however, the older patients developed significantly higher systolic blood pressures both at the initial 50-watt stage ($p < 0.01$) and during all stages thereafter ($p < 0.001$). Thus, the older group developed a very high systolic pressure of 241 ± 18 mmHg at a workload of only 80 watts, which is substantially different from the 211 mmHg recorded in the younger women. A similar pattern of systolic elevation was seen in the recovery period.

The resting diastolic pressure of the older women was 97 mmHg and thus significantly lower than the 101 mmHg recorded in the younger women. During

Table 17. Systolic (S.B.P.) and diastolic (D.B.P.) blood pressures and heart rates (H.R.) response (means ± SD) as a function of age of the female hypertensives of groups 1 and 2 at rest and during and after work (*$p < 0.05$; **$p < 0.01$; ***$p < 0.001$)

n = 49		Rest	Ergometric work (watts)						Recovery period (min)				
		Supine	50	60	70	80	90	100	1.	2.	3.	4.	5.
S.B.P. (mmHg)	Group 1 n = 30 39.9 yrs	156.7 15	184.2 18.7	194.8 21.7	202.6 18.8	210.8 19.5	216 19.5	220.4 18.9	188 19.7	170.1 15.9	159.6 15.2	158.8 13.3	156.9 11.3
	Group 2 n = 19 60.4 yrs	162 17	198.5 14.9**	218.7 16.7***	232.3 19.2***	241.3 18.2***	– –	– –	214 17.9***	188.6 15.9***	175.9 16.7***	170.2 17.6**	169.9 19.3*
D.B.P. (mmHg)	Group 1 n = 30 39.9 yrs	103.7 10	114.5 11.7	117.7 10.5	119.4 9.9	122.6 10.2	124.6 12	125.5 11.8	106.6 12.1	102.4 9.7	101.1 10.4	101.1 10.3	101 9.5
	Group 2 n = 19 60.4 yrs	97.4 7.5*	113.1 11.2	119.3 12.0	121.3 12.1	124.1 11.2	– –	– –	103.3 12.7	99.6 12.7	98.7 11.5	99.1 11.2	99.8 11.3
H.R. (bts/min)	Group 1 n = 30 39.9 yrs	79.5 16.1	112.3 17.9	121.4 17.9	128.9 19	136.1 18.6	142.6 16.3	146 15.3	110 17.1	98.4 16.9	93.3 16.6	92.2 16	90.5 15.7
	Group 2 n = 19 60.4 yrs	72.3 13.5	110 11.5	119.2 13.8	127.7 13.4	132.1 13.2	– –	– –	97.9 14.9	88.5 11.7	84.9 12.9	84.1 10.6	81.9 9.6

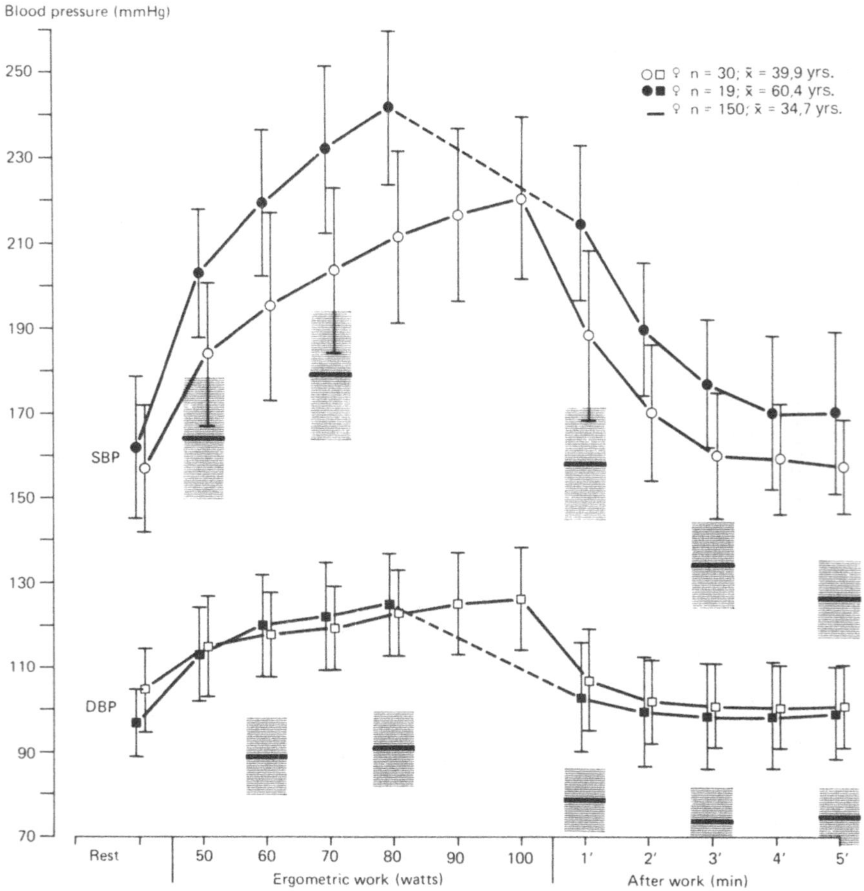

Fig. 17. Blood pressure responses of female hypertensives of different ages (average 39.9 years and 60.4 years). The shaded columns show the responses of the younger normotensive controls

exercise at 50–80 watts, however, the diastolic pressure rose to a level above that measured in the younger patients, though this increase was not confirmed statistically.

If we compare the systolic and diastolic blood pressures of the two groups after five minutes of recovery, we find that, except for the diastolic pressure in group 1, the pattern of response is similar to that observed in the male hypertensives, with pressures in the older group remaining elevated above pre-exercise levels.

The heart rates showed no significant age-specific differences before, during or after ergometry. An age comparison for the two groups was carried out only for the range of 50–80 watts, because most of the women in group 2 either stopped exercising at 80 watts, or the test had to be terminated at that point due to an excessive rise in blood pressure.

3.4. Summary and Conclusions

3.4.1. Mean Systolic and Diastolic Blood Pressure Responses

Hemodynamic studies in hypertensive patients at rest and during exercise [51, 152, 215, 216, 277, 278, 366, 367] have consistently shown that increased *peripheral vascular resistance* is a characteristic feature of arterial hypertension.

Exercise in *normotensive persons* stimulates a *metabolic vasodilatation* in the periphery which markedly lowers the total peripheral resistance [37, 152, 277]. Hence these individuals experience only a minimal rise of diastolic blood pressure during ergometry despite a high cardiac output (see Fig. 3). In hypertensives, on the other hand, this compensatory vasodilatation may be seriously restricted during ergometry [277, 278, 366, 367], allowing the diastolic blood pressure to rise sharply. Folkow [102] theorizes that this is due to a thickening of the arteriolar wall which prevents the vessel from responding normally to vasoconstrictor stimuli [328]. Other possible causes are an excessive release of endogenous catecholamines or hyperresponsiveness of the alpha adrenergic receptors. Thus, a major goal of ergometric blood pressure testing is to ascertain whether the arterioles can dilate normally in response to the increased oxygen demand of the muscles during dynamic exercise.

The results presented here prove that the pathophysiologic processes associated with arterial hypertension can be recognized on the basis of systolic and especially diastolic blood pressure elevations demonstrated during ergometry by noninvasive means.

The hypertensive patients in this study had significantly higher blood pressures than normal subjects both during and after ergometry, regardless of age, sex and severity. In addition, significant *age effects* were apparent regardless of the level of the resting blood pressure. Thus, an age-dependent increase in the systolic blood pressure was observed both during ergometry and in the recovery period. The diastolic pressures also were markedly higher in the older groups, regardless of the level of the resting diastolic pressure, though statistical significance was not shown.

If we compare the blood pressure responses of the different groups both at rest and during ergometry, we find that higher systolic and diastolic pressures in the resting state imply higher blood pressures during exercise. For example, the younger hypertensive males with a mildly elevated resting blood pressure of 152/98 mmHg had a mean blood pressure of 213/116 mmHg at 100 watts. The male hypertensives of the same age but with a higher resting blood pressure of 173/114 mmHg (group 1B) developed a significantly higher mean blood pressure of 225/126 mmHg at the same workload. A similar pattern was evident in the older groups. Thus, while the mild hypertensives of group 2A had a resting blood pressure of 159/98 mmHg and an exercise pressure of 224/119 mm Hg at 100 watts, the hypertensives of group 2B, with their higher resting pressure of 176/110 mmHg, developed 234/128 mmHg when stressed at 100 watts.

Examining the blood pressure responses of the hypertensive females, we find that the younger women (average age 39.9 years) had significantly higher systolic and diastolic blood pressures ($p < 0.001$) at 80 watts than the normal subjects:

211/123 mmHg vs. 179/92 mmHg. The hypertensive women in group 2, who were 20 years older on the average, had systolic blood pressures of 241 ± 8 mmHg at 80 watts. These were significantly higher ($p < 0.001$) than the systolic readings in group 1, despite the similar resting blood pressures in the two groups during recumbency. Thus, the age effect appears to be even more pronounced in female hypertensives than in males. Similar patterns were observed during recovery. The older hypertensive women also developed higher diastolic pressures during exercise than the younger women, despite their lower resting pressures, although the difference was not statistically significant.

It is interesting to compare the blood pressure responses of the hypertensive males of group 1A with those of the younger hypertensive women, who are comparable to the men in terms of age and resting blood pressure. Even at equal workloads we find that the women tended to develop higher systolic pressures over the range from 50 to 100 watts, with a statistically significant difference ($p < 0.05$–$p < 0.01$) observable at loads of 80 and 90 watts. At all stages the diastolic pressures of the younger hypertensive women were significantly higher ($p < 0.01$–$p < 0.001$) than those of the comparable hypertensive males, e.g., 126 mmHg in the females vs. 116 mmHg in the males at 100 watts. This statistically significant difference was no longer present in the recovery period.

Comparing the exercise blood pressure responses of the older male and female hypertensives of group 2 and 2A, who have comparable resting blood pressures, we find significantly higher ($p < 0.001$) pressure levels in the older women, e.g., 241/124 mmHg vs. 213/115 mmHg at a load of 80 watts.

The fact that the systolic and diastolic blood pressure patterns characteristic of a particular age, gender and resting blood pressure level are demonstrable both during exercise and in the recovery period serves to underscore the significant diagnostic value of blood pressure determinations during ergometry.

3.4.2. Reproducibility of the Blood Pressure

The value of ergometric testing becomes particularly evident when one considers that the reliability of any diagnostic procedure depends on the reproducibility of its data. In our comparative ergometric studies of 20 hypertensive patients, we found that blood pressure responses did not show significant variation when the tests were repeated at different times of day. It is especially noteworthy that some of these patients were mildly hypertensive (WHO Stage 1), and that others were borderline. Even in the marginal range the results of each test were conclusive and provided sufficient basis for a diagnosis of arterial hypertension to be made. The differences between individual systolic and diastolic blood pressure readings at 100 watts were smaller than the fluctuations in resting values.

These results are in good agreement with blood pressures measured directly by Krönig [259], who demonstrated excellent reproducibility of blood pressure readings taken during step exercise. Repeating the test at three different times of day, as well as on different days, did not significantly alter the exercise response. As in our investigations, Krönig [259] noted a tendency toward lower systolic and diastolic pressures during the second test conducted around midday.

Table 18. Shows the prevalence of the three hemodynamic reaction types in each of the groups tested. Patients whose systolic pressure at 100 watts exceeded the mean plus one standard deviation for that group, and whose diastolic pressure did not exceed the mean, were assigned to Type A. Patients who had a diastolic pressure greater than the mean plus 1 SD at 100 watts but a systolic pressure lower than the mean were classified as Type C. All other patients were assigned to Type B. Moreover, the prevalence by group of patients whose blood pressure at 100 watts was in the range of 190–200 mg systolic or below the upper limit of 100 mg diastolic (B. H. + exercise-positive borderline hypertensives; B. H. - exercise-negative borderline hypertensives)

	Males 37 yrs Group 1A n=132	Males 59.7 yrs Group 2A n=35	Males 40.1 yrs Group 1B n=72	Males 60.9 yrs Group 2B n=42	Males 38.3 yrs B. H. + n=49	Males 39.9 yrs B. H. – n=49	Females 39.3 yrs Group 1 n=30	Females 60.4 yrs Group 2 n=19
Type A	>235 mmHg <116 mmHg 17%	>245 mmHg <119 mmHg 22.9%	>247 mmHg <126 mmHg 8.3%	>254 mmHg <128 mmHg 14.3%	>237 mmHg <113 mmHg 8.2%	>222 mmHg <92 mmHg 16.3%	>239 mmHg <126 mmHg 10.0%	>259 mmHg <124 mmHg 15.8%
Type B	69.7%	74.2%	76.4%	83.3%	83.6%	81.6%	80%	84.2%
Type C	<213 mmHg >126 mmHg 17.4%	<224 mmHg >131 mmHg 2.9%	<225 mmHg >137 mmHg 15.3%	<234 mmHg >141 mmHg 2.4%	<216 mmHg >121 mmHg 8.2%	<204 mmHg > 99 mmHg 2.1%	<220 mmHg >138 mmHg 10%	<241 mmHg >135 mmHg 0%
S. B. P. at 100 watts between 190–200 mmHg	25%	5.7%	9.7%	0%	18.4%	49%	16.7%	0%
D. B. P. at 100 watts <100 mmHg	0%	0%	0%	0%	0%	100%	0%	0%

3.4.3. Analysis of Blood Pressure Responses by Hemodynamic Reaction Type

In analyzing individual blood pressure responses to ergometry, we can distinguish three basic patterns called "hemodynamic reaction types" (Table 18). Type A individuals develop a very high systolic pressure with only a moderate rise of diastolic pressure during ergometry. Type B is characterized by approximately equal degrees of systolic and diastolic pressure elevation, and Type C by a sharp rise of diastolic pressure with a moderate concomitant rise of systolic pressure.

Table 18 show the prevalence of the three reaction types in each of the groups tested. Patients whose systolic pressure at 100 watts exceeded the mean plus one standard deviation for that group, and whose diastolic pressure did not exceed the mean, were assigned to Type A. Patients who had a diastolic pressure greater than the mean plus 1 SD at 100 watts but a systolic pressure lower than the mean were classified as Type C. All other patients were assigned to Type B.

The results indicate that the great majority of patients had roughly equal elevations of their systolic and diastolic pressures at 100 watts, making Type B the predominant reaction type. Interestingly, a significant prevalence of Type C was found only in groups 1A and 1B of the younger hypertensive men, in the younger hypertensive women, and in exercise-positive borderline hypertensives to some degree. It is tempting to speculate that the primary abnormality in these patients is an elevated peripheral resistance, leading predominantly to an elevation of the diastolic pressure. Once the heart adapts to the high peripheral resistance through myocardial hypertrophy, these patients would experience an equivalent degree of systolic pressure elevation.

Not surprisingly, the prevalence of Type A increases with the rise of systolic blood pressure with age and was greatest in the two older groups of hypertensive males and in the older females. Besides myocardial adaptation, this may reflect a failure of the "windkessel" or expansion chamber function of the aorta with increasing age.

3.4.4. Analysis of the Upper Normotensive Limit

Table 18 shows the prevalence by group of patients whose blood pressure at 100 watts was below the upper limit of 190–200 mmHg systolic or 100 mmHg diastolic. Regardless of age, gender and severity of hypertension, we did not find one patient whose diastolic pressure was less than 100 mmHg at 100 watts, and so this limit appears to be very reliable for discriminating between a normotensive and pathologically elevated stress response. None of the hypertensive patients had a systolic pressure less than 190 mmHg at 100 watts. In 14.8% the systolic pressure was between 190 and 200 mmHg and thus below the value of 200 mmHg at 100 watts chosen for the systolic limit. Nevertheless, these patients could be readily identified as hypertensives on the basis of their diastolic blood pressure response.

Table 19 shows the prevalence by group of patients who had diastolic pressures above 100 mmHg, between 99 and 95 mmHg, between 94 and 90 mm Hg, and below 90 mmHg at 5 minutes postexercise. None of the male hypertensives and only 3 of the female hypertensives had a diastolic pressure less than 90 mm

Table 19. Shows the prevalence by group of patients who had diastolic pressures above 100 mmHg, between 99 and 95 mmHg, between 94 and 90 mmHg, and below 90 mmHg at 5 minutes postexercise

	Total study population n=379	Males 37 yrs Group 1A n=132	Males 59.7 yrs Group 2A n=35	Males 40.1 yrs Group 1B n=72	Males 60.9 yrs Group 2B n=42	Males 38.3 yrs B. H. + n=49	Females 39.9 yrs Group 1 n=30	Females 60.4 yrs Group 2 n=19
$P_d > 100$ mmHg	75.7%	74.2%	68.6%	94.4%	95.2%	57.2%	63.4%	52.6%
P_d 99–95 mmHg	11.9%	15.2%	17.1%	4.2%	2.4%	16.3%	13.3%	15.8%
P_d 94–90 mmHg	11.6%	10.6%	14.3%	1.4%	2.4%	26.5%	20%	21.1%
$P_d < 90$ mmHg	0.8%	0%	0%	0%	0%	0%	3.3%	10.5%

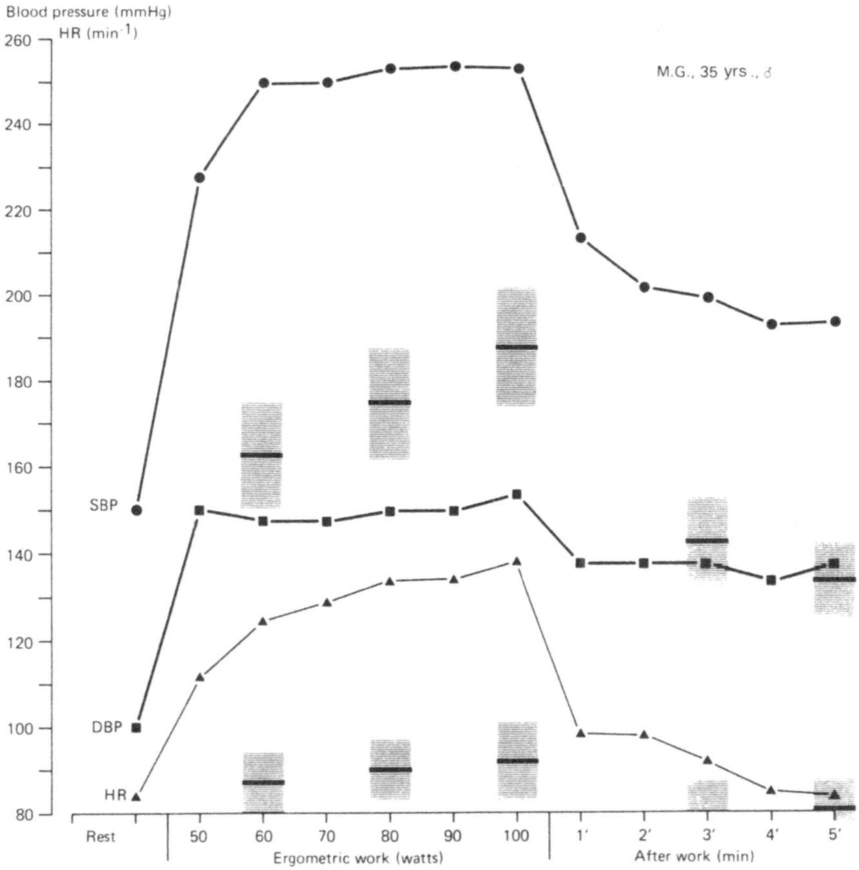

Fig. 18. Blood pressure response of a 35-year-old hypertensive male of normal body weight whose resting blood pressure of 150/100 mmHg climbed to 228/150 mmHg at 50 watts and to 250/154 mmHg at 100 watts. The shaded areas show the blood pressure responses of age-matched normotensive controls

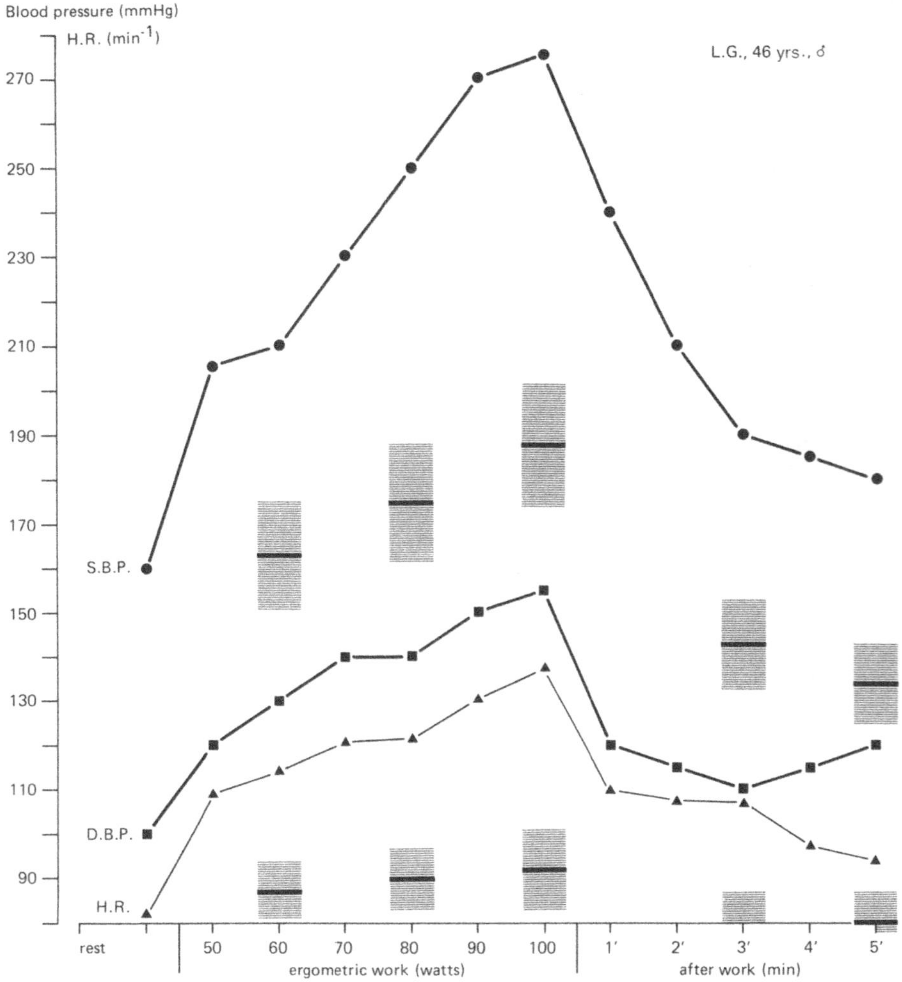

Fig. 19. Blood pressure response of a 46-year-old patient of normal body weight whose resting blood pressure rose from 165/100 mmHg to 275/155 mmHg at 100 watts of exercise

Hg at 5 minutes postexercise, and so this appears to be a rational limit for discriminating between normotensive and hypertensive individuals. This assumption is strengthened by the fact that 75.7% of the 379 hypertensive males and females enrolled in the study still had diastolic pressures of at least 100 mmHg after 5 minutes' recovery. This was true in almost 95% of the two groups of males with elevated resting blood pressures.

3.4.5. Individual Blood Pressure Response

It must be understood that our discussion of blood pressure responses is based upon mean values for groups, and that the individual blood pressure response to exercise cannot be reliably predicted from the resting blood pressure. Even

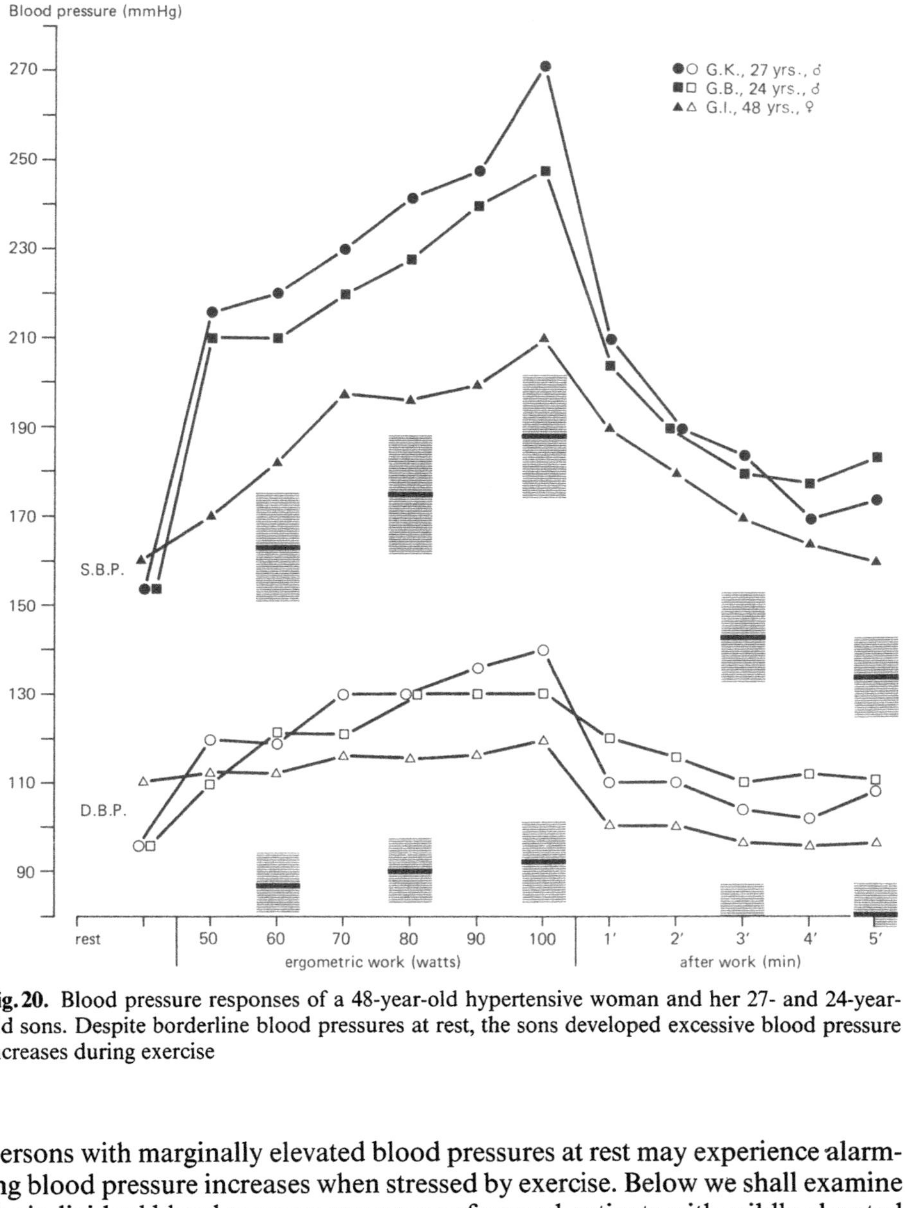

Fig. 20. Blood pressure responses of a 48-year-old hypertensive woman and her 27- and 24-year-old sons. Despite borderline blood pressures at rest, the sons developed excessive blood pressure increases during exercise

persons with marginally elevated blood pressures at rest may experience alarming blood pressure increases when stressed by exercise. Below we shall examine the individual blood pressure responses of several patients with mildly elevated resting blood pressures to illustrate how ergometric testing can aid in assessing the severity of a patient's condition and thus provide results that are of prognostic significance.

Fig. 18 shows the blood pressure response of a 35-year-old man of normal weight whose resting blood pressure of 150/100 mmHg rose to 228/150 mmHg at a workload of only 50 watts, corresponding to very low-level everyday exertion, and subsequently rose to 250/154 mmHg at 100 watts. Five minutes after ergometry a significant elevation (194/138 mmHg) was still present.

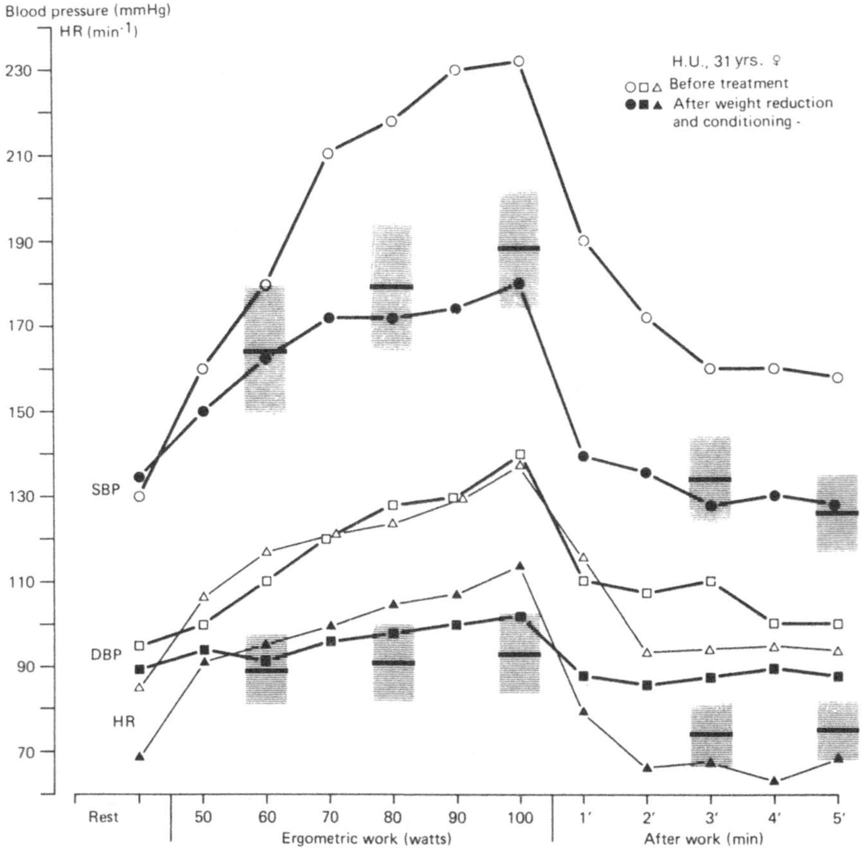

Fig. 21. Blood pressure response of a 31-year-old overweight woman whose resting blood pressure of 130/95 mmHg rose to 232/142 mmHg at 100 watts. The effect of a three-month conditioning and weight-reduction program is also shown

Fig. 19 shows the response of a 46-year-old man of normal weight whose resting blood pressure, 165/100 mmHg, rose steadily during ergometry to 275/155 mmHg at 100 watts. Again we see that the blood pressure was still markedly elevated at 5 minutes postexercise (180/120 mmHg).

Fig. 20 shows the blood pressure response of a 48-year-old mother together with that of her 27- and 24-year-old sons. The mother's resting blood pressure of 160/110 mmHg, which already was markedly elevated, rose during ergometry to 210/120 mmHg and thus showed a relatively small amount of increase. Her sons, on the other hand, who had borderline pressures of 154/96 and 156/96 mmHg at rest, developed pressures of 272/140 and 248/130 mm Hg at 100 watts with concomitant heart rates of 130 and 132 beats/min. These blood pressure increases were entirely reproducible on repeat testing. Since the maternal grandfather was also hypertensive and had died one year previously from the effects of a stroke, it may be presumed that a genetic predisposition for hypertension exists in this family. It is interesting to speculate whether the severity

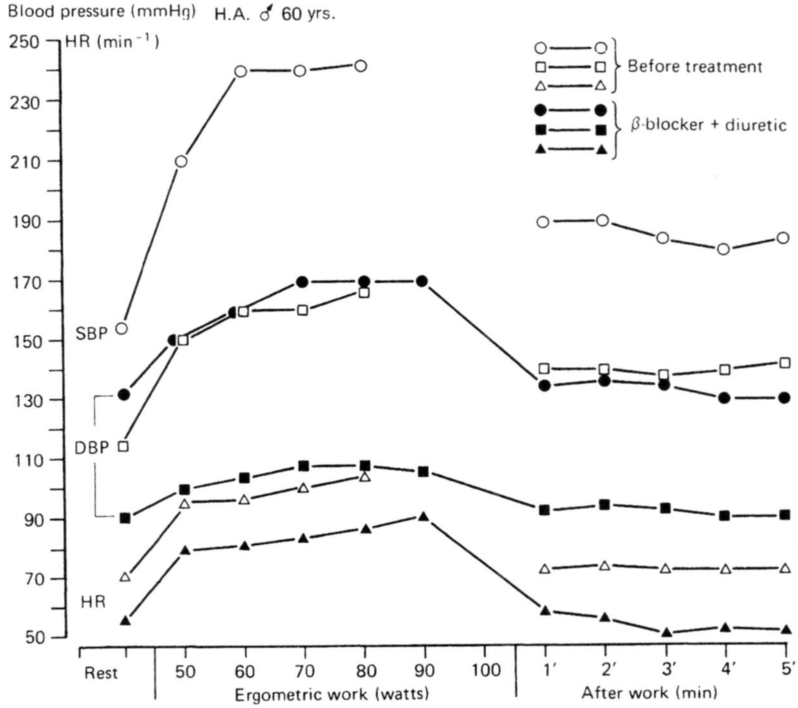

Fig. 22. Blood pressure and heart rate responses of a 60-year-old patient whose resting blood pressure of 154/114 mmHg rose to 210/150 mmHg at only 50 watts. The result of combined treatment with a beta-blocker and diuretic is also shown

of the exercise blood pressure elevation is also subject to genetic influences, as is suggested by the correlation of blood pressure responses in the two sons.

Even young women who have borderline blood pressures at rest may experience severe blood pressure elevations during exercise, as Fig. 21 illustrates. The blood pressure of this 31-year-old overweight woman rose from 130/95 mmHg at rest to 232/142 mmHg at 100 watts.

Fig. 22 and 23 demonstrate that the occurrence of pathologic exercise blood pressures is by no means peculiar to younger hypertensives. In fact, marked blood pressure peaks are particularly characteristic of hypertension in the elderly [48]. The 60-year-old hypertensive man (Fig. 22) had resting blood pressures of 160/112 mm Hg. At only 70 watts these pressures increased to 242/160 mmHg, raising the systolic pressure 42 mmHg above the age-normal level of 100 watts and the diastolic pressure 57 mm Hg above that level.

Exercise blood pressure responses in the elderly can be used as a means of identifying those patients who probably will not benefit from pharmacologic treatment. Thus, the 60-year-old patient in Figure had a resting blood pressure of 170/112 mmHg, but his blood pressure during exercise was normal for his age. Typically, the diastolic blood pressure also returns to normal during the recovery period, and so in the absence of additional risk factors or coexisting

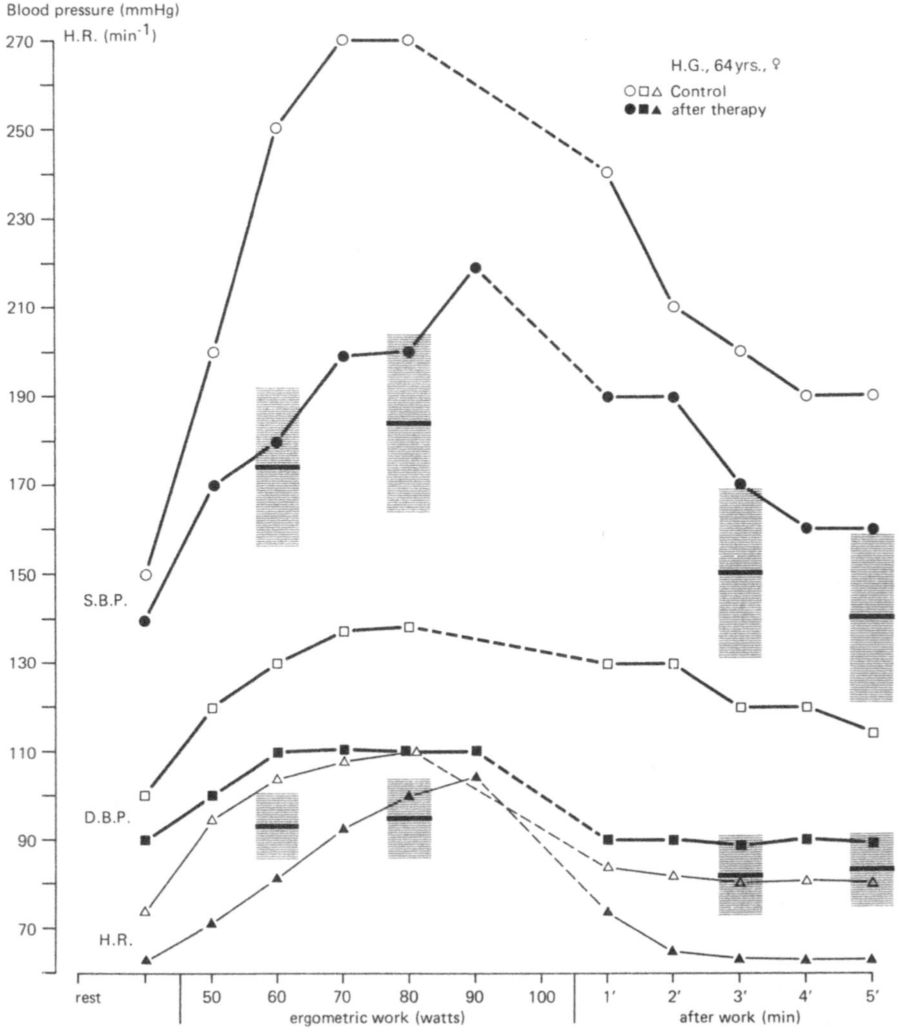

Fig. 23. Blood pressure response of a 64-year-old woman whose blood pressure rose from 150/100 mmHg at rest to 270/138 mmHg at only 80 watts. The effect of combined treatment with a diuretic and beta-blocking drug is also shown

problems such as coronary artery disease, antihypertensive drug treatment would not be indicated.

The final example in Fig. 23 illustrates once again that older hypertensive women appear to be at particular risk for developing a pathologic rise in blood pressure during exercise. The blood pressure of this 64-year-old woman rose from 150/100 mmHg at rest to 270/138 mmHg at 80 watts, although the concomitant heart rate was only 110/min. The blood pressure was still markedly elevated (190/114 mmHg) at 5 minutes postexercise. The patient reported that years of blood pressure tracking by her family physician had disclosed only mild to marginal elevations of her resting blood pressure. This appeared to conflict with ECG signs of left ventricular hypertrophy and the finding of an enlarged left heart and elongated aorta with an accentuated aortic knob on chest roentgenograms, but could be readily explained on the basis of the patient's exaggerated blood pressure response to exercise.

Thus, in both younger and older individuals with borderline or mild hypertension at rest, the demonstration of pathologic blood pressures during exercise can greatly facilitate the selection of patients for pharmacologic treatment.

Given the fact that the vascular risk of arterial hypertension is directly proportional to the level of the blood pressure during the course of the day (s. Chap. III.1.), it is reasonable to except that the severity of hypertensive disease can be evaluated more realistically by ergometric testing than by determinations of the highly variable resting blood pressure.

In addition to its diagnostic value, then, ergometry should have significant prognostic value in hypertension, especially in the mild and borderline forms.

4. Blood Pressure and Heart Rate Responses of Borderline Hypertensives

The *evaluation of borderline hypertension* in the physician's office is a difficult matter, and doubts frequently persist as to the pathologic significance of marginal blood pressure elevations and the necessity of treatment. In asymptomatic individuals and especially in juveniles, there is a tendency to attribute mild blood pressure elevations to temporary "excitement" [181, 182] and neglect further evaluation [166, 364]. In addition, most hypertensive persons have occasional periods of normotension which can mislead the examiner. According to Linss and Böthig [270] there is a very low success rate in predicting, on the basis of resting blood pressure readings, whether an individual with borderline hypertension will eventually progress to established hypertension or will become spontaneously normotensive.

Therefore we investigated the blood pressure response during and after exercise in patients with borderline hypertension. We wished to learn whether blood pressure readings taken under standardized ergometric conditions could demonstrate the dividing line between an arbitrarily defined normal and pathologic resting blood pressure and thus facilitate evaluation, and whether this type of test could provide a new, measurable clinical parameter that would be of value in the early recognition of hypertensive disease.

4.1. Blood Pressure and Heart Rate Responses of Men 20-50 Years of Age

4.1.1. Patients

We tested a total of 98 patients aged 20-50 years who presented for routine cardiac examinations. All the men had blood pressures in the borderline range according to WHO criteria [451] (140-160 mmHg systolic, 90-95 diastolic) based on casual readings taken after 3 minutes' recumbency on at least two different days.

After blood pressures were taken during ergometry and in the recovery period, the patients were divided into two groups based on their responses: an *"exercise-positive"* group with blood pressures over 200/100 mmHg at 100 watts and corresponding heart rates of 126 ± 13/min, and an *"exercise-negative"* group with blood pressures below 200/100 mmHg. Another criterion for assignment to the "exercise-positive" group was a persistence of the systolic and diastolic pressure elevation above normotensive (> 140/90 mmHg) at the end of 5 minutes' recovery. The reasons for these criteria were explained in Cap. II.2.5.

When the foregoing criteria were applied, it was found that 50% of the patients (n = 49) had to be classified as "exercise-positive" and the remaining 50% (n = 49) as "exercise-negative." The "exercise-positive" group had an average age of 38.3 ± 9.5 years, average height of 178.3 ± 6.8 cm and average weight of 79.8 ± 10.4 kg. The "exercise-negative" patients were younger on the average (30 ± 9.6 years), while other anthropometric data were comparable to the "exercise-positive" group: height 180.8 ± 6.2 cm, weight 79.6 ± 9.5 kg.

4.1.2. Blood Pressure and Heart Rate Responses

Table 20 and Fig. 24 show the mean values and standard deviations for systolic and diastolic blood pressure and heart rate in the "exercise-positive" and "exercise-negative" borderline hypertensives before, during and after ergometry. When the two groups are compared statistically, it is seen that the "exercise-negative" group has a significantly higher ($p < 0.001$) mean systolic blood pressure in the resting state than the "exercise-positive" group (153.6 mmHg vs. 144.7 mmHg), while the "exercise-positive" patients have a significantly higher ($p < 0.01$) mean diastolic pressure (92 mmHg vs. 88.3 mmHg).

During ergometry the "exercise-positive" borderline hypertensives had higher systolic pressures at all stages of exercise, and particularly at 80-100 watts, where the difference was statistically significant ($p < 0.05$–$p < 0.01$). The "exercise-negative" patients also had lower systolic pressures during the recovery period, but the difference was significant only for the 2nd minute.

The essential criterion which differentiated the "exercise-positive" and "exercise-negative" groups, however, was the behavior of the *diastolic blood pressure* during and after ergometry. The "exercise-positive" group experienced a highly significant ($p < 0.001$) rise of diastolic blood pressure at a workload of only 50 watts. This pressure rose steadily during the course of the test, attaining a level of 112.5 mmHg at 100 watts. A significantly ($p < 0.001$) different re-

Table 20. Systolic (S.B.P.) and diastolic (D.B.P.) blood pressures (means ± SD) of 98 male borderline hypertensives at rest and during and after work, who could be divided into two groups based on their blood pressure responses during and after work: an "exercise-positive" group (B.H.+), and an "exercise-negative" group (B.H.–) (*p < 0.05; **p < 0.01; ***p < 0.001)

n=98		Rest	Ergometric work (watts)						Recovery period (min)				
		Supine	50	60	70	80	90	100	1.	2.	3.	4.	5.
S.B.P. (mmHg)	B.H.+ n=49 38.3 yrs	144.7 10.6	179.7 16.6	188 15.7	194.8 17.6	202.2 20.3	207 19.5	215.9 21.2	185.2 17.7	171.2 14.6	163.4 12.3	159.6 12.5	157.1 12.3
	B.H.– n=49 30 yrs	153.6 13.5***	176.5 17.7	183.4 17.8	189 17.5	193.4 18.5*	198.8 18.5*	204.2 17.5**	178 17.7	165.6 15.5*	158.8 13.1	155.3 12.5	152.1 13.8
D.B.P. (mmHg)	B.H.+ n=49 38.3 yrs	92 3.8	104.5 7.3	107.6 7.6	108.1 6.5	110 6.9	111 7.3	112.5 8.3	101.7 6.1	100.3 5.8	98.8 6.4	99.1 6.1	99.6 5.9
	B.H.– n=49 30 yrs	88.3 7.9**	90 8.3***	90.4 7.2***	91.6 7.2***	91.5 7.6***	91.7 7.4***	91.9 7.3***	86.7 7.7***	86.1 7.1***	85.2 6.2***	85.6 5.9***	85 5.8***
H.R. (bts/min)	B.H.+ n=49 38.3 yrs	70 11.8	99.1 13.1	104 14.3	108.3 14.6	113.9 16.5	118 16.6	124.1 17.2	89.4 17.1	83.1 16.2	81 16.5	78.9 14.6	78.2 15.2
	B.H.– n=49 30 yrs	73.2 11.1	98.8 11.4	103.4 11.3	108 11.3	113 10.5	116.8 11.5	121.1 11.3	87.3 13.8	83.2 13.2	80.5 14.8	78.8 13.5	78.2 12.6

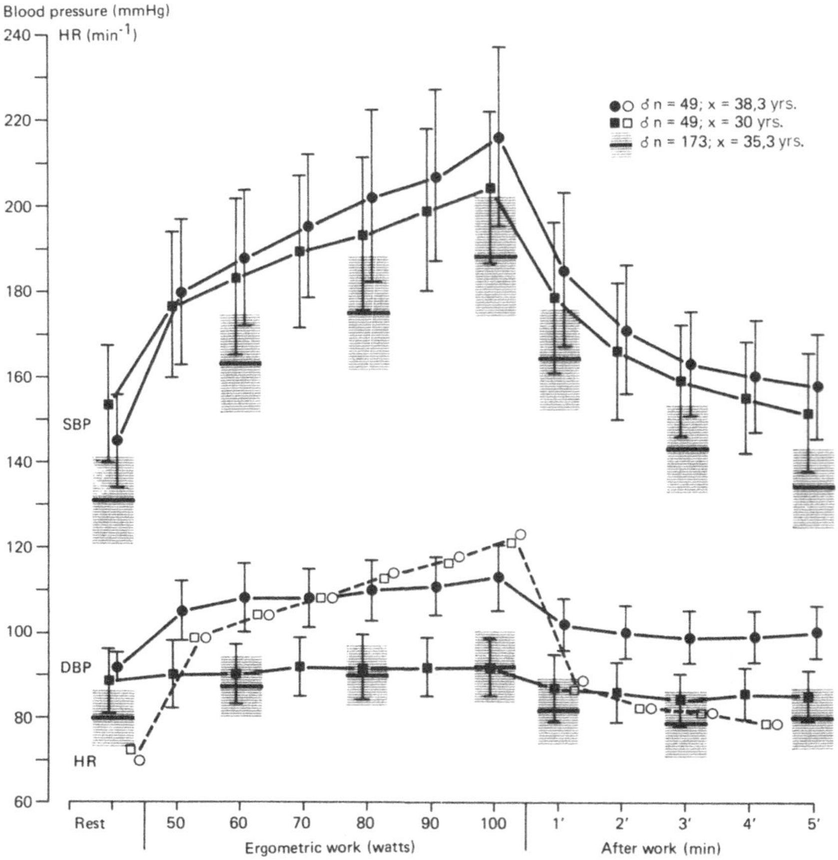

Fig. 24. Blood pressure and heart rate responses in 49 "exercise-positive" and 49 "exercise-negative" borderline hypertensives compared with normal controls (shaded columns)

sponse was observed in the "exercise-negative" group, whose diastolic pressure rose to only 91.9 mmHg during ergometry - not a significant increase.

A similar pattern of diastolic blood pressure response was seen in the recovery period. Again, the diastolic pressures in the "exercise-negative" patients were significantly lower ($p<0.001$) than in the "exercise-positives." By the 1st minute of recovery the diastolic pressure of the "exercise-negative" group had already reentered the normotensive range (86.7 mmHg), while that of the "exercise-positive" group was still markedly elevated even after 5 minutes' recovery (99.6 mmHg) and was significantly ($p<0.01$) above the pre-exercise borderline level. The groups also showed different patterns of systolic blood pressure recovery. While the "exercise-positive" borderline hypertensives had not yet reached their pre-exercise systolic reading after 5 minutes of recovery ($p<0.001$), the systolic reading in the "exercise-negative" patients had fallen slightly below the pre-exercise level, though it did not enter the normotensive range.

Comparing the blood pressure responses of the "exercise-positive" borderline hypertensives and the younger "definite" hypertensives of group 1A (s.

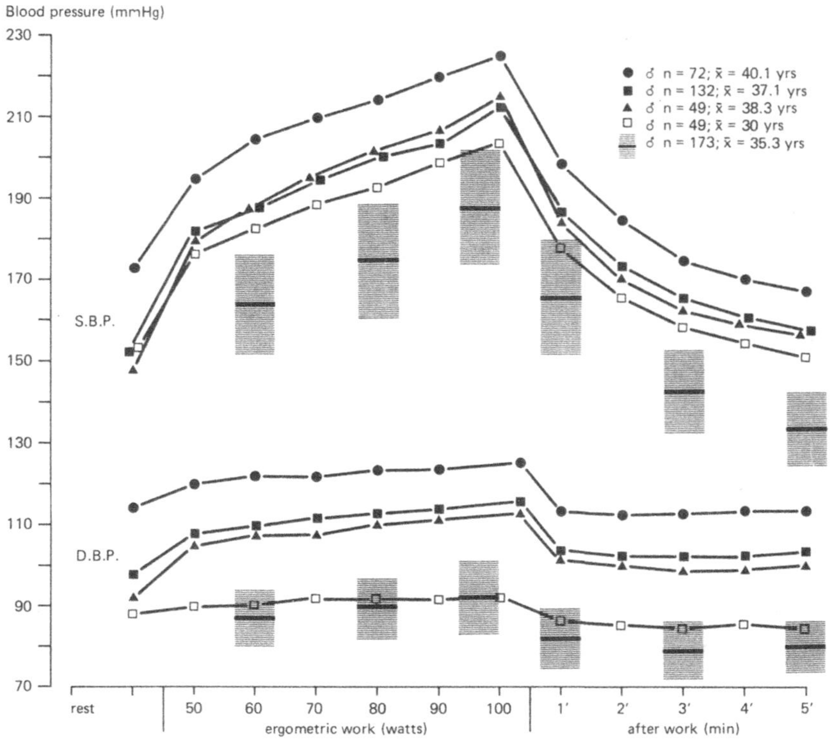

Fig. 25. Blood pressure responses of "exercise-positive" and "exercise-negative" borderline hypertensives compared with responses in mildly hypertensive patients

Chap. II.3.2., Fig. 25), we find that the mean resting systolic pressure of 145 mm Hg in the former group is significantly lower ($p < 0.001$) than the 152 mmHg recorded in the definite hypertensives. Nevertheless, these groups showed no significant difference in their systolic responses to exercise over the entire range from 50 to 100 watts (e.g., 216 mmHg in the "exercise-positive" borderline hypertensives vs. 213 mmHg in the definite hypertensives at 100 watts). Neither did the groups show significant differences during recovery.

On comparing the diastolic blood pressure responses of the two groups, we find that while the resting diastolic pressure of 92 mmHg in the "exercise-positive" borderline hypertensives was significantly lower ($p < 0.001$) than the 98 mmHg in the definite hypertensives, both groups had similar responses to workloads of 80 to 100 watts (e.g., 113 mmHg vs. 116 mmHg at 100 watts).

A similar pattern was evident in the recovery period, although the diastolic pressure of the "exercise-positive" borderline hypertensives were significantly lower ($p < 0.05$) in accordance with theier lower pre-exercise pressures.

Thus, the younger definite hypertensives and the "exercise-positive" borderline hypertensives had almost identical blood pressure patterns before, during and after ergometry, and their blood pressures were significantly higher ($p < 0.001$) than those of comparable, normotensive subjects.

When we compared the responses of the "exercise-negative" borderline hypertensives with those of normal subjects of equal age, we found significantly higher systolic pressures ($p < 0.001$) before, during and after ergometry. As for the diastolic pressure, we found that despite a significantly higher ($p < 0.001$) resting pressure of 88 mmHg in the "exercise-negative" borderline hypertensives vs. 80 mmHg in the normotensives, both groups had similar diastolic pressure responses when exercised at 80 to 100 watts (e.g., 92 mmHg for both groups at 100 watts). However, at the initial stages of 50 to 70 watts the "exercise-negative" borderline hypertensives were found to have significantly higher ($p < 0.01$–$p < 0.001$) diastolic blood pressures, presumably on account of their higher initial readings. At greater workloads these patients experienced a metabolic vasodilatation which served to normalize their blood pressure response.

At the end of the 1st minute of recovery the borderline hypertensives attained a diastolic pressure of 86 mmHg. While this was within normotensive limits, the readings at all stages of recovery were significantly higher ($p < 0.001$) than in the normal subjects.

When we examined the heart rate responses of the groups before, during and after ergometry, we could find no group-specific differences.

4.2. Comparative Study of Borderline Hypertensives, Definite Hypertensives and Normotensives of Equal Age Distribution

In 1976 we conducted ergometric tests in 52 borderline hypertensives in an effort to elucidate the value of ergometry in the evaluation of borderline hypertension (109). We also conducted tests in normotensives and definite hypertensives, because comparable studies in these groups were unavailable at that time.

4.2.1. Study Population

The study was done on a total of 156 males ranging in age from 20 to 65 years who had presented for routine cardiac examinations on a random basis (Table 21). The patients were divided into 4 groups based on casual blood pressures taken after 2–3 minutes of recumbency [186, 259, 304]. These groups consisted of a total of 47 normotensive persons, 52 borderline hypertensives, and 57 definite hypertensives with varying degrees of blood pressure elevation. The mean values and standard deviations of blood pressure for the separate groups as well as the upper and normal limits used for the group classification are shown in Table 21. The definite hypertensives had Stage 1 or Stage 2 disease according to WHO criteria.

The groups were further divided by age into subgroups of 20–40 and 41–65 years so that possible age effects could be excluded. This subdivision showed a similar age distribution within the four groups, indicating that a valid group comparison could be made.

Based on blood pressure readings taken before and after exercise, the borderline hypertensives (group 2) were subdivided into patients who had elevated blood pressures both during and after ergometry (group 2b, "exercise-positive")

Table 21. Systolic (S.B.P.) and diastolic (D.B.P.) blood pressures (means ± SD) for the separate groups as well as the upper and normal limits used for the group classification. The groups were further divided by age into subgroups of 20-40 and 41-65 years

	n	S.B.P. (mmHg)	D.B.P. (mmHg)	Age 20-40 (years)	Age 41-65 (years)
Normotensives Group 1	47	132.4 ± 7.4 (110-139)	83.9 ± 5.8 (70-90)	30.5 n = 26	52.9 n = 21
Borderline hypertensives Group 2	52	150.7 ± 6 (140-159)	92.4 ± 4.9 (91-95)	31.1 n = 30	50.7 n = 22
Hypertensives Group 3	32	157.5 ± 5.2 (150-160)	99.5 ± 1.2 (96-100)	31.6 n = 16	49.9 n = 16
Hypertensives Group 4	25	172.4 ± 6.5 (160-175)	110.4 ± 3.5 (101-115)	37.4 n = 9	54.9 n = 16

and patients who had normotensive blood pressures during these periods (group 2a, "exercise-negative"). A blood pressure of 200/100 mmHg was chosen as the upper limit at a workload of 100 watts and concomitant heart rate of 110-130/min. Another criterion for "exercise-positive" was a persistence of the systolic and diastolic pressure elevation above the normotensive range (140/90 mmHg) at 5 minutes postexercise.

4.2.2. Blood Pressure and Heart Rate Responses

Table 22 and Figs. 26 and 27 show the systolic and diastolic blood pressures of groups 1-4 determined before, during and after ergometry. Group 1, consisting of patients normotensive at rest, had a mean blood pressure of 178/91 mmHg at 100 watts. Neither the systolic nor diastolic pressure in this group differed significantly from the values of the normal population described in Chap. II.2.1. Similar agreement was found in the recovery period, when the normotensives reentered the normal diastolic range during the 1st minute (83 mmHg) and the normal systolic range during the 3rd minute (139 mmHg).

In this study 57.7% of the borderline hypertensives were classified as "exercise-positive" (group 2b) based on their exercise and postexercise blood pressures. Their responses conformed to the typical pattern described in Chap. II.4.1. relative to normotensive and hypertensive persons. Their blood pressure reached 211/115 mmHg at 100 watts, which was significantly higher ($p < 0.001$) both systolically and diastolically than that of the normotensives but did not differ significantly from the 219/118 mmHg measured at 100 watts in the group 3 hypertensives. In the 5th minute of recovery the systolic and diastolic blood pressure of the "exercise-positive" borderline hypertensives was still higher than the pre-exercise level, thus corresponding to the pattern seen in the group 3 and 4 hypertensives (s. Chap. II.3.2.).

A very different pattern was observed in the 42.3% of the borderline hypertensives who were found to be "exercise-negative." These patients had a blood pressure of 183/92 mmHg at 100 watts, a value which did not differ signifi-

Table 22. Systolic (S. B. P.) and diastolic (D. B. P.) blood pressures (means ± SD) of the groups 1–4 determined before, during and after work (***$p < 0.001$; n. s. = non significant)

n = 156	Rest		Ergometric work (watts)						Recovery period (min)					
	supine		50		70		100		1.		3.		5.	
	SBP	DBP	SBP	DBP	SBP	DBP	SBP	DBP	SBP	DBP	SBP	DBP	SBP	DBP
Group 1, n = 47	132.4	83.9	154.2	89.7	163.9	90.7	177.5	91.4	154.2	83.1	138.8	81.1	133.5	81.6
Normotensive	7.4	5.8	14.3	6.5	12.6	8.8	16 n.s.	9.1	13.2	7.8	10.8	8.2	9.8	5.8
Group 2A, n = 22	150.7	91.7	167	91.6	174.5	90	183	91.8	161.6	86.4	149.5	86.4	144	86.3
Exercise-negative borderline hypertensives	5.4	5.4	9.7	6.2	11.5	8.6	13.9 ***	8 ***	12	8.6	10.4	10.4	9.8	8.8
Group 2B, n = 30	150.8	93	183.3	106.7	196.7	109.8	210.5	114.5	188.3	102.2	165.8	100.3	160.5	99.8
Exercise-positive borderline hypertensives	6.8	4.3	13.5	10.3	15.9	12.6	20.4 n.s.	12.2 n.s.	14.6	9.5	13	12.2	13.2	8.7
Group 3, n = 32	157.5	99.5	187.5	110.5	203	115.4	218.6	118.4	192.9	105.5	172.6	104.2	166.1	105.5
Hypertensives	5.2	1.2	16.2	11.7	17.8	10.8	23.6 n.s.	11.0 ***	17.7	10.3	12.1	9.5	14.1	8.5
Group 4, n = 25	172.4	110.4	196.8	121	213.2	123.8	226.4	129.8	197	116.6	183.6	113.8	180.2	115.0
Hypertensives	6.5	3.5	16.1	7.9	21.3	10.4	18.5	11.3	19.2	11.7	13.7	9.5	15.2	9.4

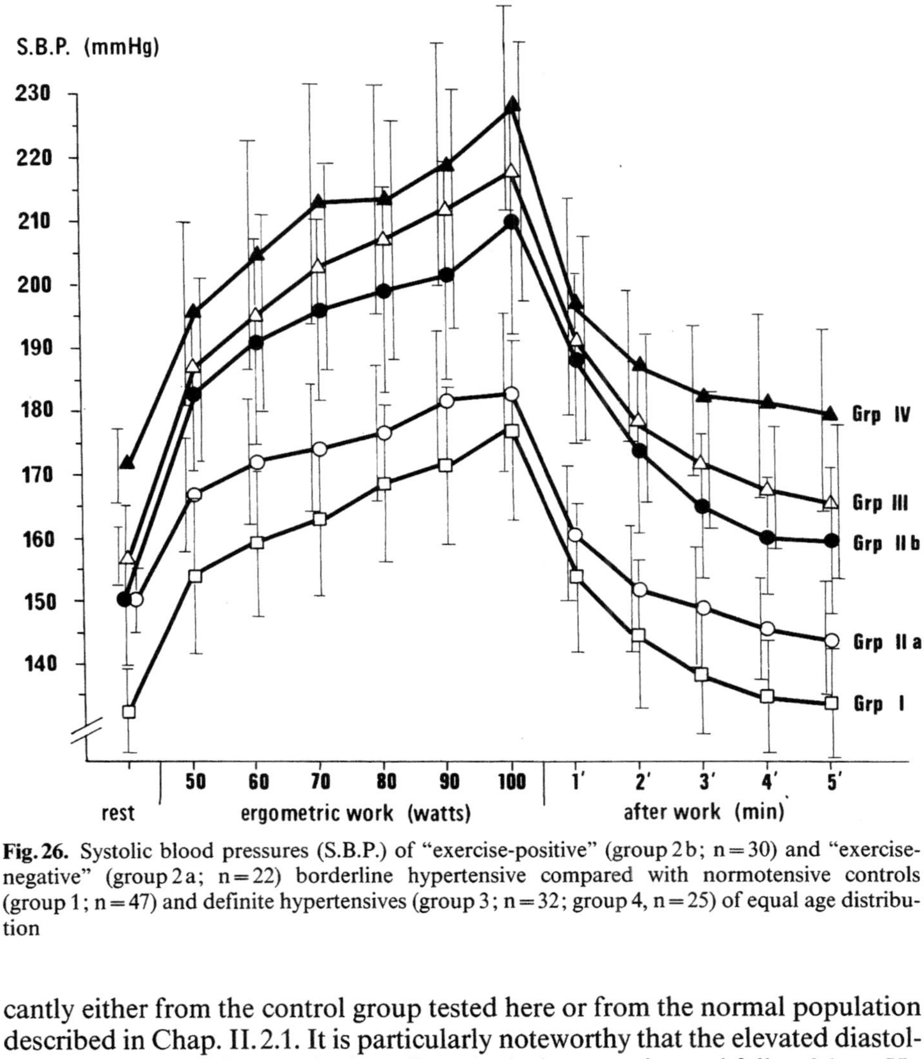

Fig. 26. Systolic blood pressures (S.B.P.) of "exercise-positive" (group 2b; n=30) and "exercise-negative" (group 2a; n=22) borderline hypertensive compared with normotensive controls (group 1; n=47) and definite hypertensives (group 3; n=32; group 4, n=25) of equal age distribution

cantly either from the control group tested here or from the normal population described in Chap. II.2.1. It is particularly noteworthy that the elevated diastolic pressure at rest did not rise inordinately during exercise and fell to 86 mmHg only 1 minute after the termination of exercise, thereby entering the normotensive range and even falling below the pre-exercise reading.

If we set an upper normal limit of 200/100 mmHg for the blood pressure at 100 watts, we find that 100% of the group 3 and 4 hypertensives had pathologic blood pressure elevations during exercise. This occurred in 57.7% of the borderline hypertensives, and in none of the normotensives.

These results make it clear that individuals with marginally elevated blood pressures at rest can be uniquely assigned to either the normotensive or hypertensive population on the basis of their response to ergometry.

Comparing the blood pressure responses of the two different age groups of borderline hypertensives (Table 21), we find that a definite age effect is apparent. Of the 30 borderline hypertensives who were in the 20–40 age range, only

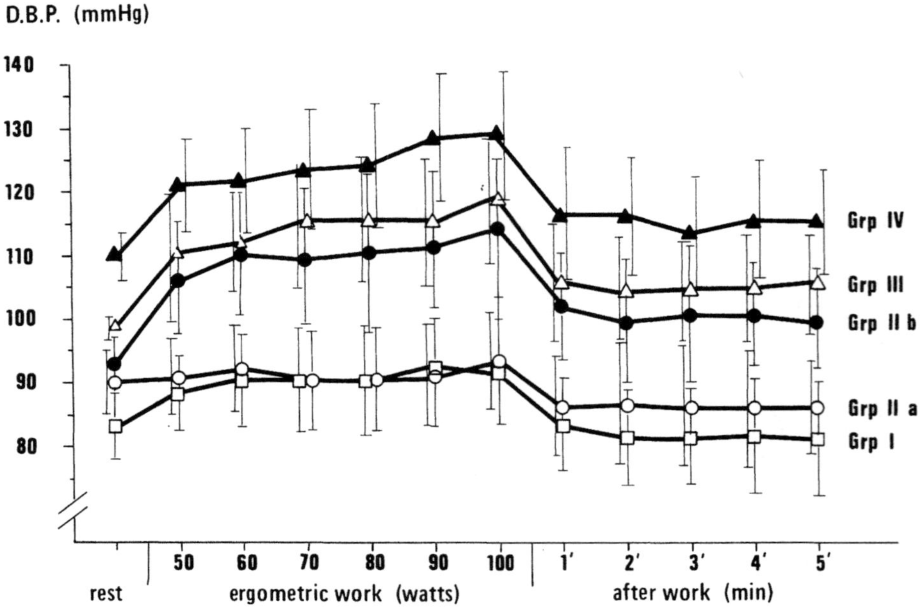

Fig. 27. Diastolic blood pressures (D.B.P.) of "exercise-positive" (group 2b; n=30) and "exercise-negative" (group 2a; n=22) borderline hypertensive compared with normotensive controls (group 1; n=47) and definite hypertensives (group 3, n=32; group 4, n=25) of equal age distribution

13 were found to be "exercise-positive." The situation is quite different in the 22 patients aged 41-65 years. Of these, 16 had elevated blood pressures during and after ergometry, and only 6 had normal blood pressures. In other words, one may expect not only a greater prevalence of borderline hypertension with increasing age [216] but also an increase in the percentage of patients who are "exercise-positive." Given the normal blood pressure responses of the 21 control subjects in group 1, this tendency cannot be explained in terms of reduced arterial elasticity with age.

On comparing the definite hypertensives of group 3 and 4, we find that higher initial blood pressures at rest tend to imply higher blood pressures during and after ergometry (Table 22), as we saw in Chap. III.3. The difference between the two groups was significant ($p<0.001$) for the diastolic pressure at 100 watts (118.4 mmHg vs. 129.8 mmHg) and for the systolic and diastolic pressure in the 5th minute of recovery (166.1/105.5 mmHg vs. 180.2/115 mmHg). This rule does not hold in every case, however, as we pointed out in Chap. II.3.4.

As part of this study we examined the correlation between the diastolic blood pressure measured at 100 watts and that measured in the 3rd and 5th minute of recovery. We found a very high correlation between these quantities, with a correlation coefficent of 0.86 ($y=0.776x+11.5$; $r=0.86$; $p<0.001$) (see Fig. 5).

Table 23. Age, height and weight measured initially and after 3.8 years of the different groups of borderline hypertensives

n=41		Age (years)	Height (cm)	Body weight (kg)
Exercise-positive borderline hypertensives	Initial examination	37.1±10.2	176.3±7.5	79.4±9.9
n=22	Follow-up after 3.8 years	40.4±10.3	176.3±7.5	77.1±9.4
Exercise-negative borderline hypertensives	Initial examination	35.9±10.7	177.3±3.3	75.9±9
n=13	Follow-up after 3.6 years	39.5±10.4	177.3±3.3	77.1±9.4
Exercise-negative borderline hypertensives who developed	Initial examination	37.2± 9	179.6±4.2	79.9±7.8
hypertension n=6	Follow-up after 4.1 years	40.5± 9.8	179.6±4.2	79 ±9.4

4.3. Follow-Up of the Borderline Hypertensives at 3.8 Years

We conducted a 3.8-year follow-up of the borderline hypertensives for the purpose of answering three essential questions (130):

1. Is the classification into "exercise-positive" and "exercise-negative" borderline hypertensives *reproducible* over a period of years?
2. Do the borderline hypertensives classified as "exercise-positive" eventually progress to established hypertension?
3. What is the natural course of "exercise-negative" borderline hypertension?

4.3.1. Patients

Of the 52 borderline hypertensives tested initially, 45 were available for follow-up after an average period of 3.8 years (3.1–4.6 years). Twenty-six of the 30 "exercise-positive" and 19 of the 22 "exercise-negative" patients were retested. Data on height, weight and age are presented in Table 23.

A comparison of the body weights of the borderline hypertensives at initial and follow-up testing clearly indicates that body weight did not significantly influence the outcome of the tests.

Table 24. Systolic (S. B. P.) and diastolic (D. B. P.) blood pressures and heart rates (H. R.) (means ± SD) of 22 exercise-positive borderline hypertensives at the initial examination and after 3.8 years (*p < 0.05; **p < 0.01; ***p < 0.001)

n = 22		Rest	Ergometric work (watts)						Recovery period (min)				
		supine	50	60	70	80	90	100	1.	2.	3.	4.	5.
S. B. P. (mmHg)	1st examination	152.7 11.3	179.8 15.6	187.5 16.5	193.7 17.1	194.1 17	198.1 18.4	205.3 21.5	186.1 20.3	193.9 17.1	167.1 13.7	163.6 13.5	163.5 14.5
	2nd examination	156.4 17	184.2 21.4	192 23.1	198.1 23.4	202.4 24.3	208.5 26.1	214.9 28	192.5 26.7	176.2 22.8	169.6 20	167.5 18.1	163.4 19.5
D. B. P. (mmHg)	1st examination	93.2 6.1	110 12.1	109.8 11.3	109.6 11.9	111.7 11.3	113.3 10.8	115 10.6	103.3 8.3	99 6.3	99.6 8.6	100.2 6.8	101.6 7
	2nd examination	103.2 11.2***	113.1 9.5	115 9.7	115.8 9.5	116.8 10	119.4 10.7	119.6 12.8	109 10.0*	108 9.2***	108.3 8.7**	107.3 9.6**	109.2 10.7**
H. R. (bts/min)	1st examination	70.5 14.3	92.2 14	97.7 14.8	102 16.3	103.2 16.4	107.7 16.3	113.1 17	88.5 17.2	83.4 16	78.7 16.4	75.3 13.3	74.9 12.9
	2nd examination	67 13.1	94.7 11.4	102.4 15.4	102.4 15.4	107.1 16.3	116.6 18.7	116.7 20	86.7 18.8	80.1 17.7	77.6 17	77.7 16	76.1 16.1

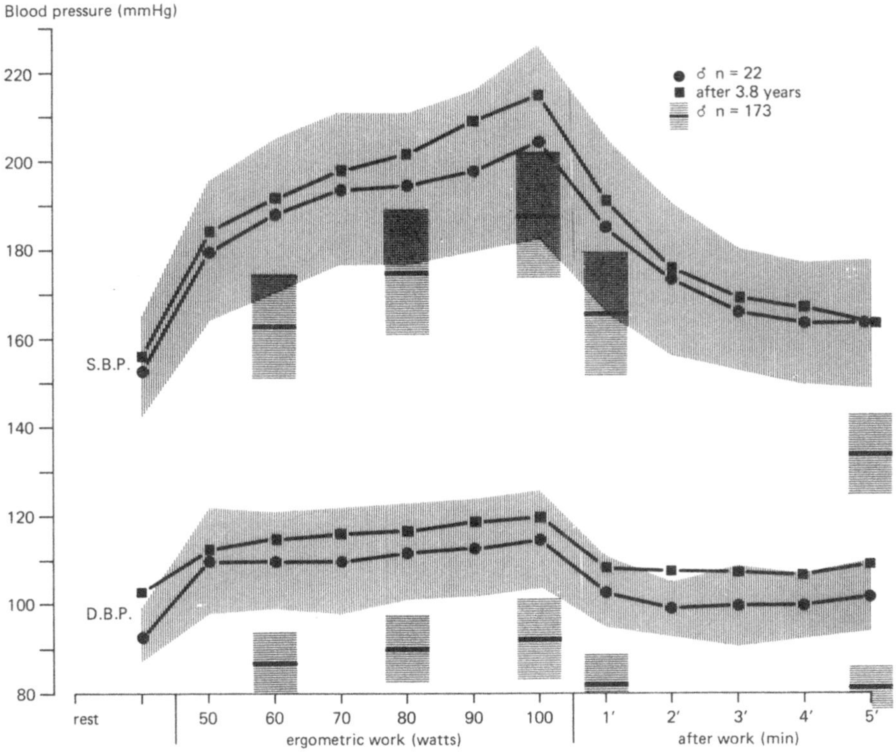

Fig. 28. Blood pressure responses of "exercise-positive" borderline hypertensives on initial testing and 3.8-year follow-up who had progressed to established hypertension. The shaded areas show the standard deviation of the initial readings

4.3.2. Follow-Up of the "Exercise-Positive" Borderline Hypertensives

At follow-up 25 of the 26 "exercise-positive" borderline hypertensives showed marked blood pressure elevations during and after ergometry. Only 1 of the 26 patients had normotensive readings before, during and after exercise. A review of his blood pressure records from 1976 revealed that his systolic and diastolic pressures were only mildly elevated at 100 watts (205/105 mmHg), and also that his diastolic pressure returned to 90 mmHg in the 1st minute of recovery and did not decline further until the 5th minute.

Of the 25 remaining "exercise-positive" borderline hypertensives, only 22 were suitable for statistical evaluation. The other three had progressed to established hypertension since their first test, prompting their family physicians to initiate treatment.

Table 24 and Fig. 28 show the blood pressure and heart rate responses of the "exercise-positive" subjects on initial and follow-up testing. A look at the resting blood pressures shows a significant ($p < 0.001$) rise of the diastolic pressure by 10 mmHg, from 93 to 103 mmHg, clearly indicating a progression toward es-

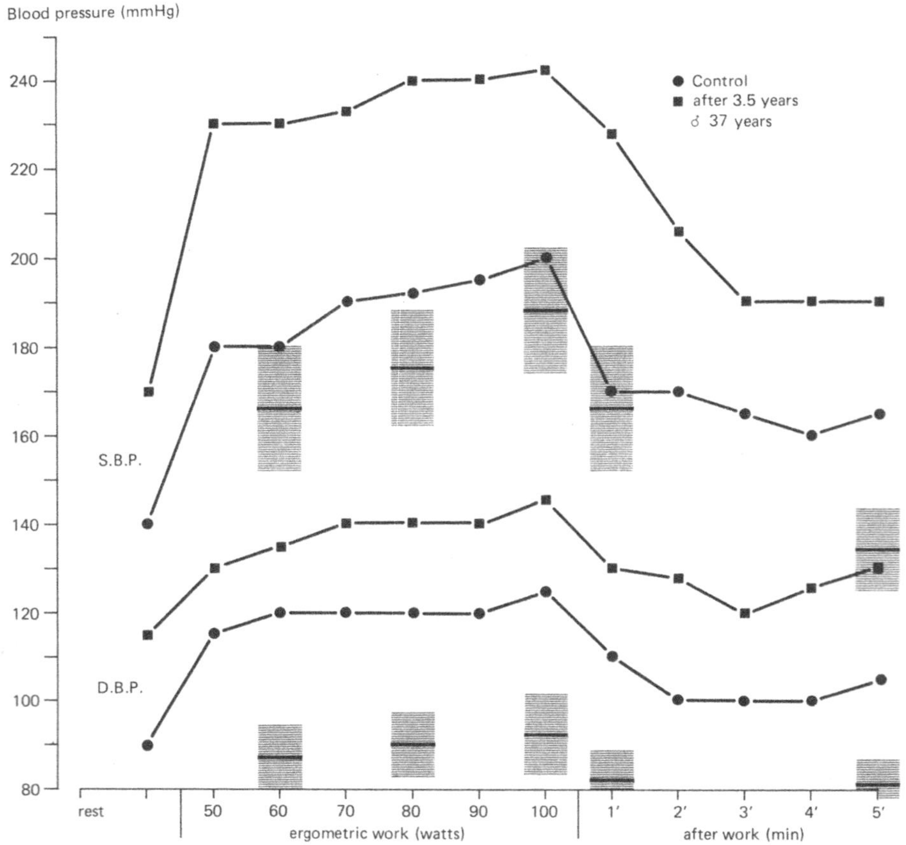

Fig. 29. Blood pressure response of a 37-year-old "exercise-positive" borderline hypertensive on initial testing and 3.5-year follow-up. The patient has developed stable hypertension since his first examination

tablished hypertension. This was the case in all exercise-positive borderline hypertensives with only one exception.

After 3.8 years both the systolic and diastolic blood pressures were higher at all stages of exercise than at the time of the first examination (e.g., 215/120 mm Hg vs. 205/115 mmHg at 100 watts), though the difference was not statistically confirmed. Statistical significance was confirmed for the recovery period, however ($p<0.05$–$p<0.001$).

Thus, at follow-up the "exercise-positive" borderline hypertensives had blood pressures before, during and after ergometry which did not differ significantly from the comparable hypertensive patients of group 1A or group 3. The resting diastolic pressure after 3.8 years offered particularly strong evidence that the "exercise-positive" borderline hypertensives had become definitely hypertensive since their first examination. Allowing for the one incorrectly classified patient, we find that ergometry was 96.2% accurate in identifying prospective hypertensive patients. This is particularly well illustrated in Fig. 29 for the case of a 37-year-old man.

Table 25. Systolic (S. B. P.) and diastolic (D. B. P.) blood pressures and heart rates (H. R.) (means ± SD) of 13 exercise-negative borderline hypertensives at the initial examination and after 3.6 years who were still obviously normotensive after the follow-up time (*$p < 0.05$; **$p < 0.01$)

n = 13		Rest	Ergometric work (watts)						Recovery period (min)				
		supine	50	60	70	80	90	100	1.	2.	3.	4.	5.
S. B. P. (mmHg)	1st examination	151.5 6.3	168.9 13.9	178.9 18.2	180 17.6	182.3 18	186.2 17.8	188.5 18.5	172.3 19.8	163.9 22.1	158.9 17.8	153.9 16.2	154.2 15.8
	2nd examination	144.5 14.2	159.8 12.8	167.1 12.9	173.4 12.8	177.7 12.9	185.4 15.3	192 15.9	169.2 19.4	153.1 15.7	147.7 15.3	143.9 13.8	140.9 10.2*
D. B. P. (mmHg)	1st examination	90.8 5.7	92.7 6.3	92.7 6.7	92.7 10.3	92.8 9.3	92.4 8.5	92.4 8.6	87.7 9.9	85.8 13.8	85.8 13.7	87.3 11.1	89.3 10.9
	2nd examination	90.2 4.8	92.5 4.0	94.8 5.2	94 4.2	94.9 4.3	97.5 4.9	97.7 5.2	88 6.6	87.9 5.9	86.9 6.9	88.2 6.1	87.1 6.7
H. R. (bts/min)	1st examination	66.8 16.2	86.3 15.3	91.8 13.7	94.2 14.1	98 14.4	102.2 14.3	104.5 13.7	81.9 17.5	76.8 17.3	74.7 15.8	75.2 15.4	73.5 13.5
	2nd examination	69.8 11.3	92.2 10.2	96.9 9.9	103.5 10.2	107.2 11	113.4 12*	120.4 12.2**	79.5 17.2	76.9 17.8	75.6 16.2	74.9 14.5	77.1 14.6

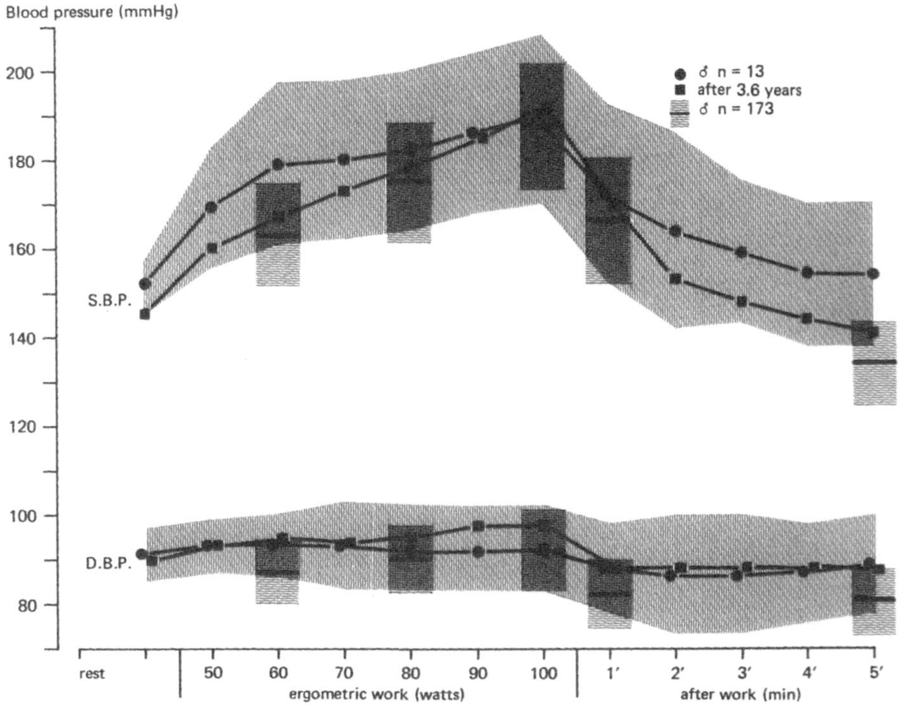

Fig. 30. Blood pressure responses of "exercise-negative" borderline hypertensives on initial testing and 3.6-year follow-up who became normotensive after the first examination. The shaded areas show the standard deviation of the initial readings

4.3.3. "Exercise-Negative" Borderline Hypertensives

Of the 19 "exercise-negative" borderline hypertensives who were retested at follow-up, 68.5% (n = 13) were still obviously normotensive after a mean follow-up time of 3.6 years (Table 25, Fig. 30). Their resting blood pressures continued to occupy the borderline range and did not differ significantly from readings obtained on initial testing, though a trend toward lower systolic readings was apparent.

The systolic pressure response to exercise at follow-up did not differ significantly from the response at first examination or from readings in normotensive individuals. An obvious trend toward lower systolic pressures was again apparent after the 2nd minute of recovery, when readings were around the upper limit of normal.

An analysis of diastolic pressure during ergometry showed that while initial and follow-up readings concurred over the range from 50 to 80 watts, the follow-up readings were 5 mmHg higher in the last two stages of exercise, though they did not reach the limit of 100 mmHg at 100 watts. The diastolic readings converged again during the recovery period.

On comparing heart rate responses, one is struck by the higher follow-up

Table 26. Systolic (S.B.P.) and diastolic (D.B.P.) blood pressures and heart rates (H.R.) (means ± SD) of 6 exercise-negative borderline hypertensives at the initial examination and after 4.1 years, who showed marked blood pressure elevations after the follow-up time (*$p<0.05$; **$p<0.01$; ***$p<0.001$)

n=6		Rest	Ergometric work (watts)						Recovery period (min)				
		supine	50	60	70	80	90	100	1.	2.	3.	4.	5.
S.B.P. (mmHg)	1st examination	151.7 2.6	170.8 10.2	174.2 11.2	175.8 13.2	180.8 12	184.2 10.7	187.5 12.6	181.7 14.7	167.5 15.4	160.8 12.8	157.5 13.7	150.8 13.5
	2nd examination	162.3 6.4**	183.8 15.1	192 16.8	197.7 14.3*	205.7 17.3*	210.3 21*	220 20.9**	186.7 17.6	174.7 14.9	168.7 11.8	164 7.6	159.7 10.7
D.B.P. (mmHg)	1st examination	91.7 6.1	92.5 5.2	92.5 8.2	91 10	91.8 10.2	94.2 11.2	97.5 8.2	92.5 6.9	93.3 7.5	92.7 8.6	93.5 6.6	92.3 7.7
	2nd examination	97.7 9.0	105.7 4.6***	104 5.5*	108.3 4.8**	110.3 6.1**	111 7*	111.7 6.4**	99.7 2.3*	101.7 2.7*	100.3 0.9	102 4.4*	101.3 2.7*
H.R. (bts/min)	1st examination	69.8 12.3	98 16	101 15.4	103 15.9	107.7 16.1	112.7 15	113.8 17.3	95.8 17.3	91.7 15.2	84.8 13.8	84.7 13.9	83.8 13.5
	2nd examination	78 11	104.8 16	110.7 16.5	115.7 16.2	120 16.6	126.5 15.5	132.2 15.6	102.8 17.2	93.5 18.6	92 16.4	88.8 14.2	89.2 15.4

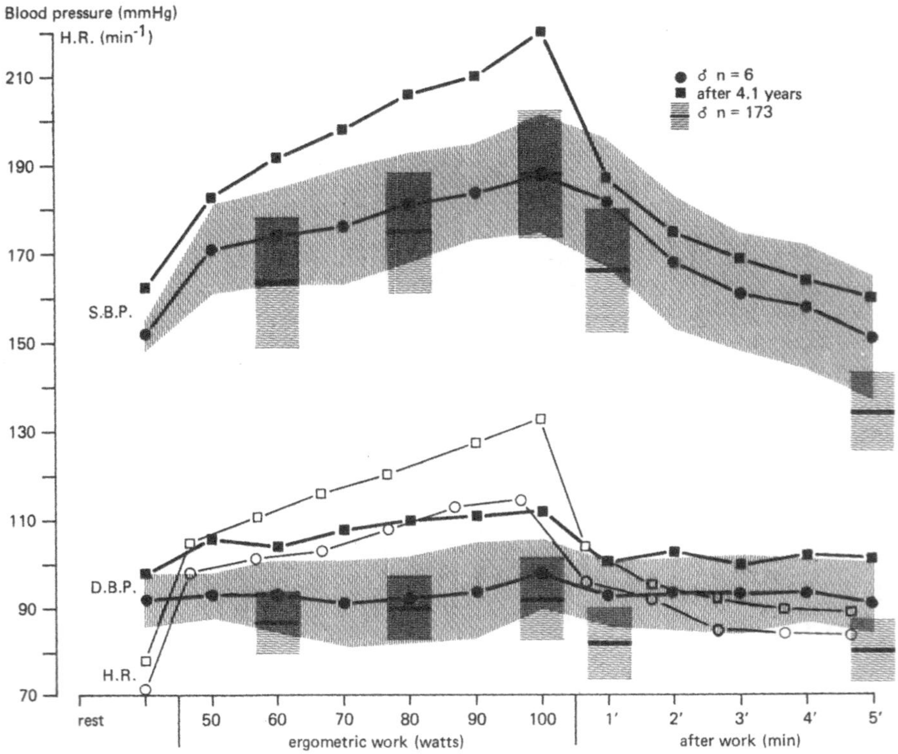

Fig. 31. Blood pressure responses of "exercise-negative" borderline hypertensives on initial testing and 4.1-year follow-up who had progressed to established hypertension. The shaded areas show the standard deviation of the initial determination

heart rates at all exercise stages and particularly at 90 and 100 watts, where the follow-up rates are significantly ($p<0.05$–$p<0.01$) higher than initial values.

After a period of 4.1 years, however, 31.5% (n=6) of the 19 "exercise-negative" borderline hypertensives showed marked blood pressure elevations during and after ergometry (Table 26, Fig. 31). Both the systolic and diastolic pressures were higher in the resting state, though only the systolic values showed a statistically significant elevation ($p<0.01$). When exercised at follow-up, these patients developed significantly higher ($p<0.05$–$p<0.001$) blood pressures (e.g., 220/112 vs. 188/98 mmHg at 100 watts), which did not differ significantly from those of the group 1A hypertensives. The follow-up also disclosed a marked elevation of the postexercise recovery pressures, though a significant difference ($p<0.05$) was confirmed for the diastolic pressure only.

A retrospective analysis of the exercise and postexercise diastolic pressures of the borderline hypertensives initially classified as "exercise-negative" shows that even on initial testing 4.1 years ago these patients had relatively high diastolic pressures, especially during recovery. The exercise and postexercise limits used here for classification apparently are not discriminating enough for these patients.

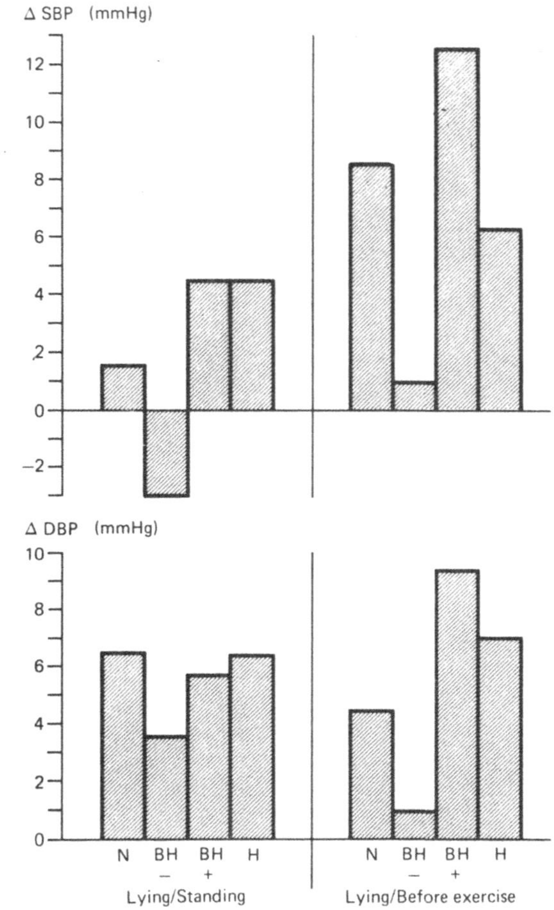

Fig. 32. Changes in blood pressure (Δ S.B.P., Δ D.B.P.) from a lying to a standing position and from recumbency to immediately before the start of exercise in borderline hypertensives (BH) compared with age-matched hypertensives (H) and normotensive controls (N)

4.4. Resting Blood Pressures of Borderline Hypertensives Compared with Hypertensives and Normotensives

Table 27 and Fig. 32 compare the systolic and diastolic blood pressures and heart rates of normal subjects, "exercise-positive" and "exercise-negative" borderline hypertensives and definite hypertensives of similar age distributions. Blood pressures were taken in three different resting states: after 3-5 minutes' recumbency, after 1 minute of standing, and immediately before the start of exercise.

4.4.1. Orthostasis

During the change from a lying to standing position, the systolic pressure of the normotensive subjects showed only a minimal rise and corresponded to the normal values reported by Schellong [372], Thulesius [420] and Currens [77]. The blood pressure responses of the "exercise-positive" borderline hyperten-

Table 27. Systolic, diastolic blood pressures and heart rates (means ± SD) of normotensives (N), exercise-negative (B.H.−) and exercise-positive (B.H.+) borderline hypertensives and hypertensives (H). Blood pressures were taken in three different resting states: after 3-5 minutes recumbency, after 1 minute of standing, and immediately before exercise. Moreover, the changes in blood pressure from lying to a standing position and between taken in recumbency and immediately before exercise are shown (***p < 0.001)

n = 375	Systolic blood pressure (mmHg)				Diastolic blood pressure				Heart rate (bts/min)			
	N n = 173	B.H.− n = 40	BH+ n = 40	H n = 122	N n = 173	BH− n = 40	BH+ n = 40	H n = 122	N n = 173	BH− n = 40	BH+ n = 40	H n = 122
Supine	125.7	153.2	145.5	150.9	80	87.7	92.1	97.8	67.9	72.3	69.9	69.5
	8.1	12.8	11.3	11.4	6.2	7.7	3.7	6.3	9.5	10.4	12.1	12.6
Standing	127.3 ***	150.2	150.1 ***	155.5 ***	86.5 ***	91.3	97.8 ***	104.2 ***	79.8	81.6	77.9	77.5
	9.7	10.1	15.7	15.7	6	8.4	7.1	8.5	10.2	12.4	13.4	14.3
Before work	134.3	154.2	158.2	157.2	84.5	88.7	101.5	104.8	67.6	68.1	68.5	68.6
	9.7	12.1	12.9	14.1	6	7.6	7.2	8.3	10.8	10.7	10.7	11.7
Δsupine/standing	+1.6	−3	+4.6	+4.6	+6.5	+3.6	+5.7	+6.4	+11.9	+9.3	+8	+8
Δsupine/before work	+8.6	+1	+12.7	+6.3	+4.5	+1	+9.4	+7	−0.3	−4.2	−1.4	−0.9

sives and the definite hypertensives were similar, showing an average rise of 4.6. mmHg systolic. In the "exercise-negative" borderline hypertensives, on the other hand, the systolic pressure fell by an average of 3 mmHg at this time.

The diastolic pressure of the normal subjects rose by an average of 6.5 mm Hg when a standing position was assumed. This increase is statistically significant ($p < 0.001$) and again is in good agreement with published data [77, 372, 420, 441]. The "exercise-positive" borderline hypertensives and the definite hypertensives show a relative diastolic pressure increase which corresponds to the normal population, a finding consistent with earlier investigations [296, 297, 424].

The average heart rate increase in the normal subjects was 11.9 beats/min and thus was consistent with the value of 11 beats/min reported by Thulesius. A smaller orthostatic heart rate increment was found in the borderline and definite hypertensives.

4.4.2. Emotional Influences

According to von Eiff [435] and Schulte et al. [379], borderline and definite hypertensives respond to emotional stress with a greater rise of blood pressure than the normal population. From this standpoint it is of interest to compare blood pressure readings taken in recumbency with those taken immediately before the start of exercise, since the latter readings presumably would be influenced by an attitude of anticipation on the part of the subjects. As one would expect, all four groups had higher systolic and diastolic blood pressures immediately prior to exercise. Interestingly, the "exercise-positive" borderline hypertensives showed by far the greatest systolic and diastolic pressure increases ($p < 0.001$), while the normotensives and definite hypertensives experienced approximately the same percentage increase. It is also noteworthy that the "exercise-negative" borderline hypertensives experienced a minimal, insignificant systolic and diastolic pressure increase of about 1 mmHg.

The results clearly show that borderline hypertensives who have been segregated into "exercise-positive" and "exercise-negative" groups on the basis of ergometric testing also exhibit different blood pressure patterns under the resting conditions investigated here. In both the orthostatic test and under conditions of emotional stress, the "exercise-positive" borderline hypertensives exhibit a blood pressure response similar to that of persons who are definitely hypertensive.

4.5. Summary and Conclusions

4.5.1. Prevalence and Course of Borderline Hypertension

The prevalence of borderline hypertension is estimated to be 10% in the United States [60], between 15.7 and 24% in Switzerland [404, 410], and as high as 25-30% in West Germany [177]. Data on the frequency with which borderline hypertension progresses to established hypertension varies between 10% [220],

25% [178] and 34% [270]. In a Japanese study published by Dock et al. in 1978 [83], 20–40% of patients who had borderline blood pressures of 140–159 systolic and 90–99 diastolic went on to develop severe hypertension over a 10-year period. This was particularly true of younger patients 30–40 years of age, with females predominating. At the same time, it is known [178, 358] that some patients with marginal blood pressure elevations will later become normotensive without treatment. The unpredictable course of borderline hypertension is well illustrated by the follow-up studies of Linss and Böthig [270], who found that 30% of borderline hypertensives had become frankly hypertensive after two years, while 20% had become normotensive. After another two years, however, 46% of the frank hypertensives had returned to the borderline range, and 10% had become normotensive. Of the persons who became normotensive initially, 30% returned to the borderline range and 15% progressed to hypertension. These findings underscore the inadequacy of resting blood pressure measurements for predicting which borderline hypertensives will develop significant hypertension.

Thus, the clinical dilemma in borderline hypertension is two-fold: First, it cannot be predicted with certainty how borderline hypertension will progress with the passage of time. Second, the extreme variability in the resting blood pressure makes it exceedingly difficult to use this parameter as a basis for early detection, prompting Taylor [416] to remark, "What high blood pressure is depends on the philosophy of each physician." We believe that the results presented here on ergometric testing for the evaluation of borderline hypertension suggest a possible solution to this dilemma.

4.5.2. The Early Diagnosis of Hypertension in Borderline Patients

The question posed initially – whether blood pressure readings during ergometry can discriminate an arbitrary dividing line between normal and elevated resting blood pressure and thus facilitate the evalution of borderline hypertension – must be answered with a definite "yes" based upon the results presented here.

This discrimination assumes particular importance when one considers the extreme heterogeneity of borderline hypertensives as a group. Hemodynamic studies have shown that borderline hypertension is associated with diverse pathophysiologic changes [103, 215, 216, 218, 324, 367]. For example, while a hyperkinetic circulatory state is characteristic of some patients, others have an elevated peripheral resistance, which is the hallmark of arterial hypertension. According to Julius [216, 218] these changes are neurogenic in nature and are caused by an abnormal integration of autonomic control, probably in the medulla oblongata. This abnormality finds its expression in increased sympathetic outflow and reduced parasympathetic inhibition.

Accordingly, it is reasonable to expect that borderline hypertension could best be evaluated by means of a standardized test of sympathetic activity, for which ergometric studies are particularly well suited. This is documented in part by studies of sympathoadrenal activity during ergometry based on plasma catecholamine assays [115, 118, 126].

The pathologic response of the total peripheral resistance to exercise described by Julius et al. [215] for certain borderline hypertensives is of particular interest in this context. These authors found that the peripheral resistance in these patients did not fall adequately during exercise to compensate for the rise in cardiac output. In this situation the high cardiac output not only raises the systolic blood pressure but also causes marked diastolic blood pressure elevations like those occurring in established hypertension.

Of the 150 borderline hypertensives tested, it was found that approximately half experienced diastolic pressure increases during and after ergometry which did not differ from those in patients with mild hypertension. When one considers that an increased total peripheral resistance at rest and during exercise is a characteristic feature of arterial hypertension [152, 216, 218, 277, 278, 366, 367, 375] and is manifested clinically by an elevation of the diastolic blood pressure, there can be no doubt that ergometric testing will enable an early diagnosis of arterial hypertension to be made in a sizable proportion of borderline hypertensives.

This is further indicated by invasive hemodynamic exercise studies performed by Lund-Johansen [278] in 17- to 29-year-old patients with mild hypertension. Over a 10-year period these patients experienced only a slight change in their resting hemodynamics, while their total peripheral resistance and diastolic blood pressure during ergometry underwent a marked increase.

In 1979 Briedigkeit et al. [49] reported on the possibility of dividing juvenile borderline hypertensives into two groups based on their response to exercise stress testing. The authors tested a total of 124 children and adolescents with borderline hypertension ranging in age from 9 to 17 years, both at rest and during ergometry. They found that 61 of the subjects could be classified as "normotensive on exercise" and 63 as "hypertensive on exercise." Thus, as in the adult subjects tested by us, approximately half of the juveniles with borderline hypertension at rest could be assigned to the normotensive range and the other half to the hypertensive range based on their response to ergometry.

A further point of agreement between the studies of Briedigkeit et al. in juveniles and our results for adult borderline hypertensives is worth nothing. Ergometric follow-up test of the children after 2-3 years showed a relative stability of the results within the two reaction types, indicating good reproducibility. Apparently a fixed pathophysiologic state is already present in juveniles found to be "exercise-positive." Follow-up tests after 3.8 years indicate that this is almost certainly true in our "exercise-positive" adults; 96% of the "positive" subjects not only continued to have elevated blood pressures during and after ergometry, but they showed strong evidence of having progressed to established arterial hypertension. In other words, it was possible to render an early diagnosis of arterial hypertension in these borderline patients based on their response to ergometry 3.8 years previously.

Further studies suggest that a pathologic rise in blood pressure during exercise is a good predictor of future hypertension. Briedigkeit et al. [50] followed 115 borderline hypertensive children with an average age of 11.3 years, as well as age-matched controls, for a period of 5 years. During that time 46.1% of the borderline hypertensives became normotensive at rest, 43.5% still had borderline blood pressures, and 10.4% became definitely hypertensive. A large percentage of the patients with sustained hypertension were "exercise-positive" children. Thus, 82.3% of the children who developed hypertension by the end of the 5-year study had experienced a pathologic rise of blood pressure during initial exercise testing. By contrast, 84,9% of the children who were normotensive at the end of the study had exhibited normal blood pressures during ergometry on initial testing.

Wilson et al. [447] reported in 1979 on 3040 men and 388 women who were followed for 30 months. In the subjects who had pathologic exercise blood pressures, the risk for developing hypertension was 2.27 times greater than in subjects with a normal blood pressure response.

In a follow-up study lasting almost 6 years, Dlin et al. [85] found no instance where a patient who was normotensive both at rest and during ergometry at first examination went on the develop hypertension. This contrasts with the 10.6% incidence of hypertension developing in patients who had normal resting blood pressures but elevated exercise pressures. Tammen and Blümchen [414] and Ammecke et al. [3] also point out that even in patients with normal resting pressures, an exaggerated rise of blood pressure during exercise is a good indication of future hypertension.

Approximately half of the borderline hypertensives tested here could be classified as "exercise-negative" on the basis of their exercise and postexercise blood pressures and could definitely be assigned to the normotensive population. Most of the 'exercise-negative" patients were persons who had an elevated peripheral resistance at rest, and thus elevated systolic and diastolic blood pressures, due to strong emotional influences. When exercised on the ergometer, however, these patients experienced a normal vasodilatation which lowered their total peripheral resistance and thus checked the rise of diastolic pressure or even produced diastolic normotension after exercise. This response of the systolic and diastolic press pressure, which differs materially from that of the "exercise-positive" borderline hypertensives, may be based upon different responses of the alpha- and beta-adrenergic receptors to sympathetic stimuli. A predominant beta-adrenergic hyperactivity would create a hyperkinetic state in which the blood pressure response would resemble that of the "exercise-negative" borderline hypertensives. A concurrent alpha- and beta-adrenergic hyperactivity, on the other hand, would produce an elevation of both the systolic and diastolic pressures, creating a pattern characteristic of the "exercise-positive" group. This disparity of blood pressure responses may be based upon a hyperactivity of central sympathetic centers (thus involving a disturbance of regulatory mechanisms), or upon a thickening of the arteriolar wall which alters its ability to respond to vasoconstrictor stimuli, as postulated by Folkow [102].

Borderline hypertensives who have been segregated into "exercise-positive" and "exercise-negative" groups will also have different blood pressure responses under conditions of rest. While the "exercise-positives" show a rise of systolic and diastolic blood pressure during orthostasis like that occurring in the definite hypertensives, the "exercise-negative" patients experience a fall of systolic blood pressure and raise their diastolic blood pressures to a much smaller degree (Table 27).

The "exercise-positive" borderline hypertensives experience a mean rise of 5.7 mmHg diastolic on changing from the recumbent to the standing position. This increase is considerably less than the 13 mmHg reported by Hull et al. [203] in 21 borderline hypertensives. These authors believe that the orthostatic test offers a simple means for the diagnosis of borderline hypertension, since the 23 normotensive subjects in their study experienced a mean rise of only 6 mmHg on standing and did not exceed the upper normal limit of 90 mmHg. The normal group of 173 subjects tested by us also showed a corresponding mean diastolic pressure increase of 6.5 mmHg and remained well below 90 mm Hg after 1 minute of standing.

Other authors found smaller diastolic pressure increases after orthostasis than Hull et al. For example, Messmann et al. [296, 297] reported a mean rise of 5.3 mmHg (from 97 to 102.3 mmHg) in 81 labile hypertensives, and a mean rise of 3.2 mmHg (from 109.7 to 112.9 mmHg) in 32 patients with stable hypertension. Trieb et al. [424] also found a mean increase of 2.4 mmHg (from 113.7 to 116.1 mmHg) between the readings obtained after 2 minutes' recumbency and 2 minutes' standing in their direct intravascular measurements in 20 hypertensive patients.

When we compare the blood pressures of the "exercise-positive" and "exercise-negative" borderline hypertensives taken in recumbency and immediately before exercise, we can appreciate even more clearly the essential difference that exists between the two groups (Table 27). While the "positive" borderline hypertensives show both systolic and diastolic blood pressure increases which are obviously greater than those of the definite hypertensives, the "negative" borderline hypertensives do not experience a further increase relative to the values in recumbency despite the presence of an emotional stress. Because the blood pressure response immediately before exercise is determined largely by emotional influences related to the test situation, these results suggest that a standardized psychological stress test would also be of value in the prediction of future arterial hypertension.

Unfortunately, some degree of adaptation is inevitable when an emotional stress test is administered a second time, and so the results of the test would not be reproducible [318]. With standardized ergometric testing, on the other hand, it is always possible to assign even borderline hypertensives to the normotensive or hypertensive range, regardless of how many times the test is repeated. This is confirmed by the results of follow-up tests after four years and by the good reproducibility of blood pressure readings in "exercise-positive" borderline hypertensives taken at different times of day (see Chap. II.3.1.). The group of borderline hypertensives could be identified as hypertensives on the basis of all three ergometric tests, although the resting blood pressure taken at midday was not a useful parameter. This result is confirmed by the telemetric studies of Krönig in hypertensives who repeatedly were normotensive in the resting state. When an exercise stress test (step climbing) was administered to these patients, however, their blood pressures became obviously pathologic [259].

In defining normal ranges, there is diversity of opinion as to whether the 1 SD or 2 SD range should be used [150]. We have found the 1 SD range to be more advantageous for evaluating the blood pressure response to ergometry.

In our classification of borderline hypertensives as "exercise-positive" or "exercise-negative," we selected a blood pressure of 200/100 mmHg at 100 watts (and corresponding heart rates) as the dividing line between the upper normal range and a pathologic blood pressure elevation. This value corresponds roughly to the mean plus one standard deviation for the overall population of 20- to 50-year-old normotensive males at 100 watts (201.8/100.7 mmHg).

Any differentiation between physiologic and pathophysiologic parameters will necessarily involve some arbitrariness. Nevertheless, our results provide ample evidence that the limit of 200/100 mmHg at 100 watts enables a reliable discrimination to be made between normal and pathologic blood pressure responses. On the one hand, none of our normotensive controls exceeded a pressure of 200/100 mmHg at 100 watts. On the other, the two groups of "exercise-positive" borderline hypertensives studied here had markedly higher pressures of 216/112 mmHg and 211/115 mmHg at 100 watts. Moreover, the diastolic blood pressures of both "exercise-negative" groups were 92 and 90 mm Hg and thus significantly below the upper limit of 100 mmHg.

A comparison with the limit of 184/94 mmHg (mean + 1 SD) determined by Krönig et al. [259] on the basis of direct intravascular measurements in 30 normal subjects aged 46 years exercised at 75 watts demonstrates the good agreement which exists between invasive data and the blood pressure of 180/95 mm Hg (mean + 1 SD) measured indirectly in our male subjects at 70 watts.

The fact that some of our "exercise-negative" borderline hypertensives raised their systolic pressure above the 200 mmHg limit did not complicate the differentiation of these subjects from hypertensives on the basis of their exercise and postexercise diastolic blood pressure readings. The assessment of the blood pressure in the recovery period is of particular value in patients whose responses to exercise are borderline. Our results clearly show that a sharp differentiation between "exercise-positive" and "exercise-negative" borderline hypertensives is possible in the recovery period. We therefore made persistence of the blood pressure above 140/90 mmHg at 5 minutes postexercise an additional criterion for inclusion in the "exercise-positive" group.

The heart rate that is attained during exercise must be taken into account when evaluating blood pressure response. As we saw in Chap. III.2.5., the male subjects on the whole attained a mean heart rate of 126 ± 13 beats/min at 100 watts. Strictly speaking, therefore, the upper limit of 200/100 mm Hg is valid only for the range from about 113 to 139 beats/min in untrained persons. This is an important consideration, because the workload relative to body weight can vary greatly from one patient to the next, and so normal values must be adjusted to the individual heart rate, especially in females. This circumstance also must be considered to avoid errors of interpretation when assessing the blood pressure response of an athletically trained patient with borderline hypertension. Frequently these patients do not raise their heart rates sufficiently at 100 watts however the same upper limit of 200/100 mmHg at 100 watts can be used for the diagnosis of hypertension (F. Boldt, I-W. Franz; unpublished data).

4.5.3. Prognostic Evaluation of Borderline Hypertension

The ability to predict accurately the future course of borderline hypertension would be a major step forward from a prognostic and preventive standpoint. The successful prevention of hypertension on a long-term basis must rely upon the early recognition of a genetic predisposition to the disease. This is particularly important in the case of borderline hypertension, where genetic influences are mediated by environmental factors such as salt intake, obesity, level of physical activity, and psychosocial conditions [35, 178, 219, 220].

If the risk for future hypertension could be accurately assessed at an early stage, it would be possible to institute specific, individualized *preventive measures* that could be implemented far more readily than large-scale measures aimed at the general population.

Successful, early intervention assumes particular importance when once considers the excess cardiovascular morbidity and mortality that are associated with borderline hypertension [87, 224, 266].

This is true even in youthful populations. In 114 adolescents aged 14 to 18 with mildly elevated blood pressures, Goldring et al. [157] found evidence of target organ damage relative to a normal population, including ECG signs of left ventricular hypertrophy with a reduction of ventricular volume from mural hypertrophy, as well as the occurrence of markedly higher peak blood pressures and heart rates.

With regard to the prognostic value of classifying borderline hypertensives as "exercise-positive" or "exercise-negative" on the basis of ergometry, the studies of Briedigkeit et al. yielded an additional important finding. On analyzing the family history of juvenile borderline hypertensives, these authors found that 35% of the parents of "exercise-positive" children suffered from cardiovascular disease (with a 13% mortality), and 87,5% of the grandparents (with a 32.5% mortality). The "exercise-negative" children had family histories which did not differ significantly from the normotensive controls, with respective cardiovascular disease rates of 10 and 15% in the parents and 30 and 23% in the grandparents [49].

In a follow-up study lasting several years, Blümchen et al. [39] were able to show that patients with coronary heart disease who had normal blood pressures at rest but elevated pressure during exercise had higher grades of coronary artery stenosis and higher morbid event rates than patients with normal exercise responses. Moreover, the patients' tolerance of ergometric testing over the period of the follow-up was found to relate strongly to the level of the exercise blood pressure. It has already been mentioned that patients in this study with elevated exercise blood pressures at first examination had a significantly higher risk of developing subsequent hypertension than patients who were normotensive on initial testing.

4.5.4. Therapeutic Implications

Because even very minor vasuclar changes are predisposing factors for degenerative disease [35], the early identification of "exercise-positive" borderline hypertensives is not only of great diagnostic value but also has major *prognostic significance*. It enables the early initiation of treatment, which can substantially lower the cardiovascular risk [205, 288]. Thus, a 10-year intervention study in 191 patients (average age 44 years) with blood pressures in the borderline range (140-149/90-95 mmHg) revealed a 29% morbidity in patients who received treatment as opposed to 52% in untreated controls [295]. In the intervention study (HDFP) conducted by the National Institute of Health [205], the mortality in mild hypertension could be significantly reduced by appropriate antihypertensive therapy. The Australian intervention study [286] likewise demonstrated a significant reduction of cardiovascular morbidity and mortality in patients with mildly elevated blood pressures who received antihypertensive drugs compared with patients who received a placebo. A similar conclusion was reached by an English study in 961 patients published by Trafford et al. in 1981 [422].

While the three intervention studies cited above have underscored the necessity of early treatment in hypertension, there is still disagreement concerning the need for drug treatment in borderline hypertension. This uncertainty is based partly on the great variability in blood pressure and partly on the extreme difficulty of predicting the future course of borderline hypertension on the basis of resting blood pressure determinations.

We believe that our 3.8-year follow-up of "exercise-positive" borderline hypertensives has demonstrated a very high probability that such patients will progress to established hypertension. Moreover, when one considers that the blood pressure responses of the "exercise-positive" borderline hypertensives were like those of the mildly hypertensive patients, they must be assumed to have an equally high vascular risk.

Thus, ergometric testing in borderline hypertensives not only aids in diagnosis but also provides a sound basis for therapeutic decision making. By enabling a definitive diagnosis to be made, ergometry helps the examining physician to convince the patient of the need for general or pharmacologic treatment. If "exercise-positive" borderline hypertensives do not respond satisfactorily to weight reduction, salt restriction to 5-8 g/day, the avoidance of emotional stress, the termination of nicotine abuse and moderate endurance training, then antihypertensive treatment should be initiated, usually in the form of a beta-blocking drug. Especially in young patients [44, 200, 371] and patients who have additional cardiovascular risk factors [183] or an hereditary predisposition [45, 211, 411], the decision to start drug treatment should not be unnecessarily deferred. The case for treatment becomes stronger when one considers that even persons who are below the upper limit for normotension recommended by the WHO may still have an excessive vascular risk [211, 223]. Treatment is essential in such cases to prevent or at least defer the onset of serious complications [48, 205, 286, 302, 430-433]. The conclusions of the follow-up study of the National Health Institute [205] prompted Relman [347] in 1980 to write an editorial in the *New England Journal of Medicine* titled "Mild Hypertension: No More Benign Neglect," urging U.S. physician to change their attitude toward the treatment of mildly hypertensive patients.

Patients who have borderline blood pressures at rest but are normotensive during and after ergometry do not require pharmacologic treatment. Nevertheless, as our follow-up of "exercise-negative" borderline hypertensives after

4.1 years indicates, repeated blood pressure determinations in standardized ergometric tests is necessary at 6- to 12-month intervals, for it cannot be predicted whether the resting blood pressure will eventually normalize, or whether the patient is indeed in an early stage of arterial hypertension.

Sixty-eight percent of the "exercise-negative" borderline hypertensives tested at 4.1-year follow-up still had borderline blood pressures at rest, but had normal systolic and diastolic blood pressures during ergometry. The normotensive status of these patients had been correctly diagnosed on initial examination.

However, 32% of the "exercise-negative" borderline hypertensives at follow-up had significantly higher and in fact pathologic blood pressures during all phases of the test. At that time their readings did not differ from those of the "exercise-positive" subjects and the group 1A hypertensives. Accordingly, even "exercise-negative" borderline hypertensives must be considered to have a non-negligible vascular risk, especially those whose diastolic blood pressures during and after ergometry are within the borderline range. Besides the necessity of follow-up examinations, the patient should be educated about the importance of general measures and regular, moderate exercise [113, 298, 444].

Another fact which may have prognostic and therapeutic significance in the older "exercise-negative" borderline hypertensives is the finding by Kannel et al. [224] that beyond age 45 the rise of systolic blood pressure constitutes an independent risk factor for cardiovascular disease. This may relate to our finding that 16 or 22 borderline hypertensives aged 41 to 65 years were "exercise-positive," as opposed to only 13 out of 30 patients in the younger age group. It would appear, then, that one may expect not only an increase in the overall prevalence of borderline hypertension with age [216] but also a greater number of "exercise-positive" blood pressure responses in individuals with borderline resting blood pressures.

5. Blood Pressure Increments from Rest to Exercise in Normotensives, Borderline Hypertensives and Hypertensives

5.1. Results and Comparison with Invasive Measurements

Besides comparing absolute values within different blood pressure groups, it is interesting also to compare the amounts by which the various groups raise their blood pressures during exercise at 50 and 100 watts compared with the supine resting state (Table 28, Figs. 33, 34). We made this comparison for normotensive males and females of different ages, hypertensive patients of different ages and degrees of severity, and for the "exercise-positive" and "exercise-negative" borderline hypertensives.

Comparing the systolic and diastolic blood pressure increments in the younger and older normotensive males, we find similar increases with respective increments of 23/6 mm Hg and 26/8 mm Hg from rest to 50 watts, and 56/12 mm Hg and 57/13 mm Hg from rest to 100 watts.

Table 28. Systolic (S. B. P.) and diastolic (D. B. P.) pressure increments from rest to 50 watts and 100 watts (females 80 watts) respectively in normotensives (N) males and females of different ages, hypertensive patients of different ages and degree of severity (groups 1A, 2A, 1B, 2B), and in the exercise-positive (BH+) and exercise-negative (BH−) borderline hypertensives. The mean increase in blood pressure and heart rate per 10 watt is also shown

	n=80	N♂ n=173 35.3 yrs	N♂ n=50 64.4 yrs	Group 1A n=132 37 yrs	Group 2A n=35 59.7 yrs	Group 1B n=72 40.1 yrs	Group 2B n=42 60.9 yrs	BH+ n=49 38.3 yrs	BH− n=49 30 yrs	N♀ n=150 35.6 yrs	H n=30 39.9 yrs	H n=19 60.4 yrs
			**		**			**				
Increments from rest supine to 50 watts	ΔSBP	23.2	25.9	30.2	31.8	22.8	24.6	35.3	24.2	31.2	27.1	36.0
	(mmHg)	11.5	11.6	16.9	19.5	17.2	16.8	18.2	15.2		15.8	21.4
				ns								
			***									
	ΔDBP	6.4	8.0	10.5	12.6	7.6	11.2	13.3	3.9	10.4	11.6	15.8
						*		*				
	(mmHg)	4.1	6.5	9.6	10.6	7.1	8.6	7.1	5.0	8.1	9.2	12.6
				*								
			*								***	
Increments from rest supine to 100 watts	ΔSBP	56.2	57	60.8	67.4	52.9	57.7	69.5	50.4	58.8	62.8	79.2+
					**			***			**	
	(mmHg)	17.4	18.4	20.2	20.3	21.3	20.6	18.1	19.2	16.4	19.6	21.5
			***									
	ΔDBP	12.1	13.1	18.1	21.9	14.2	18.7	20.5	5.1	14.8	20.3	26.7+
					*	*		***				
	(mmHg)	8.4	9.0	12.8	12.1	9.9	11.1	8.5	6.1	9.1	12.8	12.2
				***								
Increments/10 watts during ergometry	ΔSBP (mmHg)	6.6	6.1	6.3	6.8	6.0	6.9	7.2	5.5	6.6	7.2	14.3
	ΔDBP (mmHg)	1.1	1.1	1.4	1.9	1.3	1.5	1.6	0.4	1.5	2.3	3.7
	ΔHR (bts/min)	5.6	4.2	4.7	4.6	4.5	4.4	4.6	4.5	7	5.3	7.4

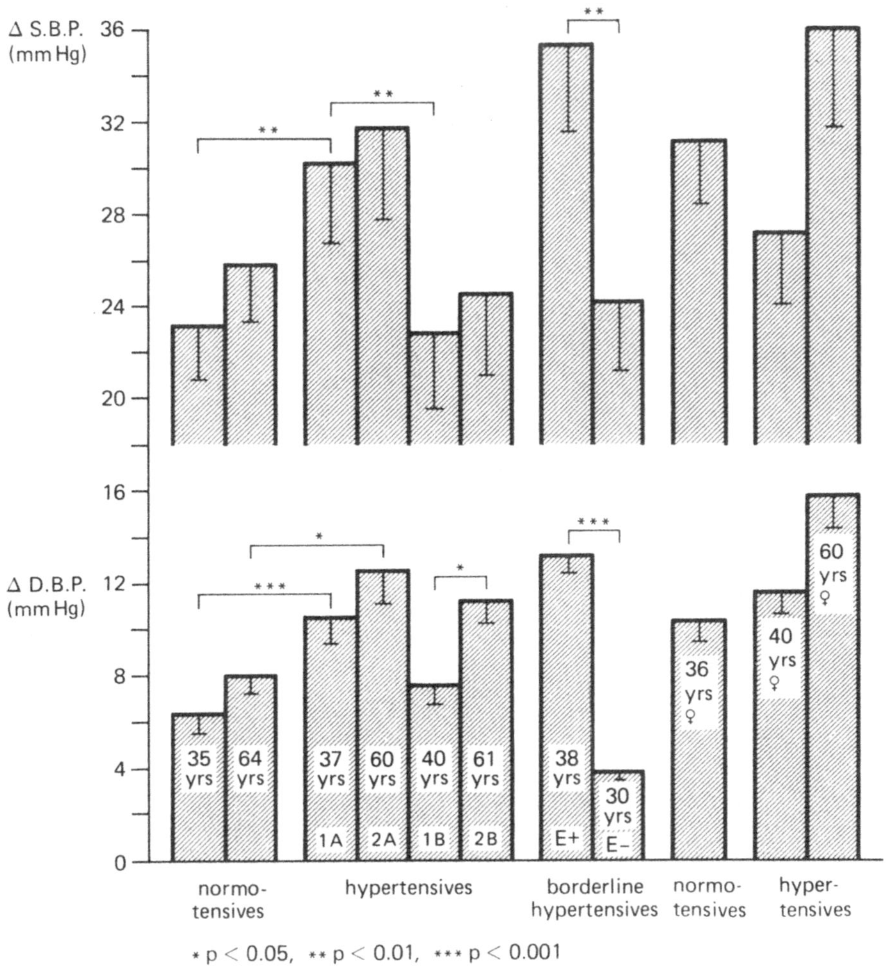

Fig. 33. Increments of systolic (Δ P_s) and diastolic (Δ P_d) blood pressure from recumbency to 50-watt exercise for hypertensives of varying age, gender and severity compared with normotensives (s. text)

Comparing the blood pressure increment from rest to 50 watts (1st stage of exercise) for the different hypertensive groups, we observe a significant difference ($p<0.01$) depending on the severity of the hypertension. Both the younger and older hypertensives (groups 1A and 2A) with lower resting blood pressures showed an excessive systolic blood pressure increment ($p<0.01$) amounting to approximately 50% of the total pressure increment from recumbency to 100 watts. By contrast, groups 1B and 2B had a substantially smaller increment corresponding to that of the normotensives, despite their higher absolute blood pressure values. The "exercise-positive" borderline hypertensives had a significantly greater ($p<0.01$) systolic blood pressure increment than even the mild hypertensives. The overall increase of 35 mm Hg at 50 watts and 69.5 mm Hg at 100 watts was the greatest observed in any of the groups tested.

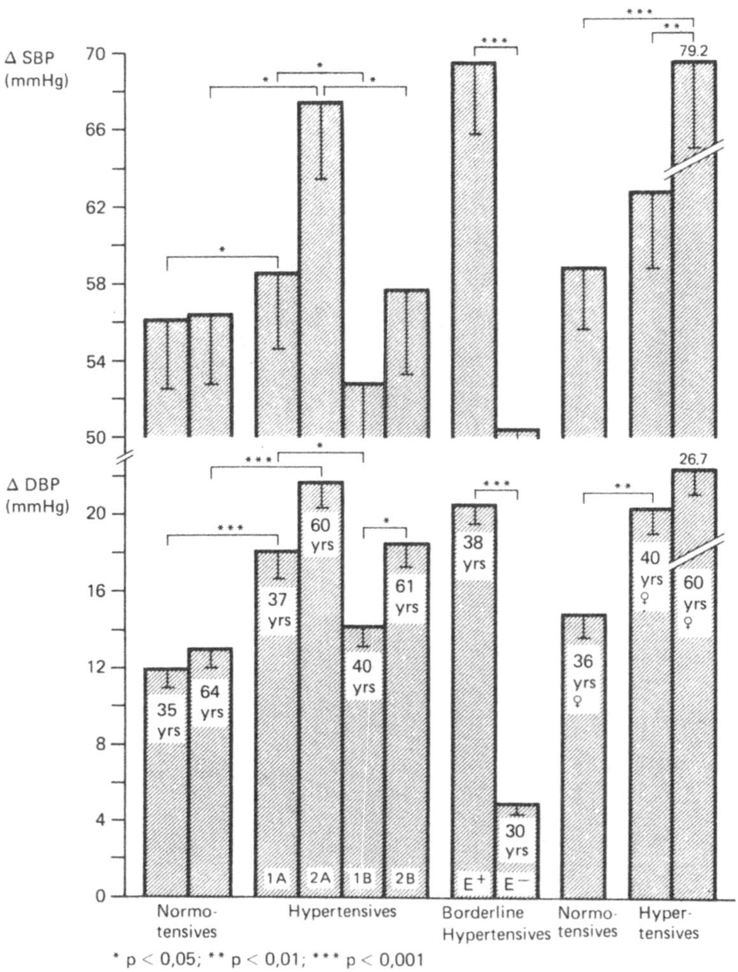

Fig. 34. Increments of systolic (Δ P_s) and diastolic (Δ P_d) blood pressure and of heart rate (Δ HR) [sic!!] from recumbency to 100-watt exercise for hypertensives of varying age, gender and severity compared with normotensives (s. text)

On comparing diastolic blood pressures, we find that the increments in groups 1A and 2A, with their lower resting pressures, were again greater than in groups 1B and 2B, regardless of age. Unlike group 2B, group 1B did not differ significantly from age-matched normotensives. As was the case for the systolic pressure, the "exercise-positive" borderline hypertensives had the greatest relative diastolic pressure increases.

The "exercise-negative" borderline hypertensives differed from all other groups tested in that they had the lowest absolute diastolic blood pressure increment from rest to either stage of exercise. Their mean increment per 10 watts (0.4 mm Hg) was also markedly below that of the other groups.

Comparing the younger hypertensive women of group 1 with the hypertensive men of group 1A, who are comparable in age and resting blood pressure, we find very close agreement between their systolic and diastolic blood pressure increments. The older hypertensive men and women are difficult to compare due to the relatively small number of women comprising the group ($n = 19$) and the fact that the women were exercised to only 80 watts. Nevertheless, it is apparent that the older hypertensive women had the greatest absolute systolic and diastolic pressure increments from rest to 50 watts of all the subjects tested, and that age was a definite factor - a trend also present in the hypertensive males. This finding is consistent with the results of Krönig [259], who found that the pressure increment from rest to stair climbing in 69 hypertensives (including 28 women) at WHO Stage 2 showed a significant ($p < 0.05$) dependence on age.

A comparison of the male and female normotensives is hampered by the fact that the men started exercising at 50 watts while the women started at 30 watts, and also by the fact that 50 watts represents a relatively greater workload for the women than the men. Consequently the normotensive women responded to the exercise with markedly greater systolic and diastolic blood pressure increments.

Bearing in mind the difficulties that are inherent in comparing different hypertensive groups, it can nevertheless be instructive to compare the results in our hypertensive subjects with the results of other studies using invasive techniques of blood pressure measurement. An excellent index for this comparison is the blood pressure increment which occurs between rest and standardized ergometry. For example, Krönig reported on a group of hypertensives whose blood pressures rose by 47.3 mm Hg systolic and 12.3 mm Hg diastolic on going from 3 minutes' rest to 3 minutes' exercise at 75 watts. Our group of 1A hypertensives, who have resting blood pressures comparable to Krönig's group, showed a pressure increment of 43.6 mm Hg systolic and 13.8 mm Hg diastolic from rest to 70 watts, indicating good agreement with the results of invasive studies [259].

Similar agreement is found for hypertensives over age 50 in whom Lund-Johansen performed intravascular blood pressure determinations during exercise stress testing. This group showed a pressure increment of 62 mm Hg systolic and 15.8 mm Hg diastolic from rest to 100 watts. These figures agree well with those for our comparable group 2B hypertensives, who had a pressure increment of 57.9 mm Hg systolic and 18 mm Hg diastolic from rest to 100 watts. A similar increment is observed in 38 hypertensives age 52 whose blood pressures were measured directly by Taylor during treadmill exercise. These subjects, who also were comparable to our group 2B patients on the basis of their resting blood pressure of $178 \pm 5/110 \pm 3$ mm Hg, had a mean pressure increment of 52.4/16.6 mm Hg.

The blood pressure increments during ergometry reported here also agree very closely with the increments measured directly by Krönig during everyday stresses in the form of stair climbing. According to his calculations, this stress was comparable to an ergometric workload of 80 watts. The total study population of 102 hypertensive patients with varying degrees of blood pressure elevation showed on overall pressure increment of 46 mm Hg systolic and 13.5 mm Hg diastolic. The pressure increment from rest to 80 watts in all the hypertensives in our study was nearly identical, with a mean value of 48.2 mm Hg systolic and 14.4 mm Hg diastolic.

5.2. Summary and Conclusions

Our results indicate that the mean *blood pressure increments* from recumbency to 50 and 100 watts are equivalent both for normotensive persons and for patients with more severe forms of hypertension. It appears, then, that the hemodynamic response to exercise in these groups is essentially the same, the only difference being the level of blood pressure at which the response takes place.

Patients with milder forms of hypertension (groups 1A and 2A) and the "exercise-positive" borderline hypertensives, on the other hand, responded to exercise with significantly higher relative blood pressure increments, both systolic and diastolic. These three groups attained at 50 watts approximately half the total pressure increment between recumbency and 100 watts. This would suggest that early arterial hypertension is associated with an increase in sympathetic activity or a heightened sympathetic responsiveness.

Particularly noteworthy is the response of the *older hypertensive women,* who showed the greatest systolic and diastolic blood pressure increment from recumbency to 50 watts of all the groups tested. Although this group consisted of only 19 subjects who were stressed only to 80 watts instead of 100, they raised their blood pressures by 79.2 mm Hg systolic and 26.7 mm Hg diastolic between recumbency and 80 watts - a remarkable amount when one considers that it exceeds the increment of the other groups stressed at a higher workload. This raises the possibility that older women may be at particular risk for developing excessive blood pressure increases in response to stress, which may account for the findings of the Framingham Study [226] on the correlation between cardiovascular mortality and age. The yearly death rate per 10,000 population was found to be 1.4 greater among women age 55 to 64 than in women age 45 to 54; in the 65-74 age group, the mortality is 5.2 times greater. A comparison of corresponding age groups in men yields an entirely different result, with factors of only 2.3 and 2.7, respectively. The markedly higher prevalence of stroke among late middle-aged and elderly women is also noteworthy in this regard.

6. Blood Pressure and Heart Rate Responses of Elderly Hypertensives

The evaluation of marginally to mildly elevated blood pressures in the elderly is difficult, and the pathologic significance of these elevations is frequently ambiguous [149, 201, 210, 230, 426]. However, given the fact that even patients with mild to moderate arterial hypertension at rest may raise their blood pressures excessively during physical exertion [108, 122, 255, 362, 416], one can readily appreciate the importance of correct *blood pressure assessment in the elderly,* in whom latent or overt hypertensive complications may already be presumed to exist [334, 405]. It is reasonable to expect that the exaggerated blood pressure responses of these patients to ordinary stresses would place them at particular risk for myocardial hypoxia [334, 405] and cerebrovascular complications [230].

6.1. Comparative Study of Elderly Hypertensives and Normotensives of Equal Age Distribution

It was our aim in this study to determine whether, as in borderline hypertensives, measurements of the exercise blood pressure could discern the dividing line between an arbitrarily defined normal and pathologic resting blood pressure in late middle-aged and elderly individuals, thereby aiding the physician in assessing the severity of the hypertension and selecting patients for drug therapy.

6.1.1. Study Population

Our study population consisted of 50 elderly normotensive men with an average age of 64.4 years (55 to 80) and 50 elderly hypertensive men (WHO Stage I-II) with an average age of 61.7 years (55 to 77) who had presented for routine cardiac examinations. We monitored the blood pressure responses of these subjects during and after ergometric exercise [123].

The average height of our normal and hypertensive subjects was 177.1 ± 8.3 cm and 173.9 ± 6.4 cm, respectively. Their average weights were 79.4 ± 8.7 kg and 79.6 ± 8.3 kg.

6.1.2. Blood Pressure and Heart Rate Responses

From a resting value of 140/83 mm Hg, the blood pressure of the elderly normotensives rose continuously during exercise from 166 mm Hg systolic at 50 watts to 196 mm Hg at 100 watts (Table 29, Fig. 35) and thus significantly ($p < 0.05$) exceeded the pressures of the 40-50 age group at all stages of exercise (s. Chap. III.2.1.). The diastolic pressures also manifested the familiar age effect and showed a significant difference relative to the 20-30 age group ($p < 0.01$) and 30-40 group ($p < 0.05$), but not relative to the 40-50 age group.

The elderly hypertensives had only a mild blood pressure elevation at rest: 168/106 mm Hg. However, their blood pressure rose to 196/117 mm Hg at only 50 watts, which was significantly elevated ($p < 0.001$) relative to the older normotensives. Their pressure was still markedly elevated at 100 watts (232/125 mm Hg), showing an increase of 36 mm Hg systolic and 30 mm Hg diastolic.

During recovery, the blood pressures of the elderly hypertensives followed the pattern characteristic of arterial hypertension, i. e., fell only to 174/109 mm Hg after 5 minutes's recovery and thus remained elevated above pre-exercise levels. This contrasted with the response of the normotensives, whose pressures reached or fell below the cut-off point of 140/90 mm Hg.

On average, then, the elderly hypertensives had significant blood pressure elevations during and after ergometry compared with normotensive controls. The most important finding of our comparative study, however, resulted from an analysis of individual values. As we noted in Chap. III.3.4.5., the response of the blood pressure to exercise cannot always be predicted on the basis of the resting blood pressure. This is particularly true of older hypertensives, in whom

Table 29. Systolic (S. B. P.) and diastolic (D. B. P.) blood pressures and heart rates (H. R.) (means ± SD) of 50 elderly male normotensives (N) and of 50 elderly hypertensives (H) before, during and after work (**p < 0.01; ***p < 0.001)

n = 100		Rest	Ergometric work						Recovery period (min)				
		supine	50	60	70	80	90	100	1′	2′	3′	4′	5′
SBP (mmHg)	N n = 50 x̄ 64.4 yrs (55–80 yrs)	140.1 15.3	165.9 16.8	173.5 18.4	178.3 19.5	184.2 19.5	191.1 20.2	196.3 19.5	173.4 23	159.1 21.3	150.4 18.9	144 18.6	140.1 19.3
	H n = 50 x̄ 61.7 yrs (55–77 yrs)	167.5 15.1***	196.2 20.4***	209.6 21.6***	214.7 20.8***	221.5 22.1***	225.6 21.7***	231.8 20.4***	204.7 22.9***	190 21.1***	181.7 19.9***	177.1 19.8***	174.3 19.7***
DBP (mmHg)	N n = 50 x̄ 64.4 yrs (55–80 yrs)	83.1 8.1	91.1 8.9	93.2 8.1	93.8 9.2	94.6 8.7	95.4 8.6	96.1 8.2	83.9 10.2	82.3 8.6	81.7 9.4	82.2 9.4	82.5 8.4
	H n = 50 x̄ 61.7 yrs (55–77 yrs)	105.6 8.4***	117.2 13.8**	120 15**	121.2 15.2***	123.1 16.2***	123.5 16.8***	124.9 16.4***	110.9 15.2***	109.6 13***	108.4 13.6***	109.1 14***	109 14.4***
HR (bts/min)	N n = 50 x̄ 64.4 yrs (55–80 yrs)	63.9 9	89.1 11.9	93.3 11.5	96.6 13.1	101.1 16.0	106.3 16.0	110.3 16.8	84.6 14.3	77.2 14.5	73.7 14.3	72.3 11.3	72.1 11.6
	H n = 50 x̄ 61.7 yrs (55–77 yrs)	71.2 10.4***	97.8 12.8***	102.8 12.1***	107.8 13.5***	113.2 14.9***	118.0 16.0***	121.9 16.2***	92.7 14.9**	85.5 15.3**	82.6 14.1**	81.5 13.1**	81.1 13.4**

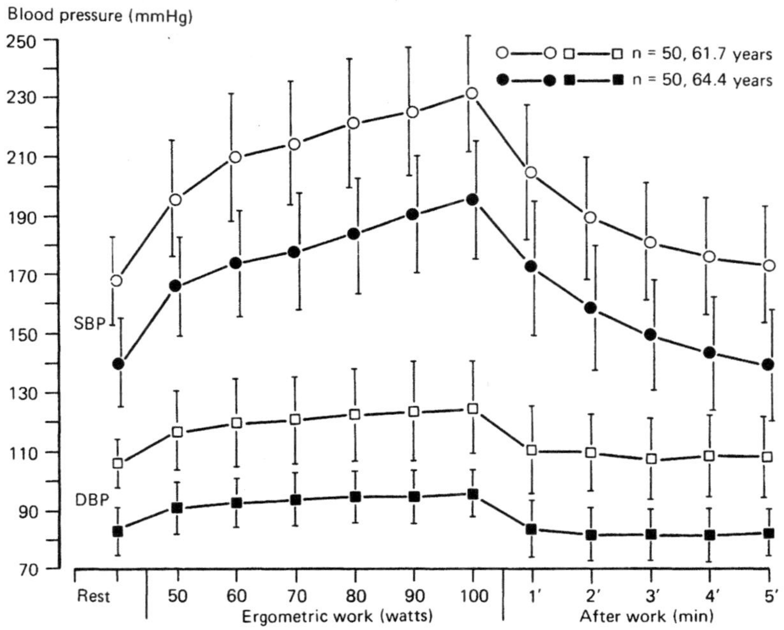

Fig. 35. Blood pressure responses of 50 elderly normotensive men (average age 64.4) and of 50 hypertensives (average age 61.7)

the level of the resting blood pressure is a poor guide to the magnitude of the exercise response and may cause the examining physician to overestimate or underestimate the vascular risk in these individuals. For example, some patients with mildly elevated blood pressures at rest raised their pressures excessively and reproducibly even at low levels of exercise, while others had blood pressure responses which were essentially normotensive both during and after exercise.

Fig. 36 shows the blood pressure response of a 70-year-old hypertensive man whose resting blood pressure of 180/100 mm Hg rose to 204/105 mm Hg at 100 watts and thus was within normal limits for this level of work, although the patient attained a heart rate of 130 beats/min. During recovery the diastolic pressure fell to 90 mm Hg in only the 1st minute, and by the 5th minute the systolic pressure reached 170 mm Hg - a value below the pre-exercise level.

Fig. 37 shows the blood pressure and heart rate response of a 60-year-old hypertensive man with pronounced sinus bradycardia and a resting blood pressure of 170/100 mm Hg. At a workload of 150 watts the blood pressure was 212/92 mm Hg and thus was age-normal. In the 1st minute of recovery the diastolic pressure fell to 80 mm Hg, while the systolic pressure remained elevated above the pre-exercise level. The elevated systolic blood pressure readings at rest are not an expression of hypertensive disease, but are causally related to the increase of cardiac stroke volume in this bradycardiac patient.

Fig. 38 illustrates how the blood pressure response to exercise can differ dramatically from resting values. Despite similar resting pressures, one elderly hy-

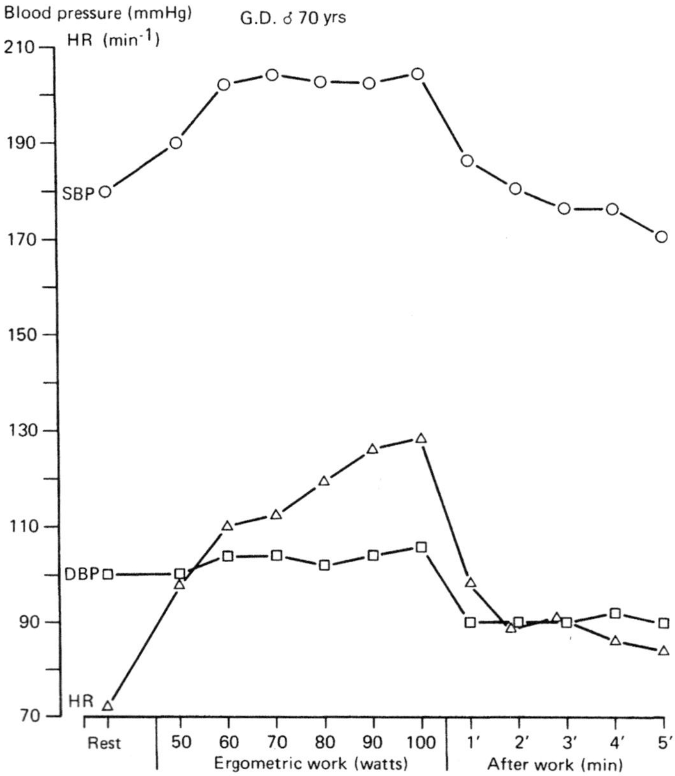

Fig. 36. Blood pressure and heart rate response of a 70-year-old man whose elevated resting blood pressure of 180/100 mg rose to a mere 204/105 mmHg at 100 watts

pertensive developed a pathologic rise of blood pressure during ergometry, while the other manifested a normotensive response.

Fig. 22 further illustrates the extreme difficulty of predicting exercise blood pressures on the basis of resting values. It shows the blood pressure response of a 60-year-old man whose resting blood pressure of 154/114 mm Hg climbed to 210/150 mm Hg at only 50 watts and then to 242/166 mm Hg at 80 watts, requiring that the test be terminated. At that time the patient showed no objective or subjective signs of myocardial hypoxia or insufficiency. It is important to note that the heart rate at 80 watts was only 100/min, suggesting that this patient will probably develop substantially higher blood pressures in response to everyday stresses, as indicated by Krönig's study of heart rate profiles in hypertensives at ordinary levels of exertion [259]. The patient's blood pressure was still markedly elevated at 5 minutes postexercise (182/132 mm Hg). The man had obvious signs of left ventricular hypertrophy in his ECG, and chest roentgenograms in two planes revealed a marked broadening of the heart shadow toward the left side with an elongated aorta.

It must be understood that the *excessive blood pressure elevations* illustrated in the last two cases are by no means exceptional. Out of the 50 elderly hyperten-

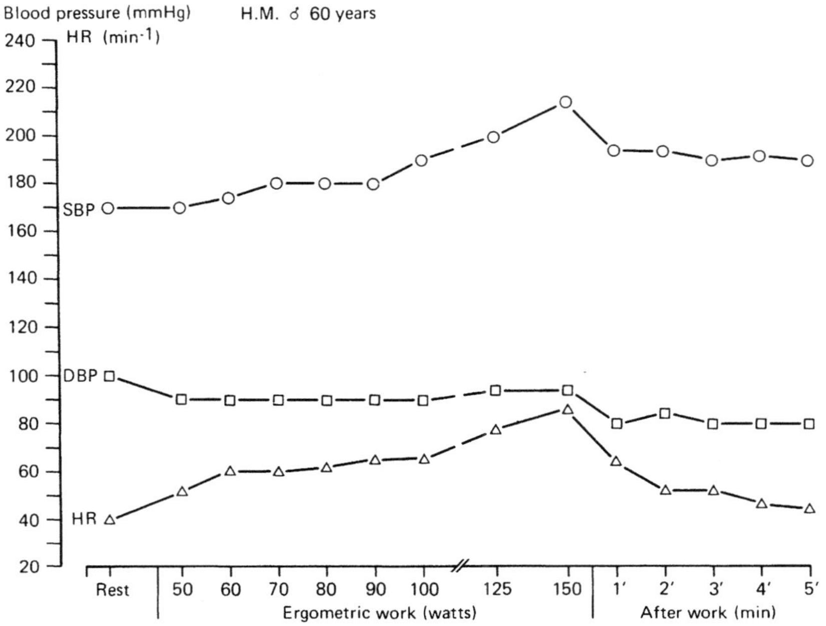

Fig. 37. Blood pressure and heart rate response of a 60-year-old bradycardiac hypertensive whose elevated resting blood pressure of 170/100 mg remained within the age-normal range during exercise

sives tested, 28 had systolic pressures greater than the value of 232/125 mm Hg determined for the total group at 100 watts, and 21 had diastolic pressures exceeding that value. The mean blood pressures of these subjects was a striking 247/138 mm Hg. The blood pressure response at 50 watts is presumably of greater prognostic significance in elderly hypertensives, since this workload corresponds to ordinary levels of mild exertion. Twenty-two of the 50 hypertensives exceeded the mean systolic pressure of 196 mm Hg at 50 watts, and 26 exceeded the mean diastolic pressure of 117 mm Hg, developing a mean blood pressure of 214/126 mm Hg. Eight of these patients exceeded the mean systolic pressure plus one standard deviation for the entire hypertensive group, 217 mm Hg, and nine exceeded the mean diastolic pressure, 132 mm Hg, showing a mean blood pressure of 230/137 mm Hg at only 50 watts.

These alarming systolic and diastolic blood pressure increases measured in some hypertensive patients even at very low stages of exercise clearly demonstrate the importance of ergometric testing for the *prognostic evaluation* of hypertension severity and *vascular risk* in the elderly. This is particularly evident when we analyze the nine patients of the hypertensive group who were identified as borderline hypertensives in the resting state. Five of these patients were definitively classified as "exercise-negative" and had blood pressure responses like those of the older normotensives. It is also noteworthy that of the four borderline hypertensives classified as "exercise-positive," three exceeded the mean pressure of 196/117 mm Hg for the whole group at 50 watts, and one borderline

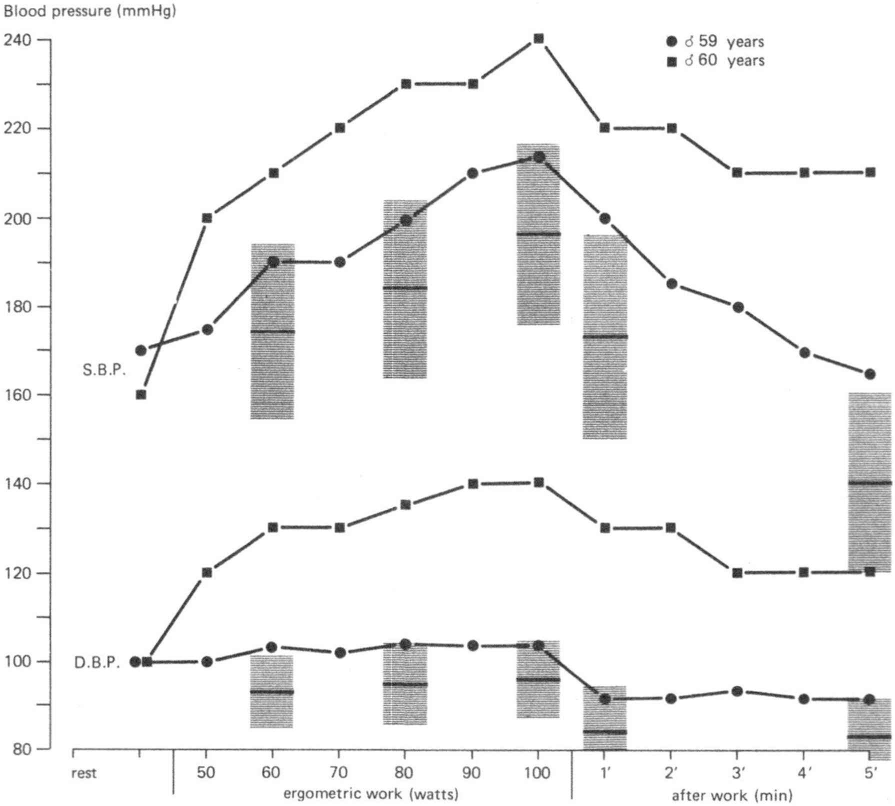

Fig. 38. Blood pressure responses of two elderly hypertensive men with approximately the same resting blood pressures. While one patient maintained age-normal blood pressures during and after ergometry, the other patient showed an exaggerated pressor response

hypertensive raised his pressure to 260/125 mm Hg at 50 watts with a concomitant heart rate of only 110/min.

The heart rates of the hypertensive patients were significantly ($p<0.01-p<0.001$) higher than those of the elderly normotensives both before, during and after exercise.

6.2. Summary and Conclusions

6.2.1. Prevalence

In a Swedish study published in 1979 [438], 19.3% of 60-year-old men were found to have arterial hypertension with diastolic blood pressures in excess of 105 mm Hg. 35.9% of these patients had previously been unaware of their hypertension, and 43.9% of the treated group had not received adequate therapy. Thus, 64,1% of the 60-year-old hypertensives investigated were either undiagnosed or poorly managed. These figures, which appear to be representative of other countries as well, underscore the alarming discrepancy between the total number of persons with hypertension, estimated at 6.3 million in the FRG, and the number of hypertensives who are receiving treatment, which is estimated at only 1.6 million.

6.2.2. *Prognosis*

Although the importance of elevated blood pressure as a risk factor for cerebral infarction and stroke in the elderly has been clearly demonstrated in the Framingham Study [225] and confirmed by other authors [388], various authorities have challenged the validity of these conclusions [149, 210]. A 36-year-old study by the Metropolitan Insurance Company [302] is frequently cited to support the argument that arterial hypertension has a progressively diminishing effect on residual life expectancy with increasing age. This statement is true as far as it goes, but it should be added that the above study found that the life expectancy of a 55-year-old man with a blood pressure of only 150/100 mm Hg is still shortened by 6 years.

The 1979 Stockholm Study [61] conducted in 3846 persons who were followed for 14 years indicates that elevated blood pressure is the preemminent risk factor for myocardial infarction in persons over age 50. The 1979 Goteburg Study [412, 413] in 855 50-year-old men followed for 13.5 years revealed a strong correlation between the level of the blood pressure and mortality from coronary heart disease, and also a close correlation between elevated blood pressure and morbidity from myocardial infarction, stroke and coronry disease. The results led the authors to conclude that "There is no indication of a decreasing importance of blood pressure as a risk factor in this age period."

This is also clear when one examines the link between high blood pressure and stroke. Thus, Neundörfer et al. [316] found that among 458 patients who had suffered a cerebral ischemic insult, 56% had arterial hypertension. This prevalence was 50% for men over age 50 and 70% for women.

6.2.3. *Diagnostic Assessment*

One reason for the uncertainty that persists in the evaluation of high blood pressure is the erroneous distinction that is often made in the literature [201, 426] between essential or secondary hypertension in the elderly and an entity called "senile hypertension." Because the systolic blood pressure is determined to a significant degree by the "windkessel" function of the aorta [34, 348], and it is known that aortic elasticity decreases with age [169, 391] while atherosclerosis becomes more prevalent [100], it is frequently argued that these changes conspire to cause hypertension in the elderly. However, the validity of this assertion is called into serious question by the findings of Franke [104], among others, who measured blood pressures of $145 \pm 4/79 \pm 2$ mm Hg in 118 persons over the age of 100. While it is true that the mean systolic blood pressure rises with age, these values are well below the 180/100 mm Hg suggested by the German League for Hypertension Prevention and Control as a useful level at which to initiate antihypertensive treatment beyond age 60–65 [81]. Thus, for example, the normotensive males investigated here, with an average age of 64 years, had a mean blood pressure of $140 \pm 16/83 \pm 8$ mm Hg, which agrees well with the mean value of $137 \pm 16/83 \pm 8$ mm Hg reported in the Swedish study [438] for 60-year-old men.

For this reason it is inappropriate to refer to the physiologic rise of blood pressure with age as "senile" or "age-dependent hypertension," and this phenomenon should be clearly distinguished from true hypertension in the elderly.

Based on the results of our exercise tests in 50 elderly hypertensives, there is little question that ergometry is a valuable adjunct in the evaluation of hypertension in the elderly. While the older normotensives exhibited significantly higher systolic and diastolic blood pressures compared with the younger decades of life, it was nevertheless possible to discriminate reliably between normotensive and hypertensive individuals on the basis of exercise response. As shown by our analysis of individual cases, some patients have an age-normal exercise response despite elevated blood pressures at rest, while others develop pathologic blood pressure elevations even at mild levels of exercise. The German League for Hypertension Prevention and Control recommends [81] that "treatment at this age (beyond 60 to 65) is beneficial above a diastolic blood pressure of 100 mm Hg and/or a systolic blood pressure of 180 mm Hg." However, our ergometric studies show that some elderly hypertensives with a resting blood pressure well below the limit recommended by the League will show definitely pathologic blood pressure elevations at only 50 watts of exercise. At the same time, the blood pressure responses of some hypertensives during exercise did not differ significantly from those of age-matched normotensives, despite their resting blood pressure of 180/100 mm Hg or higher.

Of course, it is legitimate to inquire as to the significance of exercise blood pressures in the elderly, given the reduced level of physical activity in that age group. First, it must be considered [403] that elderly persons respond to a given stress with a greater and more sustained elevation of blood pressure than younger individuals - a situation also present during and after ergometry. Second, everyday physical exertion such as walking on level ground or stair climbing may involve a considerably greater workload than 50 watts [259, 402], which, as we have seen, is itself sufficient to elicit pathologic blood pressure elevations in some persons.

Thus, an individualized program of exercise training for the treatment of hypertension in the elderly as advocated by Undeutsch and Lang [426] can be recommended only in patients whose blood pressure response to ergometry is known, or in patients who have received treatment. This is equally true for elderly hypertensives who are still physically active at home (gardening, etc.) or are engaged in a preventive or rehabilitative exercise training program. In these patients in particular, the physician is cautioned not to underestimate the potential significance of even mildly elevated resting blood pressures (s. Chap. II.7.).

The main danger of excessive *stress-induced blood pressure elevations* in elderly hypertensives does not lie in a more rapid progression of cardiovascular complications as in younger persons (despite Linzbach's finding [271] that compensatory myocardial hypertrophy is as common a response to hypertension in patients age 60-80 as in patients age 30-60). The most serious threat to the elderly, rather, is the occurrence of acute events (s. Chap. II.7.). When one considers that elderly hypertensives show a marked increase in myocardial oxygen consumption even at low levels of exercise, and that the coronary reserve is significantly decreased even in hypertensives who have adequate cardiac compensation and a normal coronary angiogram [407], one can readily appreciate the serious cardiac risk that exists in elderly hypertensives who have excessive blood pressures under stress. The increased myocardial oxygen demand, combined with a deficient oxygen supply, poses a danger of acute *myocardial ischemia,* which not only can cause necrosis of myocardial tissue but also is a major risk factor for *ventricular arrhythmias* - the mechanism of *sudden cardiac death* [36]. Thus, Kannel writes [226]: "Sudden unexpected death is sometimes the first symptom of hypertension and occurs three times as frequently in hypertensives as in normotensives." This fact, too, has a bearing on the significance of pathologic blood pressure elevations under stress as an indication for antihypertensive therapy.

It may be concluded, then, that a standardized test of the blood pressure response to exercise has greater value both diagnostically and prognostically than resting blood pressure determinations, especially when dealing with hypertension in the elderly.

The upper limits of normotension during and after ergometry, which are necessary for evaluation, are discussed in detail in Chap. III.2.5.

6.2.4. Therapeutic Implications

Trial studies in Sweden [32, 412] have demonstrated the efficacy of *antihypertensive treatment* for the reduction of morbidity and mortality from *coronary heart disease*. Moreover, the dramatic decline in the incidence of *stroke* reported in the United States [290] has been attributed at least in part to effective antihypertensive management [151, 397]. Nevertheless, there is still disagreement as to the practical conclusions to be drawn from epidemiologic and intervention studies. While some authors dispute the need to treat elevated blood pressures in the elderly [149, 210], others stress the benefits of rational therapy [67, 230, 236]. The uncertainty that exists in the literature is equally apparent on the clinical level. Thus, Kennedy et al. [230] reported in 1978 on 65 patients below age 75 who were hospitalized because of stroke. The authors found definite hypertension in 35 patients, and though all the hypertensives were under the care of a physician, there was no instance where satisfactory blood pressure control had been achieved. Either no antihypertensive drugs had been prescribed at all, or treatment had been discontinued on the physician's advice or independently. It was found that one-sixth of the strokes occurred within a month after the discontinuance of therapy.

These results underscore the need for rational antihypertensive treatment in the elderly, as well as the dangers that are posed by discontinuing treatment. The study also revealed a basic uncertainty on the part of the treating physicians concerning the prognostic significance of elevated blood pressure in the elderly. From this standpoint, the value of ergometric testing as a guide to the selection of patients for antihypertensive treatment assumes even greater significance (s. Chap. III).

7. Ergometry for Assessing the Myocardial Oxygen Consumption and Cardiocorporeal Performance Capacity of Hypertensive Patients

7.1. Comparative Determination of the Rate-Pressure Product of Hypertensives and Normotensives

The natural history of hypertension is marked by the development of cardiac complications which have major prognostic significance. On the one hand, the increased pressure load on the heart stimulates an increase in the total muscle mass which outstrips the capillary blood supply. As *myocardial oxygen consumption* rises during exercise, a disproportion develops between oxygen delivery and oxygen demand. The risk of myocardial ischemia is further aggravated by the *coronary heart disease* which frequently coexists with the hypertension. With the myocardial oxygen supply restricted in this fashion, the level of the myocardial oxygen consumption becomes a limiting factor and an extremely important clinical parameter. This consideration prompted us to conduct comparative ergometric studies to evaluate myocardial oxygen consumption in borderline hypertensives, definite hypertensives and normotensives.

We measured myocardial oxygen consumption in terms of the "rate-pressure product," which is the product of the heart rate and systolic blood pressure. This quantity is generally accepted to be a reliable indirect index of myocardial oxygen consumption [22, 214, 235, 314, 369].

7.1.1. Study Population

We first tested 132 males age 20–60 [119], who were divided into 3 blood pressure groups on the basis of casual readings taken after 2–3 minutes' supine rest. WHO criteria were used to classify the subjects as normotensive (group 1), borderline hypertensive (group 2) and hypertensive (group 3). Table 30 shows the mean age distribution of the three groups and their resting blood pressures. The similar age distributions of the groups provided a good basis for comparison.

Table 30. Age, systolic (S. B. P.) and diastolic (D. B. P.) blood pressure, heart rate (H. R.) and Physical Working Capacity 170/kg body weight (PWC 170/kg b. w.) of 57 normotensives, 24 borderline hypertensives and hypertensives (*p < 0.05; ***p < 0.001)

n = 132	Age (years)	SBP (mmHg)	DBP (mmHg)	HR (bts/min)	PWC_{170}/kg b. w. KG (Watt)
Group 1, n = 57	41.5	136.3	85.3	68.1	3.44
Normotensives	13	8.6	6.3	11.9	0.8
Group 2, n = 24	42.6	151.7	93.5	71.2	2.93
Borderline hypertensives	12.7	5.3***	2.3***	11	0.7*
Group 3, n = 51	43.6	164	105.6	72.1	2.71
Hypertensives	11.6	10.9***	7.3***	10.3	0.74***

The systolic and diastolic blood pressures showed the desired degree of intergroup variation.

We also tested 50 elderly normotensives age 55–80 (average age 64.4) and 50 elderly hypertensives age 55–77 (average 61.7) for the purpose of comparing their rate-pressure products. The resting blood pressure was 140 ± 15/83 ± 8 mm Hg in the normals and 168 ± 15/106 ± 8 mm Hg in the hypertensives.

7.1.2. Rate-Pressure Product of Younger Hypertensives, Borderline Hypertensives and Normotensives

Table 31 and Fig. 39 show the rate-pressure product as a measure of myocardial oxygen consumption for the three groups during exercise. We see that even the borderline hypertensives showed a highly significant increase ($p < 0.001$) in their rate-pressure product, which was 30.5% above normal at 50 watts and 20% above normal at 100 watts. As the figure shows, the percentage difference between the rate-pressure product of the hypertensives and normotensives was 41.7% at 50 watts and 34.7% at 100 watts and differed significantly ($p < 0.05$) from that of the borderline hypertensives at 100 watts.

The results clearly demonstrate the serious load that is placed on the hypertensive heart by excessive exercise blood pressures, and that even borderline hypertension, which frequently is attributed to transient "excitement" [181], is associated with a significant augmentation of the myocardial oxygen demand. Thus, even patients with a mild blood pressure elevation at rest are likely to have a markedly increased myocardial oxygen requirement during ordinary exercise.

Table 31. Myocardial oxygen consumption in terms of the rate-pressure product of normotensives, borderline and hypertensives of different ages during ergometric work (***$p < 0.001$)

Rate-pressure product n = 232		Ergometric work (watts)		
		50	70	100
Group 1, n = 57		13293	16085	19640
Normotensives	41.5 yrs	3958	3424	3374
Group 2, n = 24		17324	20303	23589
Borderline hypertensives	42.6 yrs	31.40***	4453***	3998***
				*
Group 3, n = 51		18841	21672	26459
Hypertensives	43.6 yrs	3332***	4924***	4868***
Group 1, n = 50		14806	17299	21582
Normotensives	64.4 yrs	2910	3655	4607
Group 2, n = 50		19158	23375	28429
Hypertensives	61.7 yrs	3332***	4041***	4979***

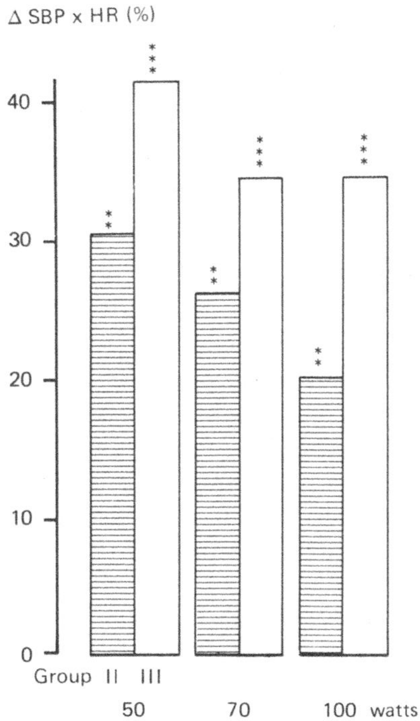

Fig. 39. Percentage increase in rate-pressure product as a measure of myocardial oxygen consumption in borderline hypertensives (group 2, shaded bars) and definite hypertensives (group 3, open bars) compared with normotensives

7.1.3. Rate-Pressure Product of Elderly Hypertensives and Normotensives

The myocardial oxygen consumption of the elderly hypertensives was significantly elevated ($p < 0.001$) relative to the elderly normotensives even in the low submaximal range (Table 31). The results for the younger and older subjects are compared in Fig. 40. We see that the elderly normotensives had a significantly higher ($p < 0.05$) rate-pressure product than the younger normotensives, and that the rate-pressure product of the elderly hypertensives also was significantly higher ($p < 0.05$) at 100 watts than that of the hypertensives 20 years younger.

Accordingly, even a slight blood pressure elevation at rest has major clinical significance in the presence of coexisting coronary disease. The therapeutic implications of this fact apply with particular force to hypertension in elderly persons, who can develop extreme systolic blood pressure elevations even at 50 watts of exercise (s. Chap. II.7.1.).

7.2. Comparative Determination of the Physical Work Capacity 170 of Hypertensives and Normotensives

As the rate-pressure product indicates, the heart rate is a major factor in determining myocardial oxygen demand in exercise. The heart rate response to exercise, and thus the degree of economization of cardiac work, depends in turn on the state of training of the working skeletal muscles.

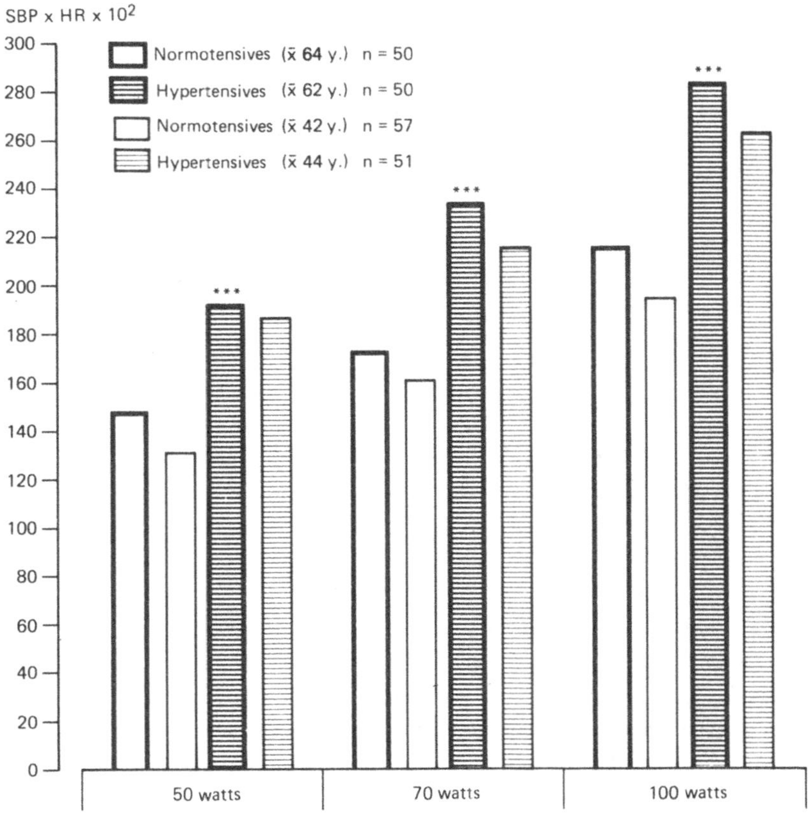

Fig. 40. Rate-pressure product as a measure of myocardial oxygen consumption in younger and older normotensives and hypertensives

7.2.1. Study Population

The Physical Work Capacity 170 (PWC 170) was determined in 57 normotensives, 24 borderline hypertensives and 51 hypertensives of equal age distribution for the purpose of assessing cardiocorporeal performance capacity [119]. Data on age and blood pressure responses are presented in Table 30.

7.2.2. PWC 170 of Hypertensives, Normotensives and Borderline Hypertensives

The PWC 170 of the hypertensives was 2.71 watts/kg body weight, which is significantly ($p < 0.001$) below the 3.44 watts/kg measured in the normal group (Fig. 41). This corresponds to a 21.2% lower aerobic capacity in the hypertensive patients. The borderline hypertensives had a 14.8% lower PWC 170/kg body weight, a difference that is statistically significant ($p < 0.05$). This uneconomical heart rate response of hypertensives has important therapeutic implications when one considers that the heart rate and thus the rate-pressure product at a given stage of exercise can be decreased by endurance training (s. Chap. III.7.2.).

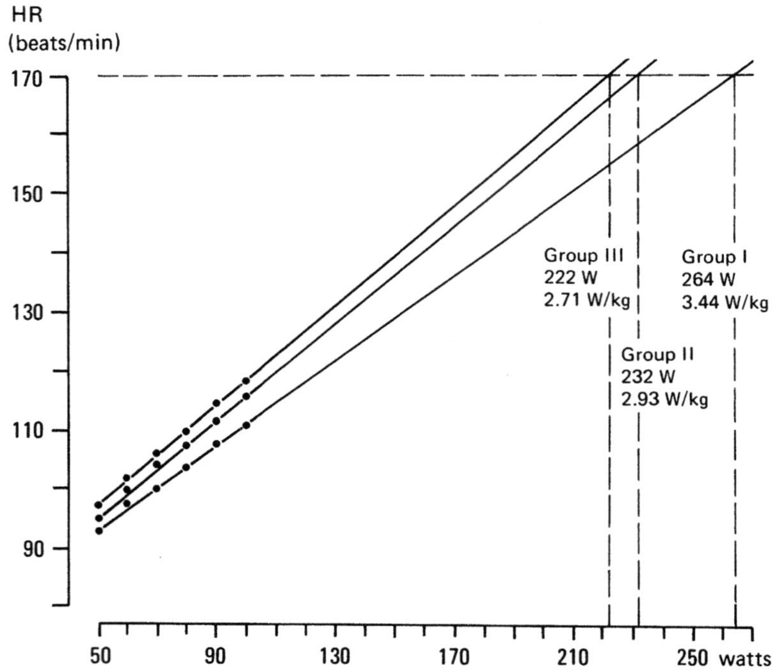

Fig. 41. Heart rate response and PWC 170 or PWC 170/kg body weight for normotensives (group 1), borderline hypertensives (group 2) and definite hypertensives (group 3)

7.3. Assessment of Myocardial Oxygen Consumption and Cardiocorporeal Performance Capacity

7.3.1. Prognostic Significance of the Myocardial Oxygen Consumption

The course and prognosis of arterial hypertension are critically influenced by the cardiac changes that occur in response to the increased pressure load on the heart. Ventricular function continues to be adequate only as long as the myocardial cell has a sufficient oxygen supply. This in turn depends on the extent and severity of myocardial hypertrophy and coronary artery disease [407]. Considering that the coronary arterial reserve is significantly decreased even in hypertensives with adequate cardiac compensation and a normal coronary angiogram [407], it is understandable that myocardial oxygen delivery cannot always be raised to the necessary extent, especially during physical exertion.

With the myocardial oxygen supply restricted in this way, the level of myocardial oxygen consumption becomes a limiting and extremely important clinical parameter. This is especially true in the presence of coexisting coronary disease. It is significant that even in borderline hypertension, so often dismissed as innocent, we demonstrated a significant elevation of myocardial oxygen consumption even at submaximal workloads corresponding to ordinary levels of exertion.

Even patients with mildly elevated resting blood pressures, then, must be assumed to have a markedly increased myocardial oxygen demand during exercise. This circumstance requires that a rational therapeutic approach must be taken in hypertensives with coexisting coronary disease, even if their blood pressure elevation is slight. This applies most particularly to elderly hypertensives, who on the one hand are already presumed to have some degree of atherosclerotic disease, and on the other tend to develop higher exercise blood pressures and thus an increased myocardial oxygen demand.

Hypertensive patients have lower *cardiac outputs* and *stroke volumes,* higher heart rates, and a markedly higher *peripheral resistance* than normotensives at the same level of exercise [4, 28, 152, 215, 278, 367, 375]. This increased resistance work in hypertensives [27, 374, 407] has the effect of raising the *myocardial oxygen consumption.* In his comprehensive studies, Strauer [407] was able to show that the total left ventricular oxygen consumption in hypertensives is 62% greater than normal and is directly proportional to the left ventricular muscle mass. Thus, the increased oxygen consumption in essential hypertension is determined by the degree of ventricular hypertrophy and the magnitude of the underlying pressure load. With the myocardial oxygen requirement increased in this fashion, the oxygen balance is further disrupted by the abnormally high *coronary resistance,* which is 38% higher in hypertensives than in normals. Strauer reports that the pharmacologically determined *coronary reserve* of the left ventricle is 72% of normal in compensated hypertensives who have no coronary disease, and only 42% of normal in compensated hypertensives with coronary disease [407]. This leads Strauer to comment that even hypertensives with a normal coronary angiogram may have clinical symptoms like those commonly associated with coronary artery stenosis. Angina symptoms in these patients can be attributed both to the reduced response range of the coronary flow and to an elevated myocardial energy demand. It is obvious that this discrepancy between cardiac oxygen supply and demand can have major clinical consequences even at low levels of exertion, especially in hypertensives with preexisting coronary artery stenosis. Because the systolic pressure load on the left ventricle is largely responsible for the occurrence of *myocardial ischemia,* it may be assumed that coronary patients with arterial hypertension are far more susceptible to ischemia than coronary patients who are normotensive. Strauer, too, notes that "essential hypertension in the presence of coronary heart disease is associated with a very high risk of myocardial ischemia." This accounts in part for the high incidence of myocardial infarction among hypertensive patients [398].

It is also interesting to note that even localized myocardial ischemia can be a major cause of ventricular arrhythmias, which are the basis for *sudden cardiac death.*

7.3.2. Economization through Endurance Training

What are the therapeutic implications of the findings described above? Earlier we stated the importance of rational antihypertensive treatment, always bearing in mind that satisfactory control of the resting blood pressure does not necessarily imply adequate control during exercise (s. Chap. III.2.2. and Chap. III.4.). In view of what has been said, however, such control is of vital importance.

Another important therapeutic implication derives from the fact that the myocardial oxygen consumption during exercise is determined to a large extent by the state of training of the peripheral skeletal muscles and thus the degree of economization of cardiac work [68, 298, 401]. The significantly higher heart rates manifested by hypertensives and borderline hypertensives compared with normal subjects, resulting in a 21.2% lower PWC 170 in the hypertensives and 14.8% lower PWC 170 in the borderline hypertensives, have a crucial bearing on myocardial oxygen demand. These significantly elevated exercise heart rates at equal levels of exertion cannot be attributed to differences in physical activity among the different groups. The uneconomical heart rate response of hypertensives has been widely described in the literature [4, 260, 335, 345, 375, 383, 384] and is a consequence of two different physiologic and pathophysiologic processes. One is the increased peripheral vascular resistance that is characteristic of arterial hypertension; the other is the state of training of the working skeletal muscles.

Thus, considering the high coronary risk in hypertensives combined with the demonstrated proneness of these patients to exercise tachycardia, one can readily appreciate the importance of *endurance training* in this group. Endurance training has proved to be of outstanding value in the prevention and rehabilitation of cardiovascular disease [78, 146, 246, 292], and as early as 1956 Mellerowicz emphasized its importance in his work "Comparative Studies on the Economy Principle in the Work and Performance of the Trained Circulation and its Relevance to Preventive and Rehabilitative Medicine" [298].

The question of whether endurance training has a positive effect on the high *peripheral vascular resistance* in hypertensives cannot be answered on the basis of our research and depends essentially on the group selected for study [42, 65, 87, 168, 212, 213, 234, 361, 444]. Nevertheless, there is no question that the response of the heart rate to exercise depends in large part on the state of training of the working peripheral skeletal muscles. Hence, endurance training in the hypertensive patient offers a means of lowering the exercise heart rate, reducing the systolic blood pressure and *myocardial oxygen consumption,* and also improving physical performance capacity, as demonstrated by our study of overweight hypertensives (s. Chap. III.7.) and by the results of Schwalb [384], Kellermann and Ben Ari [29, 229].

Physical training achieves these goals by effecting a redistribution of systemic blood flow, optimizing oxygen extraction in the working skeletal muscles [69, 197, 198], altering central circulatory regulation [68, 401], and improving metabolic oxidative capacity in the muscle fibers [17, 113]. The result is a bradycardiac state during exercise which not only lessens cardiac work but also improves the myocardial oxygen supply, since the increased duration of diastole prolongs the period of coronary flow to the myocardium.

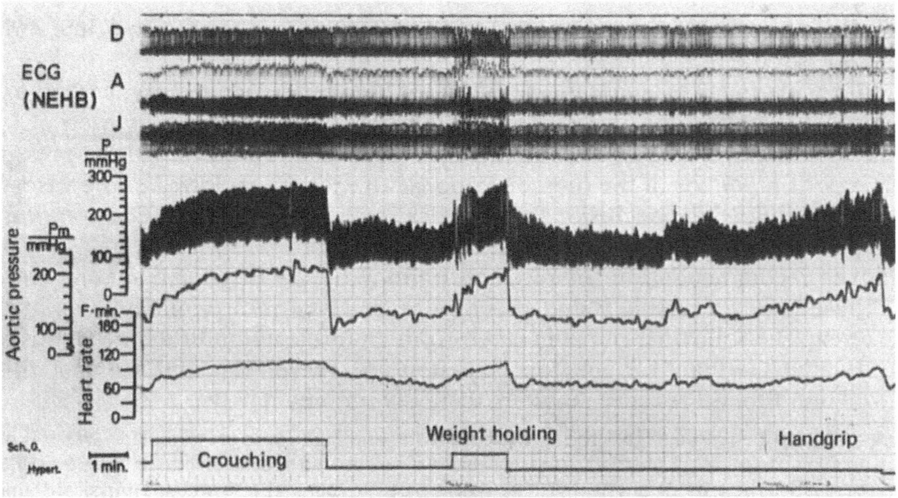

Fig. 42. Original record comparing hemodynamic responses to three different forms of isometric exercise in a 40-year-old hypertensive man (resting BP 174/82 mmHg supine, 170/90 mmHg standing). From top to bottom: three ECG leads D, A, J (Nehb's triangle), arterial blood pressure profile, mean arterial pressure, heart rate. All three exercises - handgrip, weight holding (4 kg) and crouching - raise the systolic blood pressure to 280 mmHg. The diastolic pressure response is characteristic of isometric exercise, showing an excessive rise to 148 mmHg (handgrip), 150 mmHg (weight holding) and 160 mmHg (crouching). None of the exercises raised the heart rate above 100 beats/min (after Zerzawy [455])

7.3.3. Prescribing Physical Training in Hypertensive Patients

These favorable effects on the cardiovascular system can be achieved only through an individualized program of physical endurance training [113]. Isometric exercises are of no benefit in this regard and may even be harmful due to the possible occurrence of excessive blood pressure peaks [259, 361, 416, 456] (s. Fig. 42).

While endurance training can definitely improve the ecomony of cardiac work in hypertensive patients, one must not neglect the dangers that are inherent in such therapy. For example, hypertensives frequently develop excessive blood pressures during exercise which may contribute to the progression of cardiovascular complications [456]. It must also be considered that the rate-pressure product, which reflects the myocardial perfusion requirement, is increased by 30.5% in borderline hypertensives and by 41.7% in definite hypertensives at a load of only 50 watts, signifying a risk of acute myocardial hypoxia that is particularly great in hypertensives with coexisting coronary disease. Ergometric studies by Pracher et al. [335] show that hypertensive patients with confirmed coronary disease experience marked pathologic rises of pulmonary arterial pressures during exercise due to an hypoxiainduced decrease in left ventricular myocardial contractility. Strauer [407] also performed ergometric studies which showed that even patients with a normal coronary angiogram but pronounced left ventricular hypertrophy exhibited a marked rise of left ventricular end-diastolic pressure when performing exercise which raised the tension-time index by 60% of the initial value.

Considering the significant elevations of blood pressure and myocardial oxygen consumption that have been demonstrated in hypertensives even at low submaximal workloads, and the fact that the level of the resting blood pressure is a poor predictor of the pressor response to exercise and thus of the vascular risk, the following conclusions may be drawn with regard to physical training in hypertensives:

1. The recommendation for physical training by the physician should not be based on the resting blood pressure or be given indiscriminately as in the past. The following quote is taken from an information brochure published by the German League for Hypertension Prevention and Control titled "High Blood Pressure: Answers to Ten Questions" [193]:

   > There is no reason to give up exercise because of your high blood pressure. However, it is wise to avoid strenuous physical exertion, especially if you are not accustomed to it. Your doctor can best judge the kind of physical activity that is best for you, and also whether physical training would be appropriate and what level of exercise you would be able to tolerate.

   From the results of the present study it is clear that exaggerated pressor responses to even very mild exercise represent an absolute *contraindication to physical training,* including training of the endurance type. This applies even to patients who have minimal blood pressure elevations at rest. On the other hand, the recommendation that "all untreated hypertensives with blood pressures over 180 mm Hg systolic and 120 diastolic should be excluded from athletic activities in the strict sense" is unacceptable for two reasons. First, there is no cutoff point for resting blood pressure beyond which one may or may not engage in sport. Second, the author does not ask which hypertensives should be excluded from sport, but rather how best to treat a hypertensive patient medically so that he can participate in sport safely.

   In the hypertension advice series *Sport and Movement* [190], the author not only fails to address the question of which hypertensives should or should not engage in sports, but also makes this statement: "If you have high blood pressure only, or high blood pressure not complicated by serious vascular disease, you can monitor your level of stress during exercise by taking your pulse." The author goes on the say, "This does not mean that you should become overly preoccupied with pulse-taking. It is enough to check your pulse occasionally, perhaps once or twice during each exercise period - as long as you get a feeling for the amount of stress that is present." Even if the author of this work is a strong advocate of controlled, individualized endurance training for hypertensives, he should add a stern warning against such a dangerous oversimplification of the problem of exercise vs. hypertension and hypertension vs. cardiovascular risk. In reality the patient cannot monitor or even estimate the magnitude of the pressure load acting on his vascular system simply by taking his pulse. This applies equally to the examining physician, who cannot predict how the resting blood pressure will increase when the patient is stressed. The following stipulation should be added, therefore:

2. Besides avoiding isometric exercise, it is necessary to evaluate the patient's blood pressure response and the status of his coronary flow by *ergometric*

testing before instituting a preventive or rehabilitative exercise training program so that possible acute or chronic risks associated with the training can be avoided.

3. If the test demonstrates a marked blood pressure rise at low levels of exertion, then appropriate *antihypertensive treatment* should be initiated prior to training, especially if coronary disease is also present.
4. It must be realized that a satisfactory antihypertensive effect in the resting state does not mean that the blood pressure will be adequately controlled during exercise (s. Chap. III.2.2. and 2.4.). It is necessary, therefore, to test antihypertensive efficacy by pretraining ergometry.

III. Ergometry as an Aid to Patient Management

1. Importance of Exercise Blood Pressures as a Vascular Risk Factor

1.1. Development of Atherosclerosis in Arterial Hypertension

There is no question that hypertension accelerates the development of atherosclerosis. Dustan [90], in 1970, summarized the mechanisms by which hypertension appears to act, the most important being an elevation of the *intra-arterial pressure*. Endothelial lesions produced by abnormalities of blood flow may also have causal significance. A third mechanism may involve elevated levels of circulating catecholamines or other vasoactive substances which increase endothelial permeability.

Hauss [175] was able to show that a blood pressure elevation of only 1 hour's duration significantly increases the proliferation of endothelial, medial and adventitial cells and also stimulates proteoglycane synthesis in the aorta.

In their survey article "Hemodynamics and Atherogenesis," Nerem and Cornhill [315] stressed the causal importance of intravascular *shear forces* in the pathogenesis of atherosclerosis. These shear forces may be severe enough to damage the vascular endothelium, depending on local vascular anatomy and especially on the rhythm and intensity of the blood flow. The same mechanism can adversely affect processes of vascular wall repair. Besides direct endothelial damage, moreover, shear forces may create a state of tissue hypoxia which disrupts essential physiologic and biochemical processes in the vessel wall, predisposing it to atherosclerotic change.

Berry [35] also recognized the role of even minor *vascular alterations* as a predisposing factor for degenerative disease and emphasized the importance of early treatment.

According to Epstein et al. [96], a high intra-arterial pressure appears to be the principal disease-producing factor in arterial hypertension. Assuming, then, that the pressure load itself represents the most damaging influence on the vascular system, it is reasonable to conclude that stress-induced blood pressure elevations are an important factor in the pathogenesis of complications [101, 125, 208, 259, 263, 298, 407, 413].

1.2. Severity of Stress-Induced Blood Pressure Elevations and Their Evaluation

The blood pressure response to stress assumes particular significance when we consider that hypertensives raise their blood pressures excessively even at *very low levels of exertion* [362, 456]. Thus, Bachmann et al. [21] found that 20 hypertensives with a mean standing pressure of 163/103 mm Hg raised their pressure to 214/117 mm Hg during walking and to 240/126 mm Hg when climbing 4 flights of stairs. We can appreciate the severity of these elevations when we compare them with normotensive controls, who had respective blood pressures of 144/87 and 169/93 mm Hg during walking and stair climbing. The readings of 182/102 and 225/122 mm Hg which Krönig [259] measured in WHO Stage II and Stage III hypertensives, respectively, during walking on level ground offer further confirmation of the substantial blood pressure rises that may be elicited even by mild exertion. Stair climbing raised the mean blood pressure to 212/107 mm Hg in the Stage II patients, and to 257/132 mm Hg in the Stage III patients [259].

The studies of Taylor [416] also underscore the pathophysiologic significance of the pressor response to stress. Even very mild *isometric exercise* (2-min handgrip) at only 30% of maximum capacity raised the blood pressure to 260/140 mm Hg. When isometric exercise was combined with dynamic exercise, e.g. carrying a 30-lb handbag while walking on level ground, rises up to 250/200 mm Hg were experienced. Other everyday activities, such as defecation, also elicited marked blood pressure peaks (s. Fig. 43) [259, 416].

The response of the blood pressure to exercise can vary greatly depending on whether dynamic or isometric work is being done. The difference is well illustrated by the studies of Zerzawy [455]. During ordinary cross-country running or skiing, as examples of essentially dynamic exercise (fiber shortening without significant force development), the marked increase in heart rate is accompanied by a rise in the systolic blood pressure only, while the diastolic pressure remains nearly constant. On the other hand, during isometric exercise such as assuming a skier's crouch or lifting a weight, the diastolic pressure rise to an even greater degree than the systolic. Zerzawy [455, 456] (Fig. 44) tested a group of normotensive subjects with a resting blood pressure of 135/75 mm Hg and a group of hypertensives with a supine blood pressure of 180/100 mm Hg, having them perform isometric exercises by lifting a 4-kg weight. Despite the relatively low level of exertion, the normotensives experienced marked rises in their systolic and especially their diastolic blood pressures, which attained a mean value of 185/115 mm Hg. The hypertensives raised their blood pressures to 240/145 mm Hg during the same exercise. The heart rates ranged between 125 and 135 beats/min. If we choose a workload on the bicycle ergometer which likewise raises the heart rate to 125–135/min, we find that the blood pressure increase in this submaximal range is significantly smaller in both normotensives and hypertensives than when a 4-kg weight is lifted. Thus, the normotensives raised their systolic pressure to 155 mm Hg during ergometry, while their diastolic pressure remained around 80 mm Hg. The hypertensives, meawhile, raised their blood pressure to 205/115 mm Hg. This is considerably lower than the 240/145 mm Hg developed during isometric exercise and demonstrates that

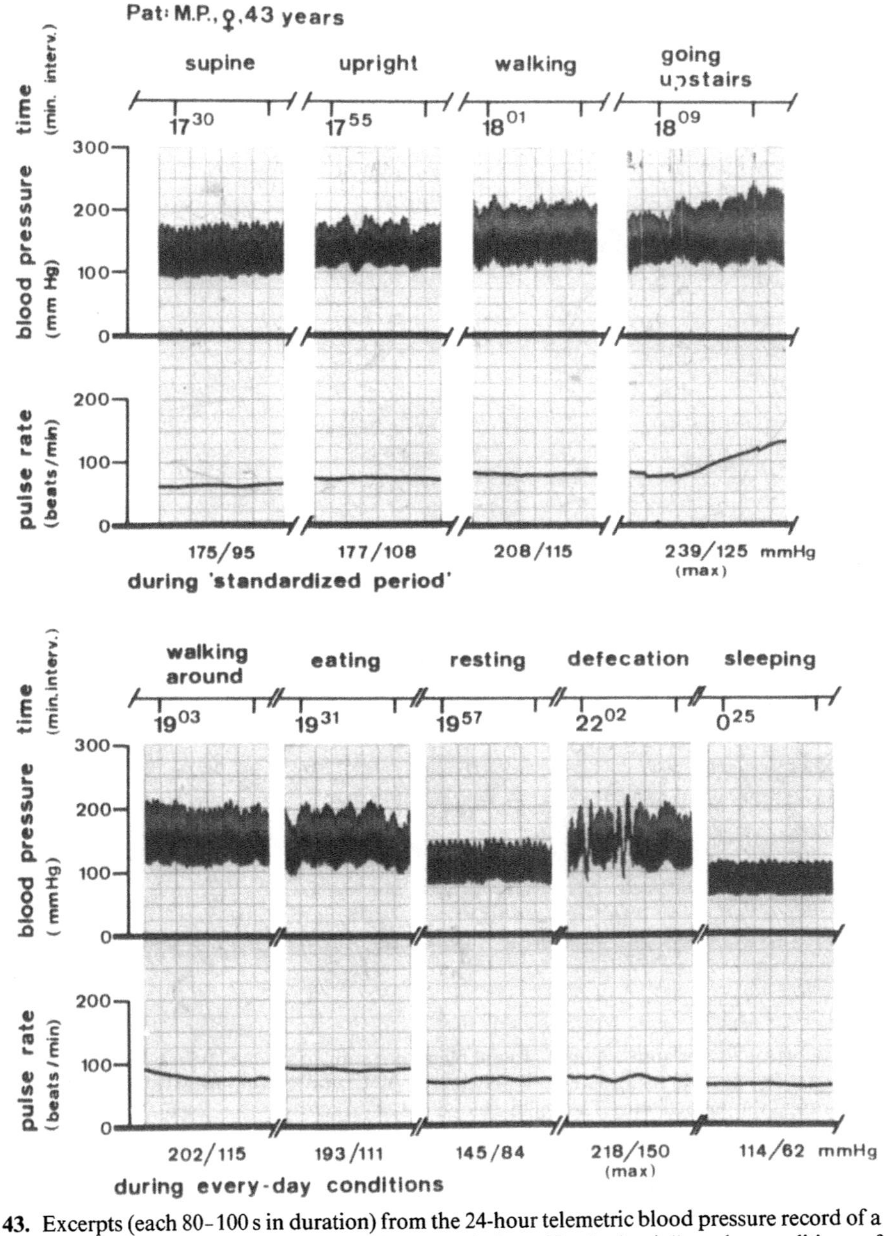

Fig. 43. Excerpts (each 80–100 s in duration) from the 24-hour telemetric blood pressure record of a 43-year-old woman with essential hypertension (WHO Stage II) obtained 1) under conditions of observation ("normalized period") with 175/85 at 5:30 p.m., 177/108 at 5:55 p.m., 208/111 at 6:01 p.m., and the maximum of 239/125 mmHg at 6:09 p.m. and 2) under general hospital room conditions with 202/115 at 7:03 p.m., 193/111 at 7:31 p.m., 145/84 at 7:57 p.m., 218/150 at 10:05 p.m. (defecation), and 114/82 mmHg at 2:05 a.m. (after Krönig [258])

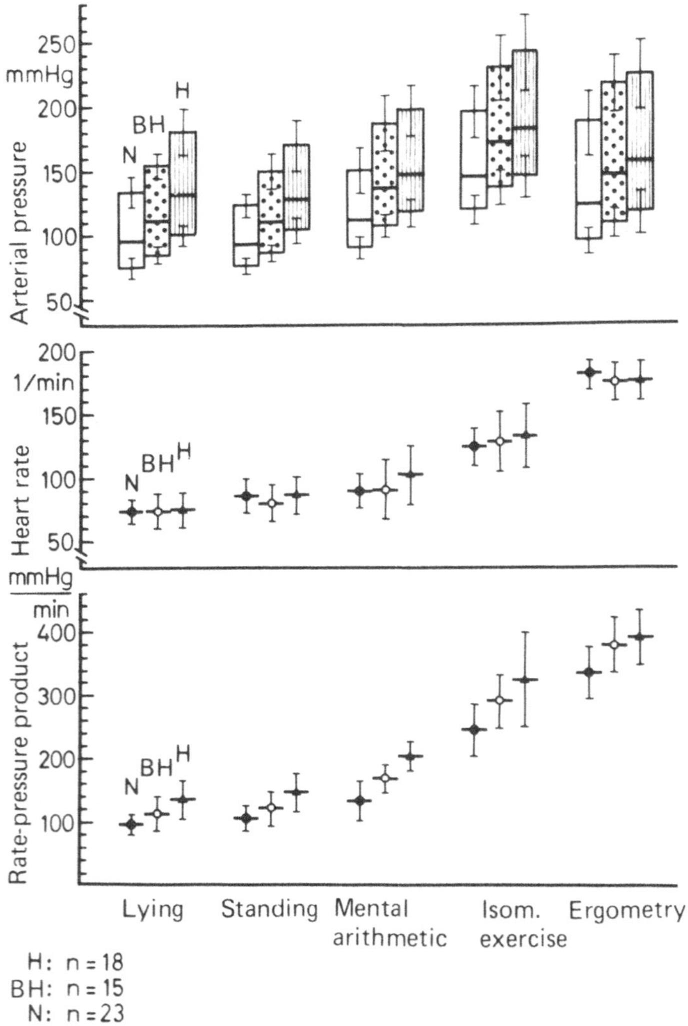

Fig. 44. Mean values and scatter of arterial blood pressure, heart rate and rate-pressure product in 18 hypertensives (H), 15 borderline hypertensives (BH) and 23 normotensive controls (N) at rest and during various activities. The relative blood pressure increases associated with mental arithmetic, isometric exercise and ergometry are approximately equal (after Zerzawy [455])

the systolic and especially the diastolic blood pressures are lower in dynamic exercise even when equal heart rates are attained.

Emotional stresses, too, can elicit significant rises in blood pressure. A mental arithmetic test conducted by Brod et al. [51] raised the blood pressure of essential hypertensives from 185/111 to 218/132 mm Hg, while the normotensive controls responded with a rise from 126/76 to only 138/87 mm Hg.

1.3. Prognosis of Acute and Chronic Complications

Considering the fact that arterial hypertension is characterized both by a blood pressure elevation at rest and most especially by an excessive pressor response to physical and emotional stress, it is reasonable to ask whether the acute and chronic complications of arterial hypertension are at all related to the severity of stress-linked blood pressure elevations.

This is plainly true with regard to the danger of acute events in hypertensives with coexisting coronary heart disease (a common finding with increasing age). It has been shown that pathologic stress-induced blood pressure elevations greatly increase the myocardial oxygen demand. At a workload of only 50 watts, representing a very low level of exertion, "exercise-positive" borderline hypertensives had a 30% higher rate-pressure product than normotensives, reflecting their higher myocardial oxygen requirement. Oxygen consumption in younger and older subjects with mild hypertension was increased by 42 and 44%, respectively.

Given the fact that a large percentage of hypertensives may be presumed to have latent or overt coronary artery stenosis, and that even hypertensives with a normal coronary angiogram have a significantly restricted coronary reserve, it can be appreciated that an excessive pressor response to stress poses a particularly serious threat to this group. The quality of life and the prognosis of coronary patients depend on the degree of disproportion that exists between myocardial oxygen supply and consumption. Even with pronounced coronary stenosis, myocardial oxygen delivery may well be adequate in the resting state. During exercise, however, it may no longer be possible to maintain an adequate coronary flow. It is easy to see that a further increase in myocardial oxygen consumption in this situation resulting from an excessive blood pressure elevation can easily shift the cardiac oxygen balance into a critical range. This has particular relevance to the issue of hypoxia-induced arrhythmias and "sudden death," especially when one considers the frequency with which coronary patients show pathologic blood pressure elevations under stress, as pointed out by Blümchen et al [39].

1.4. The Pressor Response to Stress as a Causal Factor in Chronic Hypertensive Complications

The causal role of stress-induced blood pressure elevations in the development of chronic complications is difficult to evaluate. The only available data are from a 10-year prospective study by Sokolow et al. [398], who used automatic portable blood pressure monitors to record the daily blood pressure profiles of 1076 hypertensive patients. They were able to show that patients who had a high blood pressure level during the course of the day experienced a significantly ($p < 0.001$ systolic, $p < 0.01$ diastolic) greater rate of cardiovascular complications and events than patients with lower blood pressure levels. The authors concluded that patients could be assigned to high or low cardiovascular risk groups on the basis of their daily blood pressure profiles, and that this differentiation could greatly facilitate the selection of patients for drug therapy.

Equally interesting are the studies of Floras et al. [101], who showed that patients are apt to be falsely classified diagnostically and prognostically on the basis of their resting blood pressure values. By recording the daily blood pressure profile, however, it is possible to divide the patients into two distinct groups – those with a significantly elevated blood pressure profile (group 1) and those with a normal profile (group 2) – even though the resting blood pressures of the groups were indistinguishable. First, it is interesting to note that the incidence of hypertensive complications in group 1 was greater than in group 2 with high statistical significance. Second, it is noteworthy that group 1 experienced a significantly greater rise of blood pressure during exercise at 50 and 75 watts, and that this circumstance enabled the patients to be assigned to high-risk and low-risk groups – a differentiation that could not be made on the basis of other clinical, hemodynamic and biochemical parameters. These findings also provide grounds for speculation by way of analogy – a practice which, while lacking the force of proof, is nevertheless common in medicine and can yield important insights.

Thus, it is well known that hypertension stimulates adaptive responses in the muscles of the heart and resistance vessels. Specifically, a concentric myocardial and medial hypertrophy develops which may be reversible following antihypertensive therapy [144, 363]. The progression or regression of this hypertrophy is critically influenced by the underlying "training stimulus" which acts on the cardiac and vascular muscle. It has been shown that hypertrophy in skeletal muscle is determined not by a large number of small, subthreshold stimuli, but by maximal, above-threshold training stimuli. Applying this principle to the heart and blood vessels, it is reasonable to speculate that cardiovascular adaptive responses are chiefly determined not by subthreshold stimuli, i.e. the resting blood pressure, but by maximal stimuli, i.e. the blood pressure under stress.

This appears to have been confirmed for myocardial adaptation in a recent study [310]. It was shown that persons with a normal resting blood pressure who undergo intensive power training for a prolonged period of time tend to develop a concentric myocardial hypertrophy identical to that seen in hypertensives. Such training is known to be associated with the occurrence of large blood pressure peaks.

Further confirmation is provided by the studies of Krönig [259], who found that the level of the exercise blood pressure in hypertensives increased with the WHO stage of severity. During walking on level ground, the group at WHO Stage I had a mean blood pressure of 150/84 mm Hg, the group at WHO Stage II had a mean pressure of 182/102 mm Hg, and the group at WHO Stage III had a mean pressure of 225/122 mm Hg. A similar pattern with higher absolute values was observed during the climbing of two flights of stairs. In this case the mean blood pressure was 174/90 mm Hg in the Stage I hypertensives, 212/106 mm Hg in Stage II, and 257/132 mm Hg in Stage III. One might conclude from this that higher blood pressures under stress give rise to more serious cardiovascular complications. On the other hand, it could also be argued that the excessive exercise blood pressures reflect secondary cardiac and peripheral adaptive mechanisms which vary with the degree of the pressure elevation. However, the latter interpretation conflicts with our observation of excessive blood pressure increases in some juvenile hypertensives who showed no electrocardiographic or roentgenographic signs of cardiac complications.

The results published by Irving et al. [208] are also of interest in this context. These authors used direct, continuous 24-hour monitoring to track the blood pressure variations in hypertensive patients and found that patients with left ventricular hypertrophy had a mean variability of 32 mm Hg systolic and 18 mm Hg diastolic, which was significantly greater than the 23/12 mm Hg observed in patients without ventricular hypertrophy. They concluded from these findings that the degree of *blood pressure variability* may be instrumental in determining the severity of the *complications* that arise.

We also recall the studies of Briedigkeit et al. [49], who analyzed the family history of "exercise-positive" juvenile borderline hypertensives and found that the parents and especially the grandparents of these children had a significantly higher morbidity and mortality from cardiovascular disease than the forebearers of the "exercise-negative" borderline hypertensives.

Rowlands et al. [363] found a close and significant correlation between the mean systolic blood pressure measured continuously for 24 hours and the left ventricular muscle mass in hypertensive persons. The same authors also showed that antihypertensive treatment (mainly with beta-blocking drugs or calcium antagonists) for an average period of 9.3 months led to a regression of left ventricular hypertrophy.

The importance of wall tension in vascular adaptation processes was discussed in a survey article by Berry [35]. It seems that wall tension becomes progressively greater as the blood pressure rises, the vascular radius increases, and the vessel wall becomes thinned out. By producing the greatest wall tension, high stress-induced blood pressures also impose the greatest load on the vessels. The response to this load, according to Berry [35], is an increase in the rate of division of smooth muscle cells which is proportional to the distension of the vessel wall, as well as a change from the contractile to the synthetic phase (production of scleroproteins). The studies of Hauss [175] also support this theory.

If we assume that the pressure load itself is the major causative factor for vascular disease, then stress-induced blood pressure increases may well play a significant role in the pathogenesis of cordiovascular complications. This seems especially likely when one considers that hypertensives raise their blood pressures excessively even in response to mild stresses. Littler et al. [272, 273] and Sokolow et al. [398] have pointed out that the resting blood pressure is a poor predictor of the magnitude of the blood pressure response to ordinary stresses. This fact has been amply confirmed by our own observations.

On the other hand, studies by Floras [101] and Pickering [333] indicate that the magnitude of blood pressure increases occurring during the course of the day, i.e. the daily blood pressure profile, can be estimated on the basis of ergometric testing.

A survey of the literature reveals that the blood pressure values measured during ergometry are a good measure of the response to physical stress and probably to emotional stress as well [101, 141, 259, 455]. Studies by Zerzawy et al. [455] and Neuss et al. [317] show that the relative blood pressure increases during ergometry are comparable to those elicited by psychological stress and isometric exercise (Fig. 43).

The clinical significance of the excessive blood pressure increases during ergometry demonstrated in the present investigations is that the values obtained in the range from 50 to 100 watts are representative of normal exertion levels. This is illustrated first by the heart rate response. For example, both groups of mildly hypertensive males had a mean heart rate of only 98/min at 50 watts, which is only about 55% of maximal. Yet the relative blood pressure increment was greatest from recumbency to exercise at 50 watts. Even at 100 watts the mean heart rate of 121/min still represents a decidedly submaximal stress. Assuming that these hypertensives, with an average age just under 40, have a maximum attainable heart rate of 180/min, the foregoing rate represents only about 67% of maximum performance capacity. In addition, telemetric measurements of heart rate and blood pressure during normal exertion and various athletic activities consistently show that the 50- to 100-watt range of ergometric workloads corresponds well to ordinary, submaximal performance [402, 456]. Thus, a group of 96 subjects with an average age of 31 years tested by Zerzawy attained a heart rate of 125/min during stair climbing, which corresponded to an ergometric workload of 1.2 watts/kg body weight [456]. These values coincide closely with the response of our normotensive males, who had a heart rate of 126/min at 100 watts, corresponding to a load of 1.3 watts/kg body weight.

Studies by Stein et al. [402] in 55 postinfarction patients have shown that the range of workloads from 50 to 100 watts is representative of normal submaximal exertion, even in individuals with coronary disease. Slow walking at a speed of 3.9 km/h raised the mean heart rate in these patients to 112/min, which corresponded to an ergometric load of 75 watts. Jogging at 5.3 km/h raised the heart rate to 132/min, corresponding to a workload of 125 watts on the ergometer. Swimming using the breaststroke or backstroke was comparable to 110 to 125 watts on the ergometer, and tennis was comparable to 175 watts.

From this we may conclude that the blood pressures measured during ergometry accurately characterize the hypertensive blood pressure response to ordinary stress levels.

2. The Control of Excessive Blood Pressures under Stress

2.1. Statement of Problem

Today there is no longer any question that the reduction or normalization of blood pressure is effective in reducing morbidity and increasing the life expectancy of hypertensive persons [191, 205, 286, 422, 430–433]. From the standpoint of the therapist, then, the fundamental goal of adequate antihypertensive treatment is a lowering of morbidity and mortality. One question remains to be answered, however: What blood pressure readings should serve as a basis for judging the efficacy of antihypertensive therapy?

There are two main, clinically relevant arguments in support of ergometry as a test for response to antihypertensive treatment. First, it is necessary to acknowledge that the resting blood pressure may be raised by an expectant attitude on the part of the patient, even during therapy. This may cause the evaluating physician to underestimate the efficacy of treatment. Laughlin et al. [265] report that the self-determined blood pressures in 16 of 37 patients receiving uniform drug treatment fell by more than 10 mm Hg systolic and diastolic over a period of 30 days. Thus, with no change of medication, the response to treatment improved dramatically as the patients became accustomed to the pressure-taking routine. This problem is also addressed by Gould et al. [159], who compared the effect of a placebo with that of the new antihypertensive drug indoramin. In the placebo group, the blood pressure fell by an average of 14 mm Hg systolic and 10 mm Hg diastolic based on readings taken at rest. However, the mean daily blood pressure profiles of these patients as established by intra-arterial monitoring showed that no significant blood pressure reduction had been achieved. At the same time, the resting blood pressures taken after treatment with indoramin showed only a slight, insignificant fall of 6 mm Hg systolic and 8 mm Hg diastolic compared with the placebo. But this proved to be highly misleading, for continuous intra-arterial monitoring demonstrated a highly significant reduction of the mean daily blood pressure by 18.3 mm Hg systolic and 12.7 mm Hg diastolic relative to the placebo, regardless of whether treatment preceded or followed the placebo period. Littler et al. [272], in studying the same problem, could find no target organ damage in their patients despite poor control of the resting blood pressure. This was attributed to the salutary effect of treatment on the daily blood pressure profile. The authors concluded: "Our results show how easy it could be to overtreat certain patients on the basis of casual readings."

The second argument in favor of ergometric testing is the fact that resting blood pressure determinations yield very little information on how transient, stress-induced blood pressure elevations will affect the vascular system of the hypertensive patient. Based on his comprehensive telemetric blood pressure studies in hypertensives under a variety of conditions, Krönig [259] concludes that "therapeutic measures must be geared toward mitigating the pressor response to permit effective control not only of the resting blood pressure but also of the peak elevations elicited by everyday stresses."

2.2. Requirements of Antihypertensive Therapy

The current goal of antihypertensive treatment is to lower elevated blood pressures in the resting state. However, as we have shown, this approach neglects basic pathophysiologic processes that are involved in arterial hypertension. During physical exertion or emotional stress, the work of the heart and the load imposed on the vascular bed by the stress-linked blood pressure rise are substantially increased relative to the resting state. It is desirable, therefore, to pro-

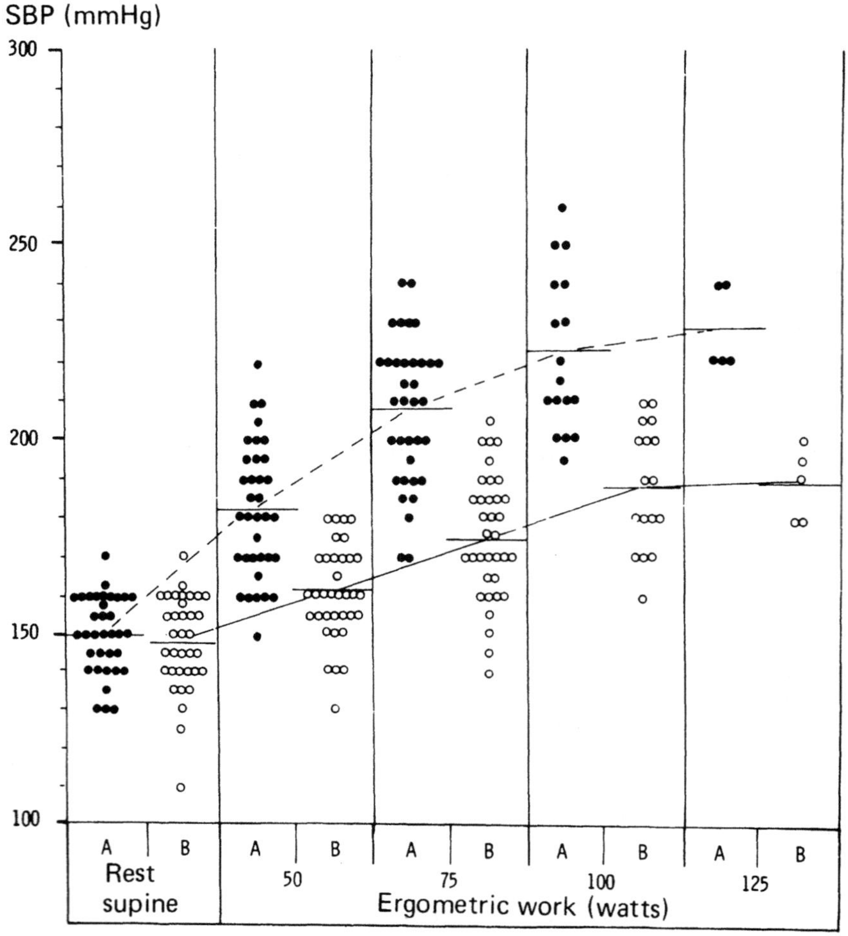

Fig. 45. Variation of the systolic blood pressure during rest and during ergometric exercise in 35 essential hypertensives being treated with a reserpine-diuretic combination (A, solid circles) or with a beta-blocking drug (B, open circles) (after Patyna [323])

tect the cardiovascular system from the elevated blood pressures that are elicited by physical and emotional stress. We must require that antihypertensive drugs not only normalize the resting blood pressure but also adequately lower the blood pressure in stressful situations [107]. This requirement is by no means satisfied by all antihypertensive drugs that are effective at rest.

Several studies have confirmed that centrally acting sympatholytic drugs such as alpha methyldopa, clonidine and reserpine, which formerly were prescribed with great frequency, can adequately lower the resting blood pressure. However, these drugs have been found to have little or no effect on blood pressure during ergometry, especially the systolic. When Stoker et al. [456] compared the antihypertensive effect of alpha methyldopa with that of the beta-blocker metoprolol, they found that despite an equivalent reduction of the blood pressure at rest, alpha methyldopa was much less effective in lowering the systolic blood pressure during exercise. The drug also had little effect on exercise tachycardia, thus allowing the rate-pressure product, as a measure of myocardial oxygen consumption, to remain high.

Lund-Johansen reports that clonidine (282), too, is unable to lower the blood pressure adequately during exercise as compared with the resting state. Thus, the systolic blood pressure at 150 watts was virtually unchanged even after one year of clonidine therapy.

Patyna [323] compared the effect of a reserpine-diuretic combination and a beta-blocking drug on the blood pressure at rest and during exercise. While these drugs had equivalent effects on the resting blood pressure, the mean systolic pressure of patients on the reserpine-diuretic combination rose to 182 mm Hg at a workload of only 50 watts, which considerably surpasses the normal limit of 167 mm Hg (Fig. 45). At 100 watts the systolic pressure reached 222 mm Hg, representing a relatively greater elevation above the upper normal limit of 200 mm Hg. The patients on the beta-blocking durg, by contast, had systolic blood pressures which were well within the normotensive range - 161 mm Hg at 50 watts and 186 mm Hg at 100 watts. The diastolic pressures showed no differences. It is also noteworthy that the patients on the drug combination had a rate-pressure product of 27 000 mm Hg/min at 100 watts, which definitely exceeded the normal limit of 23 000 mm Hg/min. The patients on the beta-blocker had a rate-pressure product of 19 000 mm Hg/min, which was within normal limits.

3. Antihypertensive Effect of Beta-Blocking Drugs

The "stepped care" approach to antihypertensive therapy provides initially for the administration of beta-blocking drugs and diuretics singly or in combination. If this does not control the blood pressure adequately, a vasodilating drug is added. It is of vital interest, therefore, to establish whether and to what extent these three classes of drugs can moderate the pressor response to stress. The first question to be answered is whether all beta-blocking drugs have the same antihypertensive effect when taken in equivalent doses. It must also be determined whether the drugs vary in their duration of action, and whether their antihypertensive effect has a tendency to decrease with chronic use.

3.1. Comparison of Atenolol/Nadolol and Metoprolol

It is clear that the beta-blocking drugs rank first among antihypertensive agents for the control of stress-induced blood pressure elevations in hypertensive patients. From a practical standpoint, however, it is necessary to answer two important questions [132]:

1. Do different beta-blockers which vary in their pharmacologic properties also vary in their duration of action, and is this related to their plasma half-life?
2. Can a single morning dose control blood pressure throughout the day, even in periods of stress?

3.1.1. Patients and Methods

To resolve these questions, we tested 20 hypertensive males age 18–43 years (average 35.8 years, 179 6.5 cm, 82.4 8.3 kg) with WHO Stage-I essential hypertension to investigate the effect of three beta-blocking drugs with different plasma half-lives on the blood pressure and heart rate before, during and after ergometry (50 to 100 watts) at different times of day. Before initiating treatment we first tested the patients at three different times on the same day. The first test was conducted between 8:00 and 10:00 a.m., the second between 10:00 a.m. and 12:00 noon (exactly 2 hours after the first test), and the third between 4:00 and 6:00 p.m. (exactly 8 hours after the first test).

Following examination at entry, the patients were arbitrarily divided into two groups. In group 1, consisting of 10 patients, we compared the antihypertensive efficacy of 200 mg metoprolol (short half-life) and 100 mg atenolol (moderate half-life) administered orally in single morning doses. Five of the patients were started on metoprolol and five on atenolol.

At initial follow-up testing after 4 weeks of treatment, we instructed the patients not to take their usual morning dose before coming in so that we could test the therapeutic effect of the drug 24 hours after the last oral dosing. On conclusion of the first test, the patients were given 200 mg metroprolol or 100 mg atenolol orally, and 2 identical ergometric tests were performed 2 and 8 hours later.

When testing was completed, the patients were switched from metoprolol to atenolol or from atenolol to metoprolol, as the case may be, and the new drug was maintained for an additional four weeks. At the end of this second course of treatment the patients were again tested 24, 2 and 8 hours after ingestion of the beta-blocker. In analogous fashion, the 10 patients in group 2 received 100 mg atenolol (moderate half-life) or 120 mg nadolol (long half-life). The test protocols in these patients were identical to those in group 1.

3.1.2. Effect 2, 8 and 24 Hours after Last Oral Dosing

In group 1 atenolol and metoprolol lowered the blood pressure and heart rate significantly ($p < 0.001$) 2 hours after oral dosing and with equal potency relative to the controls. This was true at rest was well as during and after ergometry (Table 32).

Fig. 46 and Table 33 show that the reduction of blood pressure and heart rate by atenolol and metoprolol was still significant and unabated 8 hours after dosing, and that the effect for both drugs was equivalent. At 24 hours a decline of effect especially during exercise was apparent for both agents relative to the 2-hour and 8-hour effects (Fig. 47, 48, Table 34). Considering the latter effects to be 100%, atenolol still provided a 61% reduction of systolic blood pressure during ergometry at 24 hours, and metoprolol a 51% reduction. The heart rate at

Table 32. Systolic (S. B. P.) and diastolic (D. B. P.) blood pressures and heart rates (H. R.) (means ± SD) of 10 hypertensive males before and 2 hours after last taking 100 mg atenolol or 200 mg metoprolol during chronic treatment

	n = 10	Rest	Ergometric work (watts)						Recovery period (min)				
		supine	50	60	70	80	90	100	1.	2.	3.	4.	5.
SBP	Before	158.4	177.7	180.6	184.7	192.7	197.4	204.8	177.1	166.4	162.4	158.7	154.8
(mmHg)	therapy	15.4	10.4	14.6	17.1	18.4	16.1	16.4	10.7	13.7	14.2	13.1	14.1
	2 hours after	134.1	147.5	153	158.2	164.8	169.9	175.5	150.1	144.4	140.7	136.4	135.1
	Atenolol	19.6**	22.1**	20.6**	20**	19.6**	20.5**	18.8**	18.6***	15.7**	15.5**	17**	17.4*
	2 hours after	132.9	145.9	151.2	154.4	159.8	166.2	169	155.3	147.8	142.6	141	141.4
	Metoprolol	20.6**	25**	25.5**	26.3**	26.2**	25.4**	20.3**	24.0*	21.5*	24*	24.1	24.4
DBP	Before	111.1	113.3	116.6	117.4	117.2	119.5	119.7	110.7	107.7	106.9	106.3	107
(mmHg)	therapy	5.6	10.7	10.4	10.5	11.4	11.9	10.5	8.8	9.1	8.3	9.3	9.3
	2 hours after	90.9	100.6	100.4	102.6	104.1	104.2	105.6	97	94.5	92.8	92.4	91.8
	Atenolol	18.9**	16.5	16*	14.4*	14.2*	14.3*	13.8*	13.4*	13.6*	13.9*	13.7*	14.4*
	2 hours after	91.9	97.7	99.1	100.2	101.3	104.3	105.6	96.4	95.6	93.2	93.5	92.3
	Metoprolol	14.5**	16.6*	15.7*	15.8*	16.4*	16.9*	16.9*	15.8*	16.4	17.2*	16*	16.4*
HR	Before	64.3	91.7	95.2	100.5	105.7	109.9	115	84.9	74.2	70.7	69.5	70.5
(bts/min)	therapy	4.5	9.7	11.1	12.3	12.6	13.7	16.7	15.8	13.2	12.2	10.6	10.1
	2 hours after	53.6	73.6	76.9	78.3	82.5	86.5	90.9	60.4	56.3	56.8	55.3	54.5
	Atenolol	9.0**	6.4***	6.2***	6.8***	7.2***	7.2***	8.8***	11.2***	9.1**	9.2**	7.9**	8.8**
	2 hours after	54.3	72.6	76.2	78.1	81.2	84.6	88.4	64.7	58.5	58.0	56.4	56.3
	Metoprolol	10.1*	10.0***	9.4**	9.3	10.6***	8.8***	8.8***	12.0**	10.3**	9.3*	9.8*	9.5**

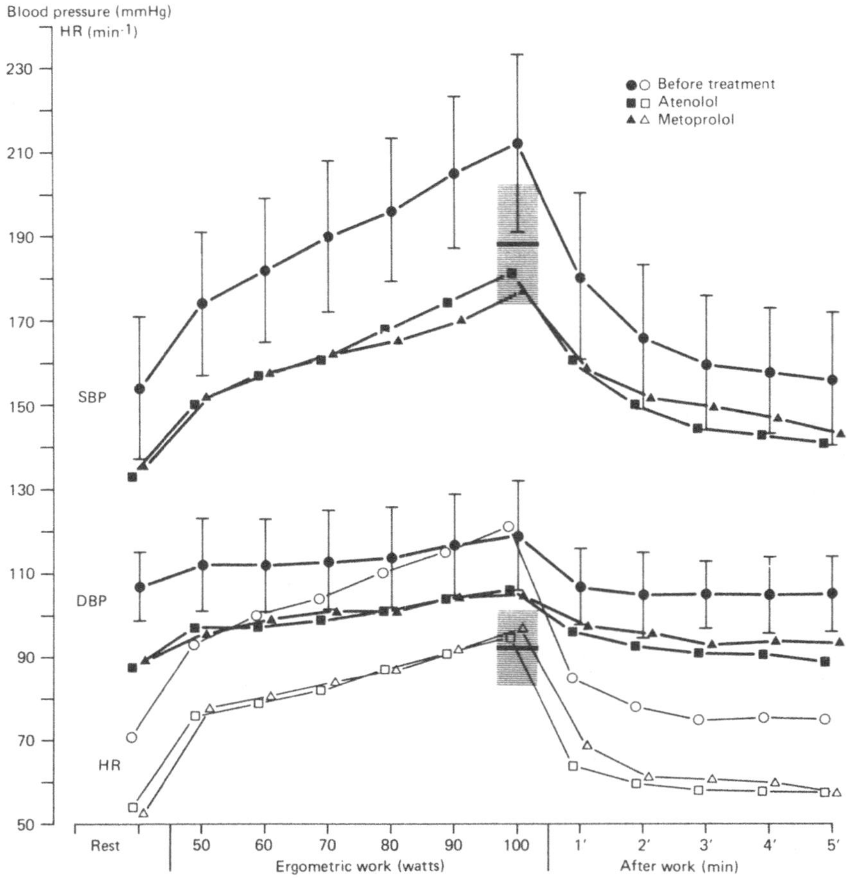

Fig. 46. Blood pressures and heart rates of 10 hypertensive males before and 8 hours after last taking 100 mg atenolol or 200 mg metoprolol. The bars indicate normal blood pressure response at 100 watts

24 hours was still reduced by 59% with atenolol and 49% with metoprolol during exercise, while the diastolic blood pressure was reduced 78% with atenolol and 71% with metoprolol.

In group 2 a comparison of nadolol and atenolol yielded results comparable to those in group 1 for the 2- and 8-hour drug effects (Fig. 49, Tables 35 and 36). At 2 and 8 hours after dosing the blood pressure and heart rate reductions were equally well maintained by both drugs and were significant relative to controls. At 100 watts 8 hours after dosing, for example, it was found that the pretreatment blood pressure of 203/114 mm Hg was reduced to 174/100 mm Hg on atenolol and to 173/101 on nadolol ($p<0.05$–$p<0.001$). The heart rate was lowered from 114 to 94 on atenolol and to 91 on nadolol.

This equally good efficacy after 2 and 8 hours is illustrated in Table 38 and Figs. 50, 51. After 24 hours, however, only nadolol continued to provide 100% control of heart rate and systolic blood pressure (Table 37, Fig. 50) during exer-

Table 33. Systolic (S. B. P.) and diastolic (D. B. P.) blood pressures and heart rates (H. R.) (means ± SD) of 10 hypertensive males before and 8 hours after last taking 100 mg atenolol or 200 mg metoprolol during chronic treatment (*p < 0.005; **p < 0.01; ***p < 0.001)

	n = 10	Rest	Ergometric work (watts)						Recovery period (min)				
		Supine	50	60	70	80	90	100	1.	2.	3.	4.	5.
SBP	Before	153.6	173.8	181.8	189.5	195.7	204.7	212.1	180.1	165.8	159.5	158.2	155.6
(mmHg)	therapy	16.8	16.6	17.3	17.5	17.0	18.3	21.3	20.0	17.4	16.1	15.1	15.9
	8 hours after	132.9	150.1	156.7	161.3	167.5	173.9	181.0	159.3	149.6	143.8	142.5	140.8
	Atenolol	20.4*	24.2*	24.1*	22.6**	21.4**	21.8**	21.4**	20.0*	18.3	19.9	18.8	18.5
	8 hours after	134.3	152.2	157.1	161.9	165.4	170.3	176.8	159.0	151.7	146.7	147.7	143.1
	Metoprolol	22.5*	27.9*	25.7*	26.7*	23.7**	21.7**	23.4**	22.3*	21.4	21.6	22.5	22.1
DBP	Before	107.0	111.6	111.8	112.8	114.0	116.5	118.7	107.4	104.8	104.7	104.5	104.5
(mmHg)	therapy	8.4	11.2	10.8	12.1	11.7	12.4	13.2	9.4	9.6	8.3	8.9	9.2
	8 hours after	87.6	96.7	98.2	98.7	100.6	102.0	104.1	94.1	92.6	91.2	91.0	89.2
	Atenolol	16.9**	17.1*	16.3*	15.8*	14.8*	14.2*	13.6*	15.3*	14.3*	13.6*	13.3*	12.9*
	8 hours after	89.4	95.5	97.2	98.6	101.0	102.4	104.0	94.8	95.9	93.0	92.2	92.1
	Metoprolol	16.8**	16.2*	16.5*	16.8*	17.9	16.7*	16.3*	15.9*	17.2	17.2	15.1*	15.0*
HR	Before	71.3	92.7	99.7	103.8	110.3	114.9	120.8	85.6	78.0	74.7	75.7	74.7
(bts/min)	therapy	11.4	11.2	11.5	13.6	13.7	13.5	15.2	15.6	16.2	13.9	13.1	13.4
	8 hours after	53.8	76.0	79.2	81.8	86.7	91.4	95.3	64.3	60.1	58.3	58.2	58.2
	Atenolol	8.6**	6.1***	6.7***	6.0***	7.2***	7.7***	7.7***	7.8**	8.1**	7.4**	6.2**	8.1**
	8 hours after	53.1	76.5	79.8	83.6	86.7	92.9	96.3	68.7	60.9	60.8	58.6	57.6
	Metoprolol	9.3**	8.3**	8.1	8.3	9.1	8.4	8.0	12.2*	10.0*	8.4*	8.2**	9.4**

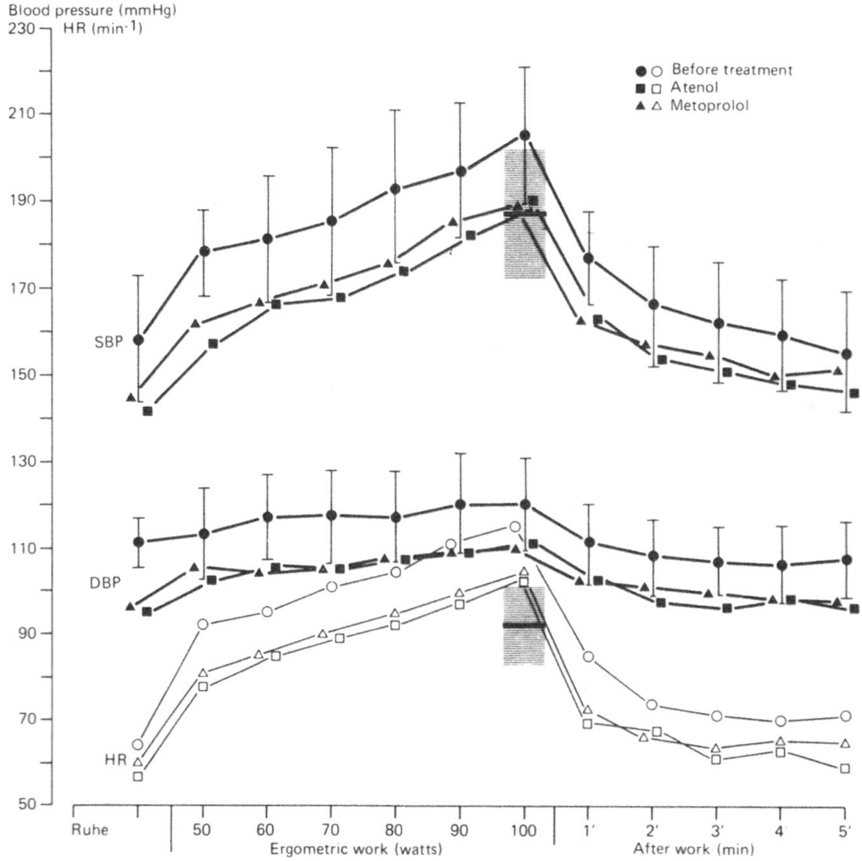

Fig. 47. Blood pressures and heart rates of 10 hypertensive males before and 24 hours after last taking 100 mg atenolol or 200 mg metoprolol. The bars indicate normal blood pressure response at 100 watts

cise. At that time atenolol provided 60% control of the heart rate, and 68% and 90% control of the systolic and diastolic blood pressures, respectively (Fig. 51).

No relationship was found between the *plasma levels* of the beta-blockers atenolol, metoprolol and nadolol 2, 8 and 24 hours after dosing and their antihypertensive effect.

Thus, our study of 20 patients treated with equipotent doses of three *beta-blocking drugs* showed that all drugs produced an equivalent *antihypertensive effect* and heart rate reduction after 2 and 8 hours, regardless of their pharmacologic characteristics (e.g., plasma half-life). Twenty-four hours after dosing, however, atenolol and metoprolol failed to maintain the reduction of heart rate achieved at 2 and 8 hours, while the effect of nadolol was undiminished.

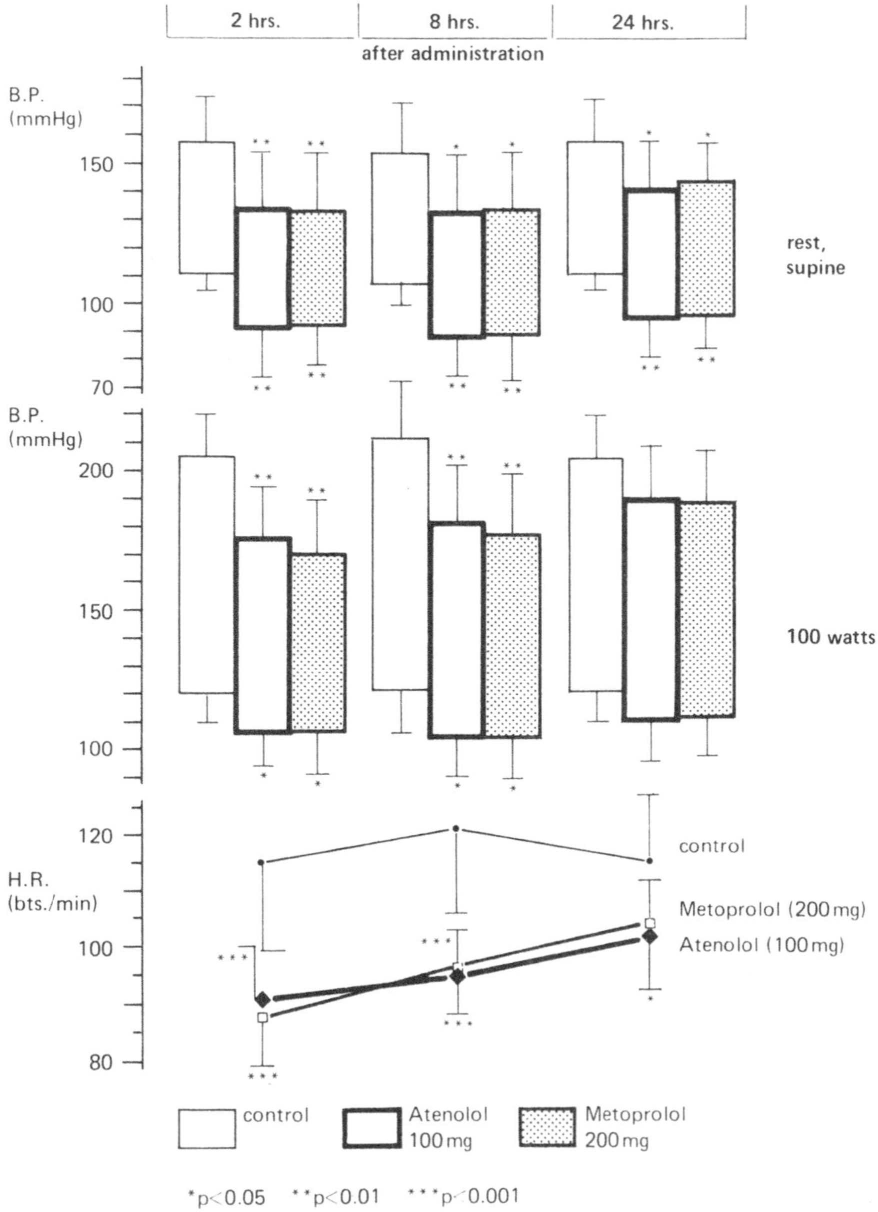

Fig. 48. Blood pressures and heart rates of 10 hypertensive patients before and 2, 8 and 24 hours after last taking 100 mg atenolol or 200 mg metoprolol at rest and during 100 watts

Table 34. Systolic (S. B. P.) and diastolic (D. B. P.) blood pressures and heart rates (H. R.) (means ± SD) of 10 hypertensive males before and after 24 hours after last taking 100 mg atenolol or 200 mg metoprolol during chronic treatment (*$p < 0.05$; **$p < 0.01$; ***$p < 0.001$)

	n = 10	Rest	Ergometric work (watts)						Recovery period (min)				
		Supine	50	60	70	80	90	100	1.	2.	3.	4.	5.
SBP (mmHg)	Before therapy	158.4 15.4	177.7 10.4	180.6 14.6	184.7 17.1	192.7 18.4	197.4 16.1	204.8 16.4	177.1 10.7	166.4 13.7	162.4 14.2	158.7 13.1	154.8 14.1
	24 hours after Atenolol	141.4 17.5*	157.3 18.3**	166.1 18.4	167.9 19.0*	174.4 20.5	181.8 18.4	189.6 20.2	163.1 17.5*	154.2 16.8	151.2 16.5	147.8 16.5	145.5 16.0
	24 hours after Metoprolol	143.9 13.6*	160.8 20.7*	166.2 20.5	169.5 21.2	175.4 19.9	184.6 20.7	189.2 20.5	162.7 21.4	156.5 19.2	153.5 17.7	149 18.2	150.5 18.5
DBP (mmHg)	Before therapy	111.1 5.6	113.3 10.7	116.6 10.4	117.4 10.5	117.2 11.4	119.5 12	119.7 10.5	110.7 8.8	107.7 9.1	106.9 8.3	106.3 9.3	107 9.3
	24 hours after Atenolol	95 14.6**	101.5 11.5*	104.9 12*	105.2 11.8*	106.5 13.8	107.7 14.6	110.8 13.8	101.9 11.2	97.6 11.7*	96.4 10.9*	97.6 12.0	96.4 12.0*
	24 hours after Metoprolol	96.4 12.5**	104.7 13.9	104 15.1*	105.3 15.2	107 13.1	107.6 16.1	109.5 14.6	101.8 13.7	100.1 13.7	98.8 12.8	97.7 12.9	97.1 13.2
HR (bts/min)	Before therapy	64.3 4.5	91.7 9.7	95.2 11.1	100.5 12.3	105.7 12.6	109.9 13.7	115 16.7	84.5 15.8	74.2 13.2	70.7 12.2	69.5 10.6	70.5 10.1
	24 hours after Atenolol	56.9 6.7**	77.7 8.3**	85.2 7.6*	89 9.7*	91.5 9.8*	97.3 9.8*	102 10.1*	68.9 10.2*	66.8 9.0	61.2 7.3*	62.7 6.6	59.3 8.2*
	24 hours after Metoprolol	59.7 9.4	81.3 10.7	85.4 10.8	90.2 10.9	95 11.5	98.8 11.9	103.6 12.4	72 11.5	66 10.4	68.7 11.7	65 12.3	65.2 12.2

Table 35. Systolic (S. B. P.) and diastolic blood pressures and heart rates (H. R.) (means ± SD) of 10 hypertensive males before and after 2 hours after last taking 100 mg atenolol or 120 mg nadolol during chronic treatment (*p < 0.05; **p < 0.01; ***p < 0.001)

	n = 10	Rest	Ergometric work (watts)						Recovery period (min)				
		Supine	50	60	70	80	90	100	1.	2.	3.	4.	5.
SBP (mmHg)	Before therapy	148.3 14.3	164.3 11.5	167.9 14	176.7 10.5	182.9 10.6	189.5 11.0	200.4 13	169.9 15.8	157.5 13.8	153.9 13.4	148.8 13.3	146.3 12.7
	2 hours after Atenolol	121.8 11.4***	144.3 7.7**	148.2 7.2**	150.4 9.7***	155.7 7.4***	161.4 9.2***	167.5 9.2***	150.4 10.9***	141.3 9.8**	140.4 11.5**	135.9 12.1**	133.9 12.1*
	2 hours after Nadolol	121.2 10.6***	141.2 13.4***	148.4 12.8***	149.9 9.4***	157.4 10.9***	162.6 11.1***	167.8 10.6***	150.4 12.7***	143.4 13.1*	138.2 13.3*	135.9 12.5*	132.0 9.9*
DBP (mmHg)	Before therapy	103.5 10.6	107.2 12.4	107 11.4	108.4 12.2	111.2 12.2	112 12.1	114.3 12.7	105.1 10.8	104.0 10.7	102.6 10.3	102.3 10.6	101.4 11.1
	2 hours after Atenolol	83.3 8.3***	92.4 7.4*	95.3 10.0*	96.4 10.5*	98 10.7*	99.2 10.5*	101.1 12.3*	92 8.7*	90.6 8.5*	88.1 9.3**	86.8 10.1**	87 9.7**
	2 hours after Nadolol	81.4 8.5***	93.4 12.3*	95 11.9*	95.7 10.0*	96.9 9.8*	99 10.5*	101.4 11.1*	88.8 10.2**	89.1 10.0*	86.8 9.0**	86.6 9.3**	86.1 9.6**
HR (bts/min)	Before therapy	58 6.8	88.9 10.2	89.7 9.6	93.1 10.1	98.4 10.4	103.4 10.5	108 9.9	69.5 13.3	65.3 9.2	63.1 10.4	65.2 10.2	64.3 10.5
	2 hours after Atenolol	47.1 8.8**	71.3 6.9***	75.1 7.7**	77.5 8.1**	83.6 7.0**	87.3 6.6***	91.8 7.3***	59.9 9.0	55.0 11.4*	53.4 9.8*	52.7 9.7*	52.8 8.8*
	2 hours after Nadolol	45.6 7.8**	69.6 6.3***	73.1 8.3***	76.3 8.4***	79.2 8.3***	84.6 8.1***	87.3 8.2***	57.1 14.2	54.7 11.8*	52.8 10.9*	50.9 9.3**	50.8 8.9**

Table 36. Systolic (S. B. P.) and diastolic (D. B. P.) blood pressures and heart rates (H. R.) (means ± SD) of 10 hypertensive males before and after 8 hours after last taking 100 mg atenolol or 120 mg nadolol (*$p<0.05$; **$p<0.001$; ***$p<0.001$)

	n = 10	Rest	Ergometric work (watts)						Recovery period (min)				
		Supine	50	60	70	80	90	100	1.	2.	3.	4.	5.
SBP (mmHg)	Before therapy	149.3 16.6	165.8 11.9	177.4 12.6	181.9 10.6	189.3 13.1	197 10.5	202.9 10.3	174.9 11.3	162.7 12.2	155.9 12.4	153.1 14.1	151.7 14.6
	8 hours after Atenolol	125.5 11.3**	145.2 8.1***	154.4 9.9***	158.6 9.0***	161.6 10.3***	166.6 10.6***	174.4 11.7***	151.0 12.0***	141.6 9.6***	137.5 9.1**	132.4 7.2***	130.8 8.2***
	8 hours after Nadolol	122.5 13.8***	140.0 9.9***	n.s. 147.7 9.9***	155.2 10.7***	160.3 9.4***	165.1 10.6***	173.4 12.2***	150.8 11.2**	146.6 11.3**	139.6 12.5**	135.4 8.3**	131.4 9.0**
DBP (mmHg)	Before therapy	101.8 11.0	105.7 13.7	106.8 14.2	108.0 14.4	110.1 15.0	111.2 14.5	114.0 13.9	102.4 12.4	101.0 11.4	99.8 12.6	99.7 12.5	100.7 13.0
	8 hours after Atenolol	82.0 11.8**	91.0 9.4*	92.3 12.8*	94.2 12.9*	95.5 11.8*	98.3 11.0*	100.3 13.4*	89.4 9.5*	86.9 8.3**	85.4 8.7**	85.5 7.5**	85.1 8.5**
	8 hours after Nadolol	78.6 8.0***	88.8 8.0**	91.5 9.6*	94.1 10.7*	95.2 10.8*	98.7 10.3*	100.6 13.7*	88.5 8.4**	86.8 8.2**	85.6 6.7**	84.1 6.7**	83.0 6.9**
HR (bts/min)	Before therapy	67.6 12.0	95.3 8.0	97.7 9.7	100.6 9.1	106.2 8.7	110.0 8.6	114.0 9.6	76.6 11.1	74.0 11.4	72.3 11.2	73.8 11.2	73.5 13.3
	8 hours after Atenolol	52.8 6.6**	77.2 5.8**	79.2 5.6***	81.9 6.3***	86.9 4.8***	90.6 5.5***	94.1 5.4***	62.7 11.2*	57.6 9.2**	57.0 9.0**	57.4 9.5**	57.4 8.3**
	8 hours after Nadolol	51.8 8.0**	73.8 6.7**	77.2 6.8***	80.8 7.0***	83.8 7.3***	86.7 7.4***	91.0 7.9***	62.2 11.2*	57.8 10.5***	57.2 9.2**	56.9 10.5**	56.9 9.2**

Table 37. Systolic (S. B. P.) and diastolic (D. B. P.) blood pressures and heart rates (H. R.) (means ± SD) of 10 hypertensive males before and after 24 hours after last taking 100 mg atenolol or 120 mg nadolol (*p < 0.05; **p < 0.01; ***p < 0.001)

	n = 10	Rest	Ergometric work (watts)						Recovery period (min)				
		Supine	50	60	70	80	90	100	1.	2.	3.	4.	5.
SBP	Before	149.3	173.6	178.3	184.4	189.3	196	201.2	170.7	163.7	158.2	155.3	153.6
(mmHg)	therapy	16.6	9.7	11.0	12.1	12.4	10.7	10.7	12.5	10.4	13.3	12.3	12.7
	24 hours after	133.8	152.9	160.5	166.1	171.7	179	187.4	161.4	154.3	147.4	144.4	146.1
	Atenolol	15.7*	16.3**	16.7*	17.2*	16.8*	19.1*	19.6	16.9	15.1	14.2	14.3	16.6
	24 hours after	131.8	145.3	153.4	157.1	163	168.9	175.9	156.5	148.5	142.9	142.9	139.9
	Nadolol	12.4*	13.6***	17.1***	16.9***	15.4***	16.0***	14.8***	11.3*	15.2*	13.4*	11.8*	14.5*
DBP	Before	101.8	110	112.2	112.4	113.8	115.3	116.2	108.2	104.3	103.4	103.2	103.2
(mmHg)	therapy	11.0	13.3	14.0	13.9	13.5	14.6	13.7	11.4	10.9	10.9	11.3	12.5
	24 hours after	85.9	98.6	98.7	98.6	100.7	102.4	104.5	95.3	91.9	91	90.2	91.4
	Atenolol	9.6**	12.4	13.7*	13.1*	13.1*	14.9*	13.6	12.5*	13.1*	11.4*	11.2*	13.0
	24 hours after	88.3	95.7	98.3	101.6	101.8	102.5	103.7	94.6	92.4	89.9	90.5	90.1
	Nadolol	10.7*	12.1*	11.4*	11.7	11.7*	11.4*	11.8*	11.4*	10.9*	10.8*	10.6*	10.7*
HR	Before	60.7	88.9	92.8	98	102	105.2	110.2	75.6	69.5	67.9	67.1	65.8
(bts/min)	therapy	7.6	9.2	9.7	10.9	8.7	9.6	9.3	11.1	9.9	11.6	12.0	9.9
	24 hours after	54.5	80.9	83.4	84.9	90.9	95.9	99.9	66.1	61.7	60.1	60	57.8
	Atenolol	12.2	9.4	8.6*	8.7*	9.0*	8.5*	9.1*	13.4	12.7	11.5	11.1	10.7
	24 hours after	48.1	70.0	75.3	79.2	81.6	86.7	91.5	58.9	53.8	54.6	52.1	52.7
	Nadolol	8.3**	9.9***	8.0***	8.6***	8.7***	8.7***	8.0***	12.3**	12.4**	11.5**	10.5**	10.4**

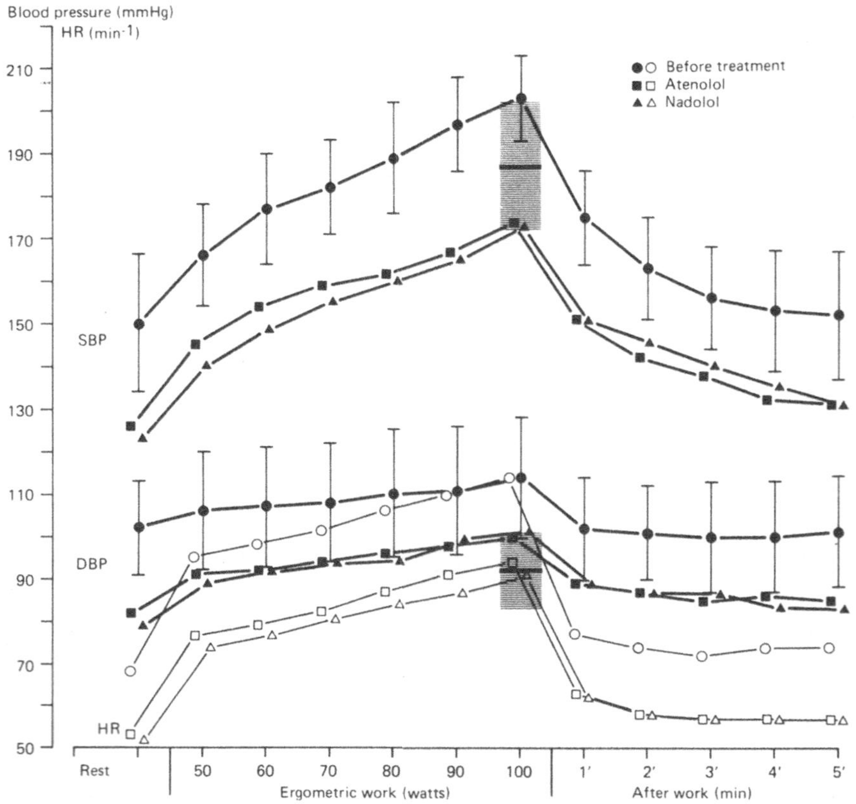

Fig. 49. Blood pressures and heart rates of 10 hypertensive males before and 8 hours after last taking 100 mg atenolol or 120 mg nadolol

3.2. Comparison of Pindolol, Metoprolol and Acebutolol

The purpose of this study was to determine whether cardioselective (β_1) and noncardioselective (β_1–β_2) beta-blocking drugs could lower the blood pressure and heart rate to the same degree on equivalent dosing during sustained, submaximal ergometric exercise. Sustained exercise induces a strong metabolic vasodilation [113] which conceivably could be inhibited by a concurrent β_2-blockade. We also studied the effect on maximal exertion. In addition, we sought to determine whether changes took place in blood pressure and heart rate responses during long-term treatment under the test conditions employed.

3.2.1. Patients and Methods

We first made a comparative study of the antihypertensive efficacy of pindolol and metoprolol in 9 male patients with essential hypertension (WHO Stage I–II) ranging in age from 27 to 51 (average 36) [111]. Following examination at entry the patients were arbitrarily divided into two groups, and each was

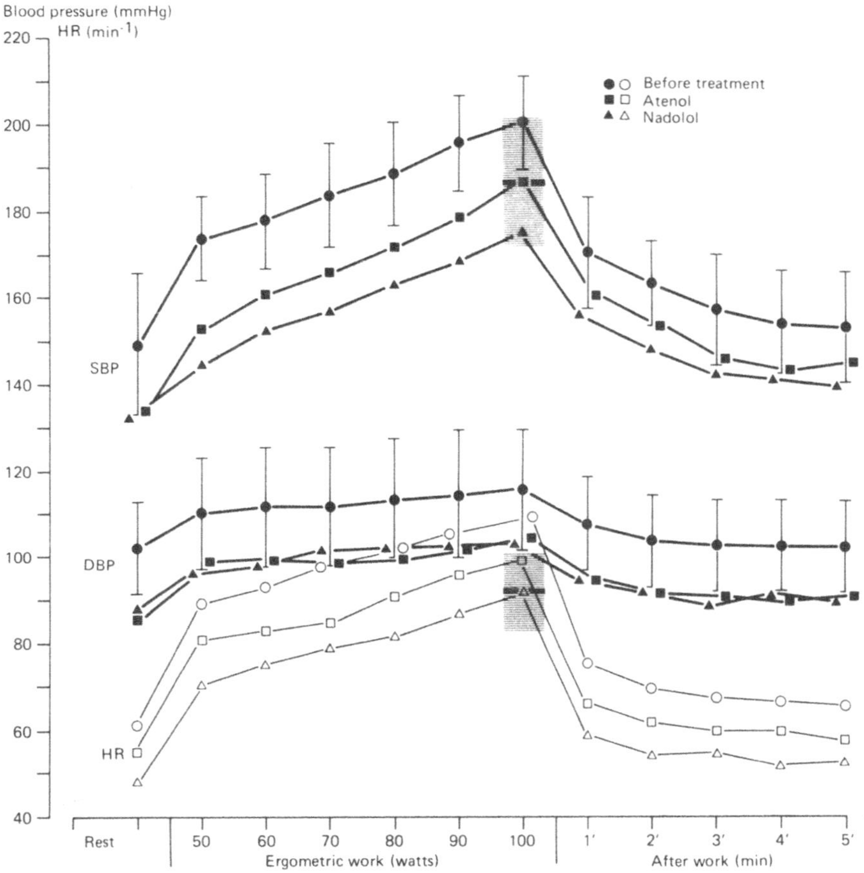

Fig. 50. Blood pressures and heart rates of 10 hypertensive males before and 24 hours after last taking 100 mg atenolol or 120 mg nadolol

initially treated for 4 weeks with an oral dose of 200 mg metoprolol or 15 mg pindolol taken once in the morning. After 4 weeks the drugs were switched. At the end of each course of treatment an identical ergometric test protocol was administered approximately two hours after the last tablet had been taken, using the same, individualized exercise stages.

The same methodology was applied to another 11 male patients with essential hypertension (WHO Stage I-II) ranging in age from 26 to 40 (average 37) to compare the effects of 15 mg pindolol and 500 mg acebutolol [120, 126].

In view of the long test duration (up to 40 minutes), we exercised the patients on the Siemens type 380 B bicycle ergometer in the upright position to make the test as comfortable as possible. Starting at 50 watts and a constant pedaling speed of 60 rpm, the workload progressed in stages of 10 watts/min until a heart rate of approximately 130-140 beats/min was attained. At this stage, which was determined individually for each patient, the workload was held constant, and the subject performed sustained exercise under steady-state con-

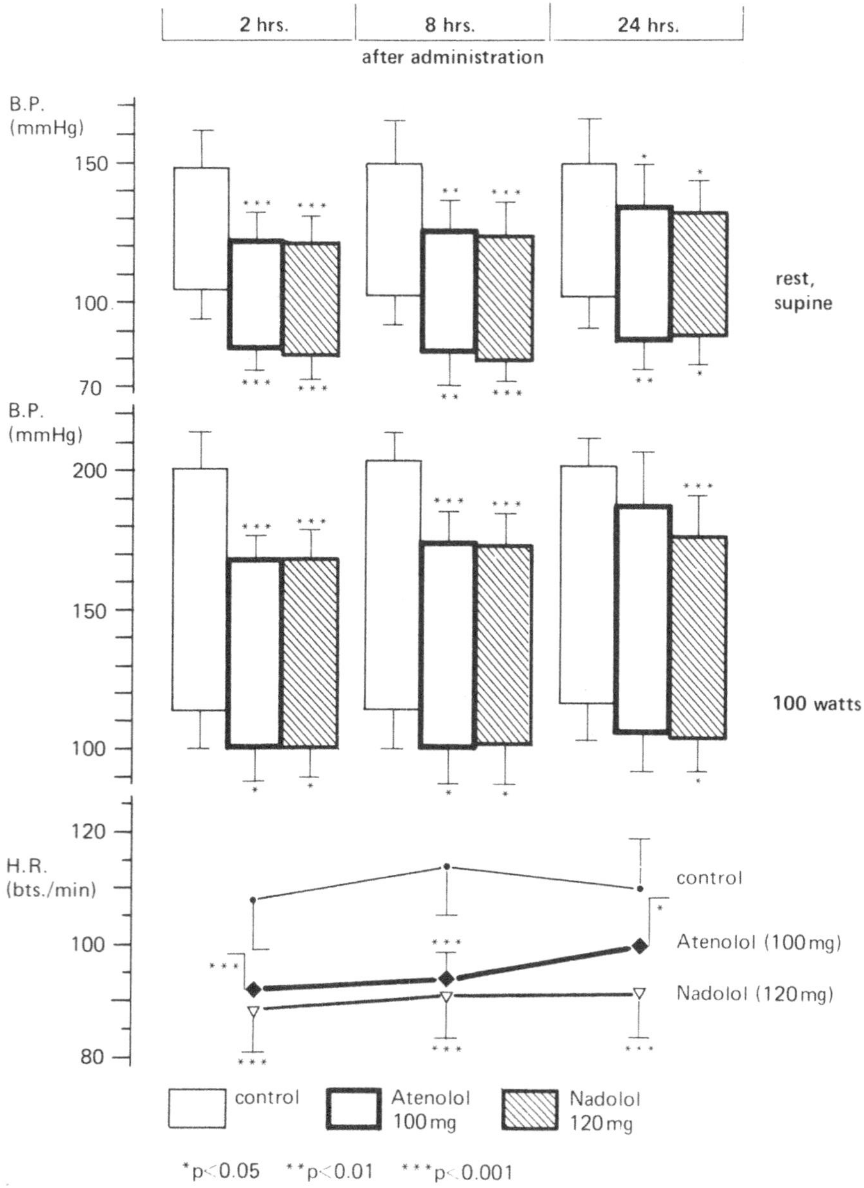

Fig. 51. Blood pressures and heart rates of 10 hypertensive patients before and 2, 8 and 24 hours after last taking 120 mg nadolol or 100 mg atenolol at rest and during 100 watts

ditions to a total exercise duration of 30 minutes. At that point the workload was increased in stages of 25 watts/min to the point of maximum tolerance or until the systolic blood pressure reached 270 mm Hg, whichever came first.

During blood pressure measurements strict care was taken that the patient's arm was relaxed and was elevated to the level of the heart.

Table 38. Therapy-induced reduction in % of the systolic (Δ S.B.P.) and diastolic (Δ D.B.P.) blood pressure and heart rate (Δ H.R.) during ergometry at 50 to 100 watts 2, 8 and 24 hours after the last dose of 100 mg atenolol or 120 mg nadolol or 200 mg metoprolol

n=20	SBP (%)			DBP (%)			HR (%)		
	2 hrs	8 hrs	24 hrs	2 hrs	8 hrs	24 hrs	2 hrs	8 hrs	24 hrs
Atenolol	14.2	13.7	9.5	11.8	12.9	11.1	16.4	18.3	10.4
Nadolol	14.2	15.5	14.2	11.9	13.3	11.1	19.2	21.0	19.6
Metoprolol	16.8	14.6	8.1	13.6	12.7	9.3	22.1	19.7	10.3
Atenolol	14.9	14.4	8.9	12.3	12.3	9.6	20.9	20.5	12.2

50–100 watts

Table 39. Blood pressures and heart rates (means ± SD) of 9 hypertensive males before and during 4-week beta blockade at rest, in min. 6 of exercise (100 W), in min. 35 of steady state exercise, at maximal work load and during recovery (*p < 0.05; **p < 0.01)

n=9		Rest	Ergometric work		Recovery period	
		Supine	6 min	30 min	max.	5 min
SBP (mmHg)	Before therapy	151.1 ± 6.5	205.0 ± 29.9	203.9 ± 26.2	238.3 ± 26.8	151.7 ± 17.3
	Pindolol	131.7 ± 12.5**	163.9 ± 19.8**	170.6 ± 23.6**	191.7 ± 23.9**	128.3 ± 22.1**
	Metoprolol	121.6 ± 5.5**	156.1 ± 20.1**	166.1 ± 18.5	205.6 ± 23.6**	126.1 ± 11.7**
DBP (mmHg)	Before therapy	100.1 ± 5.2	116.7 ± 13.9	107.8 ± 8.3	113.9 ± 12.7	93.9 ± 11.9
	Pindolol	87.2 ± 5.1**	100 ± 8.7**	98.3 ± 9.0**	110 ± 13.5	81.7 ± 15.4**
	Metoprolol	83.3 ± 6.1	96.7 ± 8.3**	98.3 ± 10.0**	110 ± 12.8	84.4 ± 9.2**
HR (bts/min)	Before therapy	73.4 ± 6.1	116.7 ± 11.9	136.3 ± 4.1	174.2 ± 11.7	105 ± 17.0
	Pindolol	66.7 ± 9.2*	96.7 ± 11**	107.4 ± 9.3**	128 ± 8.7**	83.4 ± 15.3**
	Metoprolol	56.7 ± 9*	92.7 ± 10.2**	100.9 ± 8.3**	125.6 ± 9.7**	77.4 ± 8.4**

3.2.2. Effect during Sustained Submaximal and Maximal Exertion

Both pindolol and metoprolol lowered the blood pressure significantly ($p < 0.01$) before, during and after ergometry (Table 39). In the 6th minute at 100 watts, both drugs produced approximately equal systolic and diastolic blood pressure reductions. This also applied to the 30th minute of steady-state exercise at a mean workload of 124 watts. At the maximal workload, however, it was found that pindolol and metoprolol lowered the systolic pressure significantly but could not check the rise of diastolic pressure.

Both beta-blocking drugs lowered the heart rates significantly ($p < 0.01$) and to an approximately equal degree during ergometry, with metoprolol producing a greater reduction at rest.

Table 40 shows that both acebutolol and pindolol lowered the systolic and diastolic blood pressures significantly ($p < 0.01$) and with equal potency before and after ergometry. This also applied to values measured in the 6th minute at

Table 40. Blood pressures and heart rates (means ± SD) of 11 male hypertensives before and during 4-week betablockade at rest in min. 6 of exercise (110 W), in min. 35 of steady-state exercise, at maximal workload and during recovery (*p < 0.05; **p < 0.01)

		Rest	Ergometric work		Recovery period	
		Supine	6 min	30 min	max	5 min
SBP (mmHg)	Before therapy	149 ± 10	194 ± 24	203 ± 24	236 ± 25	153 ± 19
	Acebutolol	131 ± 9**	160 ± 14**	166 ± 15**	198 ± 16**	133 ± 11**
	Pindolol	129 ± 14**	166 ± 14**	166 ± 17**	192 ± 18**	135 ± 11**
DBP (mmHg)	Before therapy	104 ± 7	114 ± 9	108 ± 7	114 ± 10	103 ± 13
	Acebutolol	89 ± 8*	98 ± 7**	96 ± 7**	110 ± 9	87 ± 9**
	Pindolol	85 ± 10**	101 ± 10**	100 ± 3**	110 ± 6	90 ± 9**
HR (bts/min)	Before therapy	64 ± 5	113 ± 10	141 ± 5	182 ± 12	107 ± 14
	Acebutolol	55 ± 7*	93 ± 6**	103 ± 7**	135 ± 14**	79 ± 12**
	Pindolol	62 ± 9	97 ± 6**	109 ± 9**	138 ± 9**	83 ± 13**

100 watts and after 30 minutes of steady-state exercise at a mean workload of 116.4 watts. As in our revious comparison of pindolol and metoprolol, only the systolic blood pressure was significantly reduced at the maximal workload, while the diastolic pressure was essentially unaffected.

Both beta-blockers lowered the heart rate significantly ($p < 0.01$) and to roughly an equal degree during and after ergometry. Only acebutolol produced a significant ($p < 0.05$) fall of the heart rate at rest.

Our comparative study of the antihypertensive efficacy of β_1-selective and β_1-β_2 blocking drugs clearly shows that the drugs are equally effective in lowering blood pressure on equivalent dosing despite differences in their pharmacologic properties. All the drugs exert a significant antihypertensive effect during both short-term and sustained submaximal exercise, and none are capable of significantly lowering the diastolic blood pressure at maximal workloads.

3.2.3. Effect of Long-Term Treatment for 12–16 Months

Table 41 and Fig. 52 show the results of long-term treatment with *beta-blocking drugs* over a period of months compared with a 4-week course of treatment. Nine patients received 200 mg metoprolol for 12 months [118], and nine received 500 mg acebutolol for 16 months [143]. It is interesting from a physiologic standpoint to note that, prior to treatment, the patients experienced a fall of both systolic and diastolic blood pressure with increasing duration of steady-state exercise. Comparing the blood pressure in the 6th minute at 100 watts, 204/116 mm Hg, with the value in the 30th minute of steady-state exercise, 206/109.3 mm Hg, we find no change in the systolic pressure and a fall of the diastolic pressure despite a mean heart rate increment of 24 beats/min ($p < 0.01$). It may be concluded that the hypertensives experienced a marked metabolic vasodilation during the course of exercise which offset the increased car-

Table 41. Blood pressures and heart rates (means ± SD) of 18 hypertensives before and during 4-week and 16-month betablockade with 200 mg metoprolol (n = 10) or 500 mg acebutolol (n = 8) at rest, in min 6 of exercise (100 W), from min 15 to 30 of steady-state exercise, at maximal workload, and during recovery (*$p<0.05$; **$p<0.01$; ***$p<0.001$)

n = 18		Rest	Ergometric work						Recovery period	
		Supine	6 min	15 min	20 min	25 min	30 min	max.	1 min	5 min
SBP (mmHg)	Before therapy	152.8	204.4	218.1	218.1	212.2	206.3	240.9	197.6	158.1
		12.6	22.8	25.3	23.9	21.5	26.4	25.3	24	14.4
	4-weeks beta-blockade	135	158.3	167.4	167.6	169	165.5	201.0	161.4	130.2
		15.2***	16.6***	19.8***	18.0***	17.5***	17.2***	19.5***	17.3***	13.2***
	16 months beta-blockade	136	158.5	167.1	164.1	163.4	164.7	195.8	166.9	133.3
		11.4	16.1	20.6	22.2	20.1	19.6	24.5	22.9	12.9
DBP (mmHg)	Before therapy	103.9	115.8	116.6	113.6	110.2	109.3	116.1	102.7	98.4
		6.9	11.2	10.0	7.4	8.3	7.1	11.5	12.7	15.2
	4 weeks beta-blockade	91.6	98.3	100	99.3	97.6	96.7	108.9	96.3	86.2
		10.3***	7.4***	8.4***	9.8***	8.4***	7.8***	11.3	10.7 *	9.7***
	16 month beta-blockade	92.6	97.4	99.4	96.8	94.3	93.4	109.0	93.1	84.4
		7.2	9.5	10.6	10.6	10.2	9.6	12.8	7.3	6.3
HR (bts/min)	Before therapy	70.9	114.3	133.4	136.8	137.0	138.1	176.2	131.4	103.2
		6.1	11.3***	6.4	5.2*	5.2	4.3	13.6	21.2	16.0
	4-weeks beta-blockade	59.1	93.7	101.9	100.9	100.9	101.3	126.8	93.3	78.6
		7.5***	8.6***	8.8***	8.0***	6.7***	6.8***	10.1***	11.2***	10.5***
	16 months beta-blockade	58.1	93.1	103.1	102.7	103.3	102.8	131.0	94.6	77.2
		8.5***	12.0***	13.1***	12.0***	11.5***	11.2***	14.5***	21.2***	14.8***

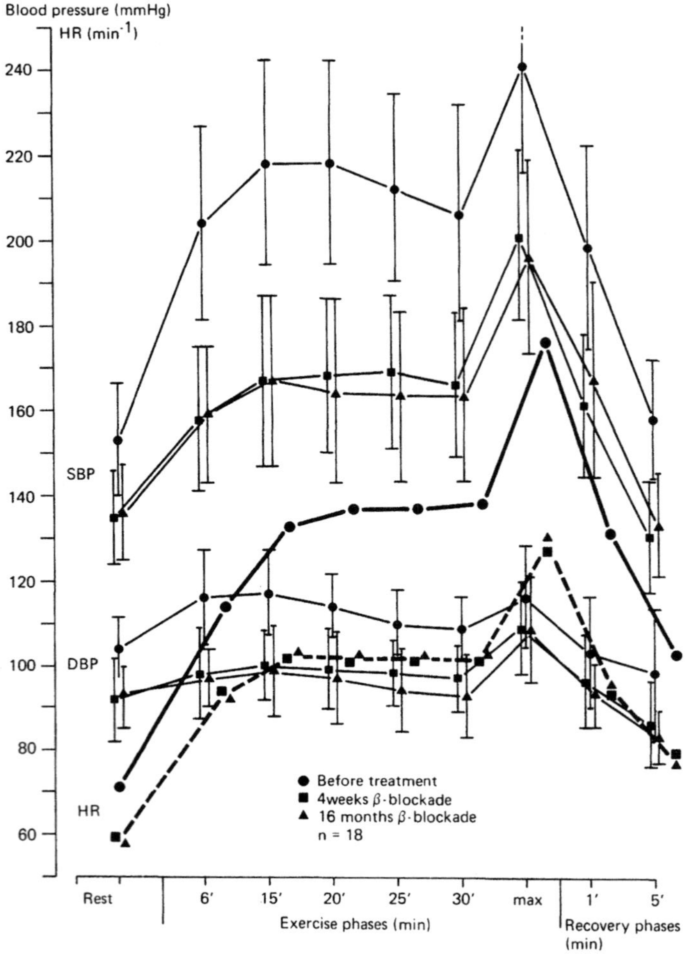

Fig. 52. Blood pressures and heart rates of 18 hypertensives before and during 4-week and 16-month beta-blockade with 200 mg metoprolol (n = 10) or 500 mg acebutolol (n = 8) at rest, in min 6 of exercise (100 W), from min 15 to 30 of steady-state exercise, at maximal workload, and during recovery

diac output, resulting in a constant systolic pressure and even a significant fall of the diastolic pressure ($p < 0.05$).

When we analyze the antihypertensive effect of the betablocking drugs, we find equal degrees of systolic and diastolic blood pressure reduction after four weeks and after longer-term therapy.

Even during the beta blockade, the diastolic blood pressure fell during the course of ergometry despite a rising heart rate, though this fall was not as pronounced as before treatment.

The heart rate response after shorter- and longer-term treatment with beta-blocking drugs is of particular significance from a clinical pharmacologic standpoint. The nearly identical heart rate responses observed during the two treatment periods underscore the excellent reproducibility of ergometric data and the potentially important role of ergometry in testing the effects and side-effects of beta-blockers [118, 122, 123, 129, 131, 137] as well as other classes of drugs. This particularly applies to *long-term tests* [126], which often are very difficult to standardize under conditions of rest.

4. Antihypertensive Effect of Diuretics Compared with Beta-Blocking Drugs and their Combinations

Diuretics and beta-blocking drugs are widely used in the therapy of essential hypertension. Numerous comparative studies have shown that the different beta-blockers and diuretics are more or less equally effective in bringing down the resting blood pressure of mildly hypertensive patients [14, 72, 75, 116, 136, 145, 222, 242, 301, 337]. However, when one considers the disproportionate blood pressure elevations that are produced even by mild physical exertion [109, 113, 259, 416], one can appreciate the great clinical importance of determining whether diuretics and beta-blocking drugs are also equally effective in lowering the blood pressure during exercise. Another salient question is whether diuretics can enhance the antihypertensive effect of beta blockers during exercise.

4.1. Comparison of Hydrochlorothiazide/Amiloride Hydrochloride and Acebutolol

In an effort to answer these questions, studies were done to compare the antihypertensive effect of the beta-blocker acebutolol with that of a fixed diuretic combination composed of hydrochlorothiazide and amiloride hydrochloride during ergometric exercise.

4.1.1. Patients and Methods

Twenty-four hypertensive persons (20 men, 4 women) age 24–57 years (average age 42) with WHO Stage I–II essential hypertension were tested [116]. None of the patients had previously received antihypertensive therapy.

Following preliminary testing, the patients were randomly assigned to two groups. Group 1 was treated with 500 mg acebutolol per day, taken once in the morning, while group 2 was given a fixed diuretic combination containing 50 mg hydrochlorothiazide and 5 mg amiloride hydrochloride. After 6 weeks of therapy the drugs were switched between groups 1 and 2, and the new regimen was maintained for an additional 6 weeks.

At the end of the study 12 hypertensives (5 from group 1 and 7 from group 2) who had not responded adequately to beta blockade alone were treated concomitantly with 500 mg acebutolol and the hydrochlorothiazide-amiloride hydrochloride combination for another 6 weeks.

Identical ergometric tests were administered to all patients at the end of each treatment period. All blood pressures were taken by the same examiner using the same calibrated mercury manometer.

4.1.2. Comparison of Monotherapies

Acebutolol and the diuretic combination produced a significant ($p<0.01$, $p<0.001$) and roughly equivalent fall in systolic and diastolic blood pressure with the patient supine (Table 42). During standing, both drugs produced a significant and equivalent reduction of the systolic pressure, but only the beta-blocker lowered the diastolic pressure to a significant degree.

Despite the similar effects of these drugs in the resting state, very different responses were observed during *ergometry* (Fig. 53). The *diuretics* did not produce a significant fall in *systolic blood pressure,* while the beta-blockers lowered the systolic pressure highly significantly compared with control readings ($p<0.001$) and with diuretic therapy ($p<0.001$), bringing it into the high normotensive range. The diastolic pressure was also lowered significantly ($p<0.05$) by the diuretic combination, although the beta-blocker had a more pronounced effect ($p<0.05$, $p<0.001$). During the recovery period only the beta-blocker lowered the diastolic pressure significantly, while the systolic pressure was significantly influenced ($p<0.05$, $p<0.01$) by both drugs, with acebutolol again showing greater efficacy.

The heart rate was not affected by *diuretic therapy* either at rest or during ergometry. *Acebutolol,* however, produced a significant fall of the *heart rate* ($p<0.01$), lowering it by 18.7% at rest and by 19.4 and 22.4% during and after ergometry, respectively.

Fig. 54 clearly shows that the different antihypertensive potencies of the beta-blocker and diuretics under conditions of exercise were independent on the sequence of drug administration and were not the result of a carry-over or training effect. Nine of the 12 patients in group 1 who were started on acebutolol again showed excessive blood pressure elevations at 100 watts after they were switched to the diuretic combination. A similar response was seen in 10 of the 12 patients in group 2, who were started on the diuretic. They showed an appreciable fall in blood pressure only after they had been switched to acebutolol. Thus, 19 of the 24 patients who took acebutolol responded better to that drug, while 5 patients showed an approximately equal response to both drugs. All of the latter patients were ones who experienced only slight to moderate blood pressure increases during ergometry. The failure of diuretics to control the exercise blood pressure was most evident in patients who experienced severe blood pressure elevations during cycling.

4.1.3. Efficacy of the Combination

In half the patients ($n=12$) the beta-blocking drug alone failed to lower the blood pressure to a satisfying degree, although a significant hypotensive effect was apparent (Table 43). However, the addition of the fixed diuretic combination significantly lowered the systolic pressure ($p<0.05$) and especially the dia-

Table 42. Blood pressures and heart rates (means ± SD) of 24 hypertensives before and during 6 weeks' therapy with a betablocker (500 mg acebutolol) or diuretic combination (50 mg hydrochlorothiazide, 5 mg amiloride) (*$p < 0.05$; **$p < 0.01$; *** < 0.001)

		Rest		Ergometric work (watts)			Recovery period (min)		
		Supine	Standing	60	80	100	1 min	3 min	5 min
SBP (mmHg)	Before therapy	164.4 14.9	166.8 18.9	207.1 22.5	221.7 23.9	233.9 22.6	199.6 18.6	177.5 15.1	166.8 14.3
	Diuretics	152.0 14.8**	147.4 16.8***	195.7 20.1	210.9 22.5	223.0 22.4	188.8 16.8	165.4 16.5*	155.4 14.0**
	Beta-blocker	148.9 10.5***	145.5 10.7***	176.4 15.3***	188.5 19.1***	198.6 17.2***	174.5 15.3***	156.0 12.0***	150.0 8.3***
DBP (mmHg)	Before therapy	106.2 10.8	111.3 11.3	121.7 11.4	124.4 11.5	127.3 12.4	109.1 10.9	107.6 10.9	108.7 11.9
	Diuretics	98.1 9.6**	109.4 10.4	113.7 10.6*	116.6 10.2*	119.3 10.2*	107.7 9.9	106.0 11.2	106.4 11.0
	Beta-blocker	94.6 8.3***	101.4 7.6**	107.6 8.4***	109.3 11.4***	112.4 11.0***	99.8 7.6**	98.2 7.7**	97.2 7.1***
HR (bts/min)	Before therapy	74.0 16.2	83.5 18.8	115.4 19.2	125.8 21.8	136.1 21.4	103.9 24.1	92.1 21.5	89.7 19.6
	Diuretics	75.3 14.7	92.0 16.2	112.7 19.3	122.4 21.0	131.8 20.5	101.3 25.0	92.2 19.6	89.5 16.6
	Beta-blocker	61.7 9.2**	66.1 9.6***	94.5 13.8***	101.6 15.9***	108.3 13.6***	77.8 15.2***	72.1 14.5***	72.9 14.4***

Table 43. Blood pressures and heart rates (means ± SD) of 12 hypertensives before and during 6 weeks' therapy with a betablocker (500 mg acebutolol) alone and combined with a diuretic (50 mg hydrochlorothiazide/5 mg amiloride) (*p < 0.05; **p < 0.01; **p < 0.01; ***p < 0.001)

		Rest		Ergometric work (watts)			Recovery period (min)		
		Supine	Standing	60	80	100	1.	3.	5.
SBP (mmHg)	Before therapy	165.3 14.7	167.7 21.2	213.8 22.1	228.0 22.4	241.2 23.0	203.8 20.0	177.7 18.1	168.8 16.2
	Beta blockers	149.7 8.9** *	147.2 7.5** *	178.3 12.7***	192.6 16.9***	204.8 17.8***	175.7 16.1***	160.0 11.3*** **	154.3 7.2***
	Beta blockers and diuretic	140.0 11.3***	130.6 13.4***	170.8 12.7***	185.3 19.6***	199.2 20.2***	166.4 16.4***	150.5 13.4***	142.2 12.7***
SBP (mmHg)	Before therapy	107.7 11.0	113.2 12.1	126.1 8.3	129.2 9.2	132.3 9.1	115.7 9.1	113.2 10.4	114.9 11.2
	Beta blockers	96.2 8.4** *	103.3 8.6* *	109.8 6.7*** *	112.2 6.9*** *	115.0 7.1*** *	103.5 5.5*** **	102.5 6.2*** **	101.2 6.0*** **
	Beta blockers and diuretic	88.8*** 8.8	95.8** 10.9	103.2*** 8.5	105.3*** 9.2	105.7*** 8.3	91.8*** 9.6	92.0*** 8.3	92.6*** 5.3
HR (bts/min)	Before therapy	76.3 16.4	86.1 16.3	118.0 12.6	128.8 14.0	138.0 11.2	104.1 23.0	94.0 19.8	90.7 16.8
	Beta blockers	61.4 4.4**	65.9 6.7***	94.8 8.9***	102.8 10.4***	110.1 10.1***	78.0 15.9**	69.4 8.6***	67.9 8.7***
	Beta blockers and diuretic	60.8 7.1**	69.3 7.5**	92.6 8.1***	100.6 9.5***	108.2 11.3***	78.9 13.0**	73.2 8.8**	70.9 8.2**

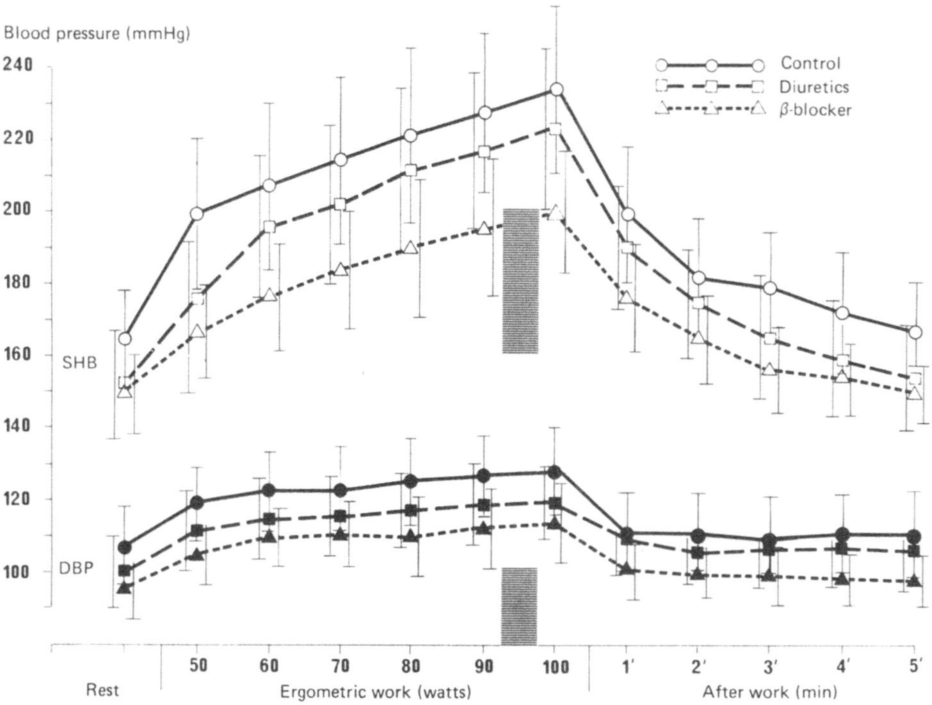

Fig. 53. Blood pressures of 24 hypertensives before and during 6 weeks' therapy with a beta-blocker (500 mg acebutolol) or diuretic (50 mg hydrochlorothiazide, 5 mg amiloride). The bars indicate the normal range of blood pressure at 100 watts

stolic pressure ($p < 0.01$), producing normotensive readings at rest. During ergometry, the addition of the diuretic produced a further significant ($p < 0.05$) fall in diastolic pressure, e.g. from 115 to 105.7 mm Hg at 100 watts. The effect on systolic pressure was less pronounced (Fig. 55).

Side-effects were mild and infrequent and were characteristic of those associated with the use of beta-blockers and diuretics. None were serious enough to warrant a reduction of dosage or discontinuation of treatment.

4.2. Comparison of Mefruside and Acebutolol

Because different diuretics may possibly have different effects on the exercise blood pressure [279], we conducted another study to determine how other diuretics compared with beta-blockers in their antihypertensive efficacy during stress, and whether diuretics would again enhance the antihypertensive effect of beta-blockers, this time in a larger study population.

We also investigated the effect of the different drugs and combinations on the rate-pressure product as a measure of myocardial oxygen consumption [22, 214, 314, 369].

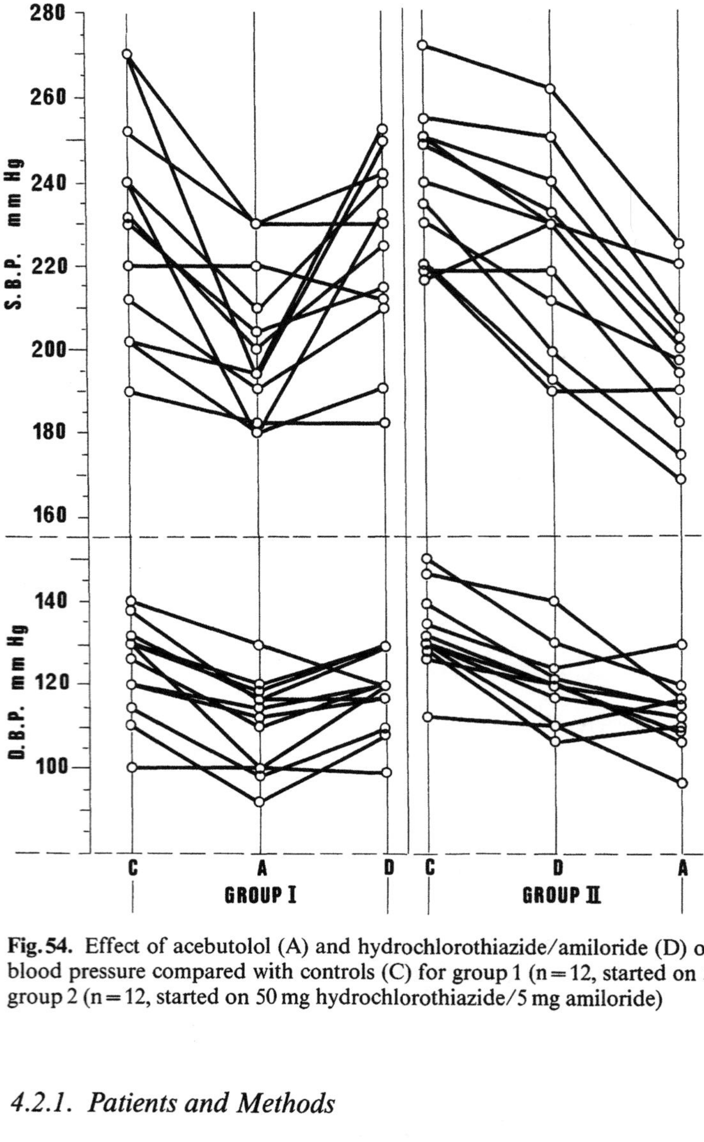

Fig. 54. Effect of acebutolol (A) and hydrochlorothiazide/amiloride (D) on systolic and diastolic blood pressure compared with controls (C) for group 1 (n = 12, started on 500 mg acebutolol) and group 2 (n = 12, started on 50 mg hydrochlorothiazide/5 mg amiloride)

4.2.1. Patients and Methods

A total of 42 hypertensive outpatients took part in the study [127]. We first tested 30 patients age 18 to 50 (average age 38.3; 26 men, 4 women) with WHO Stage I-II essential hypertension. Besides having elevated blood pressures in multiple resting determinations, all the patients had markedly elevated pressures during ergometry. None of the patients had received prior antihypertensive therapy.

Following initial testing without antihypertensive medication, we started all patients on a 4-week course of the diuretic mefruside, 25 mg taken once in the morning. Following this initial treatment period we randomly divided the patients into two groups of 15 each. For another 4 weeks the hypertensives in

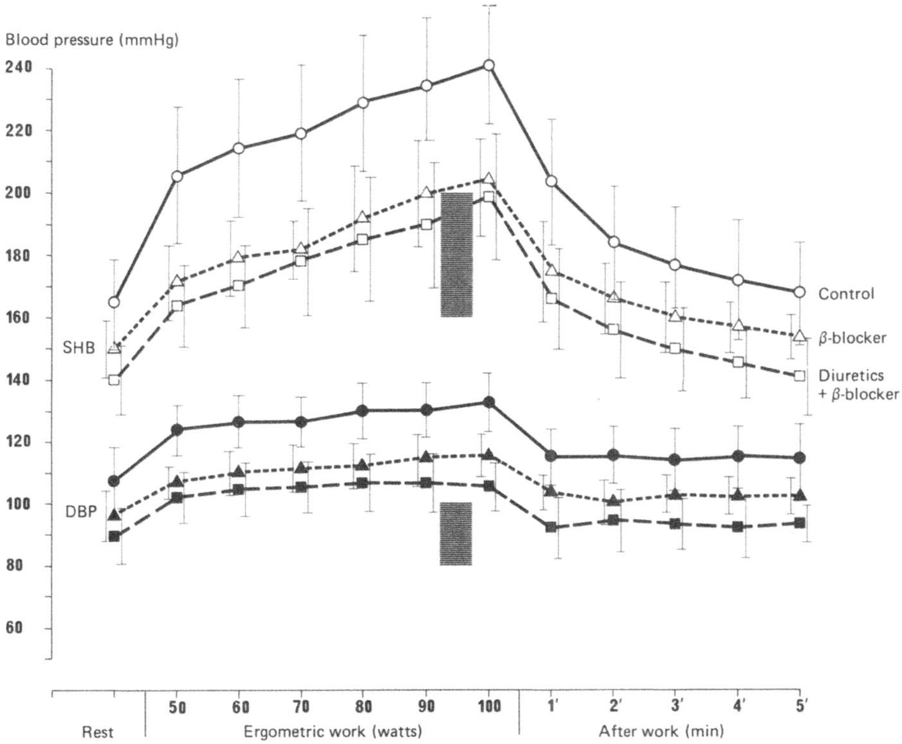

Fig. 55. Blood pressures of 12 hypertensives before and during 6 weeks' therapy with a beta-blocker (500 mg acebutolol) alone and combined with a diuretic (50 mg hydrochlorothiazide/5 mg amiloride). The bars indicate the normal range of blood pressure at 100 watts

group 1 were taken off mefruside and were switched to the beta-blocking drug acebutolol, 400 mg taken once in the morning, so that we could compare the effects of this drug with the diuretic taken previously. The result of such therapy is not affected by the sequence of the treatment periods [116]. Group 2 took the 400 mg acebutolol concurrently with their usual morning dose of mefruside. This permitted both an intraindividual comparison of a diuretic alone and a diuretic combined with a beta-blocker, and an interindividual comparison (with group 1) of a beta-blocker alone and a beta-blocker combined with a diuretic.

Exercise stress tests were administered at the conclusion of both 4-week treatment periods. All tests were done at the same time of day as the preliminary test performed at entry, i.e., between 3:00 and 6:00 p.m.

We also tested another 12 hypertensives age 30–48 (group 3, average age 41.9) with WHO Stage I–II essential arterial hypertension to compare the antihypertensive efficacy of the free combination of 400 mg acebutolol and 25 mg mefruside with that of a fixed combination composed of 400 mg acebutolol and 20 mg mefruside [139].

Table 44. Blood pressures and heart rates (means ± SD) of 30 hypertensives before and during 4 weeks' therapy with 25 mg mefruside

	n = 30	Rest			Ergometric work (watts)						Recovery period (min)				
		Supine	Standing	Before work	50	60	70	80	90	100	1	2	3	4	5
SBD (mmHg)	Before therapy	155.6 15.2	157.3 17.2	160.4 17	181.0 19	186.4 18.5	193.5 19.1	199.6 19.6	203.7 17.9	209.9 17.1	180.7 16.5	168.2 14.5	161.5 14.0	160.6 14.8	158.6 14.3
	Mefruside	146.7 13.1*	143.4 15.3**	147.7 15.0**	170.5 18.1*	177.2 18.9	182.5 16.8*	187.9 18.4*	194.0 19.1*	201.6 18.4	169.5 17.9*	160.3 15.5*	152.7 17.1*	150.8 16.5*	150.5 16.3*
DBP (mmHg)	Before therapy	102.9 10.0	107.2 11.0	106.9 8.8	109.1 8.6	110.4 9.9	112.0 10.5	112.9 10.3	113.1 10.2	114.9 9.5	104.3 9.3	102.9 8.6	104.7 9.3	105.7 9.9	105.3 9.4
	Mefruside	94.6 10.3**	95.8 9.7***	99.3 9.1**	103.1 10.5*	104.1 9.2*	105.3 11.0*	106.1 9.9*	108.2 10.1	109.4 10.3*	100.2 9.2	99.7 9.9	99.5 9.8*	99.0 10.1*	100 9.5*
HR (bts/min)	Before therapy	64.5 12.9	71.6 15.4	64.7 11.4	94.7 15.3	99.1 15.7	104.2 16.4	108.7 17.6	114.2 18.2	118.8 18.3	82.8 18.4	77.3 16.7	75.1 16.3	76.1 15.1	74.8 14.5
	Mefruside	66.7 14.3	75.2 17.8	64.4 11.9	92.9 15.0	97.8 14.7	101.7 15.7	106.3 16.6	111.9 17.7	117.1 20.3	81.8 18.7	79.2 17.9	76.7 16.0	76.6 14.6	76.2 15.2

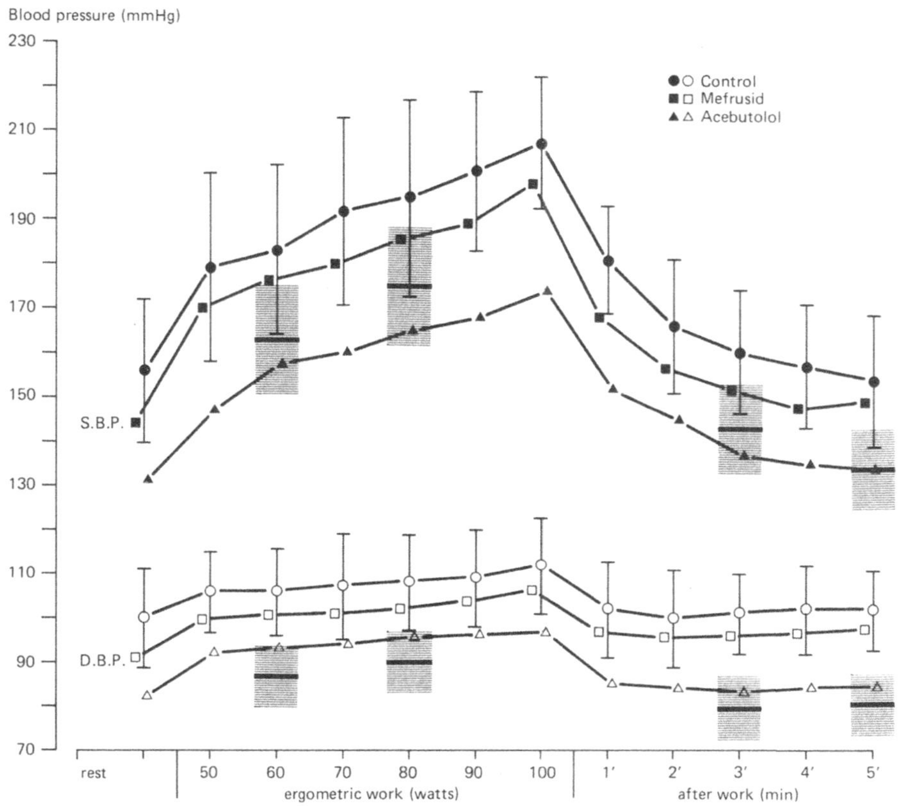

Fig. 56. Blood pressures and heart rates of 15 hypertensives before and during 4 weeks' therapy with 25 mg mefruside followed by treatment with 400 mg acebutolol (group 1, n = 15) for an additional 4 weeks. The bars indicate normal blood pressure ranges.

4.2.2. Comparison of Monotherapies

Table 44 shows the overall response of the 30 hypertensives to 4 weeks of mefruside therapy. The drug produced a significant fall in the resting systolic and diastolic blood pressure ($p<0.05$–$p<0.01$) with the patient supine, standing, and immediately before starting exercise.

As in the previous study, the diuretic also produced significant diastolic pressure lowering ($p<0.05$) during exercise. The degree of systolic pressure lowering during exercise corresponded to the effect of hydrochlorothiazide-amiloride hydrochloride, with a significant ($p<0.05$) reduction observed at 50 and 70–90 watts with mefruside owing to the larger number of patients in the study. A similar pattern was seen during the recovery period.

In group 1 it was found (Table 45, Fig. 56) that both the diuretic and the beta-blocker significantly lowered the systolic and diastolic pressure ($p<0.05$–$p<0.001$) at rest prior to ergometry, with acebutolol exerting a significantly greater effect ($p<0.05$). During ergometry, however, *mefruside* plainly was unable to lower the elevated *exercise blood pressures* significantly. Acebutolol, on the oth-

Table 45. Blood pressures and heart rates of 15 hypertensives before and during 4 weeks' therapy with 25 mg mefruside followed by treatment with 400 mg acebutolol (group 1) (*p < 0.05; **p < 0.01; ***p < 0.001)

	n = 15 Group 1	Rest			Ergometric work (watts)						Recovery period (min)				
		Supine	Standing	Before work	50	60	70	80	90	100	1	2	3	4	5
SBD (mmHg)	Before therapy	155.9 16.0	157.4 18.4	157.4 15.9	178.6 20.8	182.7 19.1	191.6 20.6	195.0 21.6	201.2 18.1	206.9 15.6	180.7 13.4	165.7 14.5	159.5 14.0	156.6 14.3	154.1 14.6
	Mefruside	143.6 12.6* *	144.3 14.0* *	147.2 17.2 *	170.3 23.2 **	175.6 23.6 **	179.5 23.5 **	185.1 21.9 **	189.2 21.7 **	197.3 20.0 ***	168 21.4 **	157.3 18.2 **	151.9 19.7 **	148 19.5 **	149.1 19.4 **
	Acebutolol	131.3 12.1***	129.5 13.1***	133.1 10.1***	147.3 11.9***	157.1 11.9***	159.5 10.8***	164.5 8.7***	167.7 9.8***	173.5 10.6***	151.8 14.9***	144.7 12.3**	137.1 9.8***	135.1 10.0***	133.7 10.4***
DBP (mmHg)	Before therapy	100.3 10.9	103.7 12.9	103.9 10.0	105.7 8.9	106.3 10.2	107.2 11.5	108.3 11.2	108.9 11.1	111.7 11.1	101.5 10.5	99.6 9.1	101.1 9.8	102.4 10.1	102.1 9.4
	Mefruside	91.3 9.3* *	93.7 9.9* *	97.9 9.7 **	99.9 11.6 *	100.9 10.2 *	100.9 10.6 *	102.4 9.6 *	103.5 10.2 *	105.6 10.7 *	96.9 9.8 **	96.4 11.3 **	96 10.1 **	96.8 9.9 **	97.9 9.7 ***
	Acebutolol	82.0 9.5***	85.6 9.3***	86.7 7.9***	92.2 7.7***	93.1 7.9***	94.3 7.6**	*94.9 8.3***	95.9 7.9***	97.2 7.2***	84.5 10.0***	83.7 7.3***	83.3 6.9***	83.7 7.1***	83.5 7.5***
HR (bts/min)	Before therapy	63.8 16.0	71.1 18.6	63.6 12.0	93.5 17.6	98.4 17.7	102.4 17.2	106.7 17.6	112.3 19.3	117.1 19.4	80.1 20.6	74.9 18.1	74.7 17.1	73.7 17.2	73.3 15.6
	Mefruside	66.1 17	75.5 19.9	67.5 14.5	93.0 18.4	96.9 18.8	101.1 19.8	105.3 20.9	111.5 22.6	118.1 24.6	78.9 22.2	77.2 22.0	75.3 18.7	75.1 17.5	75.8 18.5
	Acebutolol	54.3 8.2*	59.7 10.3*	53.9 6.6**	78.4 10.4**	81.3 11.3**	84.3 11.5	88.9 12.6**	91.7 12.4**	95.4 13.1**	63.8 12.2*	61.1 10.9*	60.1 10.2	59.1 8.9*	59.1 9.1*

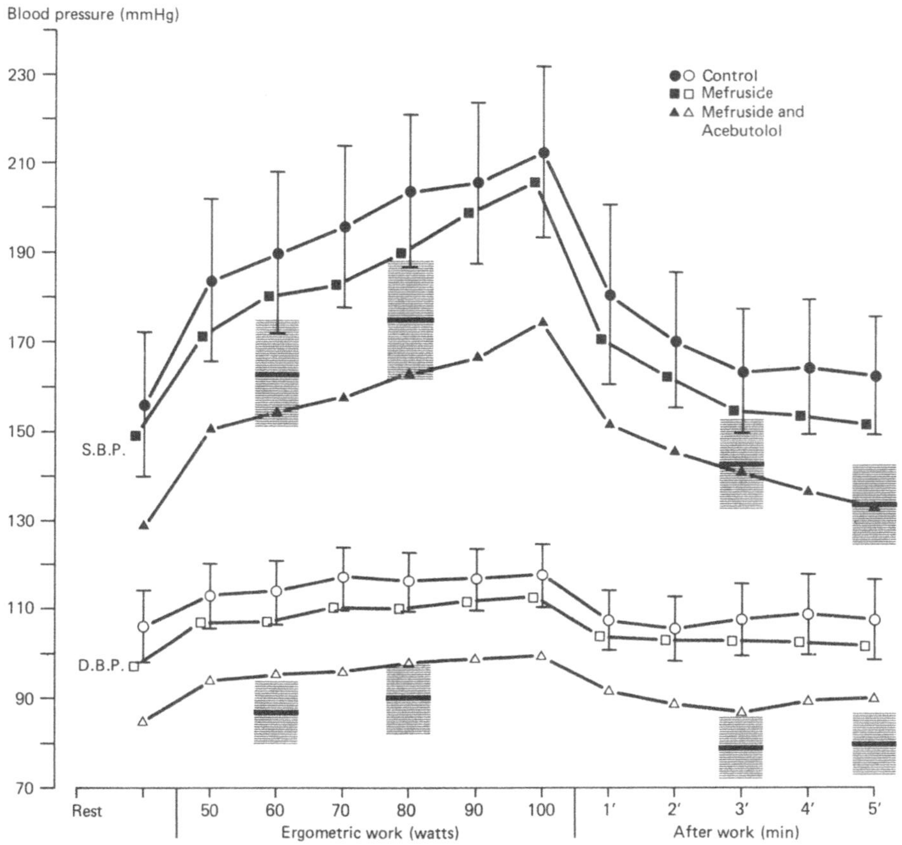

Fig. 57. Blood pressures and heart rates of 15 hypertensives before and during 4 weeks' therapy with 25 mg mefruside followed by treatment with 25 mg mefruside and 400 mg acebutolol (group 2, n = 15) for an additional 4 weeks. The bars indicate normal blood pressure ranges

er hand, produced significant systolic ($p<0.001$) and diastolic pressure lowering ($p<0.001$) compared with control tests and mefruside therapy (systolic $p<0.01$-$p<0.001$, diastolic $p<0.05$). Similar differences in blood pressure patterns were present during the recovery period.

The *heart rate* was not affected by mefruside, while *acebutolol* lowered the heart rate by 19.6% at rest and by 16.8 and 20.7% during and after ergometry.

In group 2 (Table 46, Fig. 57) mefruside also significantly lowered the systolic ($p<0.05$) and diastolic pressures ($p<0.01$) at rest. However, the *combination* of acebutolol and mefruside was significantly more effective in lowering both the systolic ($p<0.01$) and diastolic pressures ($p<0.001$). During ergometry, the diuretic alone was unable to lower the systolic or diastolic blood pressure significantly, just as in group 1. The same applied to the immediate postexercise period. By contrast, the combination of acebutolol and mefruside produced a highly significantly fall in systolic ($p<0.001$) and diastolic ($p<0.001$) pressure during exercise in comparison with control readings and mefruside therapy alone (systolic $p<0.001$, diastolic $p<0.001$). Both the systolic and diastolic pressures

Table 46. Blood pressures and heart rates (means ± SD) of 15 hypertensives before and during 4 weeks' therapy with 25 mg mefruside followed by treatment with 25 mg and 400 mg acebutolol (group 2) (*p<0.05; **p<0.001; ***p<0.001)

	n=15 Group 2	Rest			Ergometric work (watts)						Recovery period (min)				
		Supine	Standing	Before work	50	60	70	80	90	100	1	2	3	4	5
SBP (mmHg)	Before therapy	155.8	157.3	163.3	183.5	190.1	196.4	204.3	205.9	212.9	180.7	170.7	163.7	164.7	163.1
		15.6	15.8	18.0	17.5	17.7	17.7	16.7	17.9	18.5	19.6	14.6	14.2	14.6	12.9
	Mefruside	148.9	142.1	148.3	170.7	179.5	182.8	190.4	198.8	205.5	171.1	163.2	154.5	153.6	152.0
		14.0*	17.1*	13*	11.7*	12.0	11.3*	14.3*	15.2	15.6	14.2	12.3	13.8	13.0	12.9
		**	**	*	***	***	***	***	***	***	***	**	*	**	***
	Mefruside and acebutolol	129.4	124.3	135.5	150.9	154.5	158.0	163.1	168.1	175.2	151.6	145.7	141.7	136.9	134.4
		10.4***	12.8***	12.6***	11.7***	12.6***	12.7***	13.8***	14.6***	14.6***	15.2***	19.9***	14.3***	13.4***	12.3***
DBP (mmHg)	Before therapy	106.1	110.6	109.3	112.5	114.4	116.8	116.0	117.3	118.3	108.0	106.0	108.3	109.1	108.4
		8.4	7.9	6.5	6.7	7.2	6.8	7.1	7.4	6.8	7.3	7.2	8.4	8.8	8.6
	Mefruside	96.5	97.9	101.5	107.2	107.2	109.7	110.3	112.1	113.2	103.5	103.2	102.8	102.9	102.1
		9.2**	9.4***	9.0*	9.2	7.7*	9.8*	8.8	8.6	8.7	7.6	7.2	8.7	9.5	9.2
		***	***	***	***	***	***	***	***	***	***	***	***	***	***
	Mefruside and acebutolol	85.1	84.3	90.0	94.3	95.3	95.7	97.6	99.7	99.9	91.5	89.2	88.4	89.9	89.5
		6.0***	6.4***	7.4***	9.9***	9.2***	9.7***	9.1***	8.3***	8.6***	8.8***	9.0***	8.5***	7.5***	8.7***
HR (bts/min)	Before therapy	65.3	72.1	65.8	95.7	99.9	106.2	110.7	116.1	120.6	83.4	81.6	75.6	76.5	77.3
		9.5	12.1	11.1	12.9	13.9	15.6	17.0	17.6	17.2	17.4	15.0	16.1	13.1	13.3
	Mefruside	67.2	74.3	68.7	91.9	98.4	102.3	107.3	112.7	117.3	84.8	81.1	78.2	78.2	76.7
		11.6	16.2	10.0	9.6	9.5	10.7	11.5	12.8	15.0	14.4	13.2	13.2	11.4	11.6
	Mefruside and acebutolol	55.7	61.8	55.0	79.1	83.4	86.6	90.9	94.7	99.5	70.1	64.5	64.3	63.0	62.4
		9.2**	9.7**	8.2**	10.1***	10.7***	10.6***	10.9***	11.8***	13.1***	13.9*	10.7***	10.6*	9.2*	10.4*

Table 47. Percentage reduction of systolic (Δ S.B.P.) and diastolic (Δ D.B.P.) blood pressures and heart rates (Δ H.R.) by 4 weeks' therapy with 400 mg acebutolol (group 1) and a combination of 400 mg acebutolol and 25 mg mefruside (group 2)

n=30		Rest	Ergometry	Recovery period
		Supine/standing	50-100 W	1-5 min
Δ SBP	Group 1	16.3	16.1	13.9
	n=15	1.2	1.2	1.3
	Group 2	18.3	18.7	15.7
	n=15	2.3**	1.0***	1.7**
Δ DBP	Group 1	17.4	12.4	17.4
	n=15	0.9	0.9	1.0
	Group 2	20.4	16.2	17.0
	n=15	3.1**	1.1***	1.1
Δ HR	Group 1	19.6	16.8	20.7
	n=15	2.1	1.0	2.0
	Group 2	15.1	17.3	17.8
	n=15	1.2	0.9	2.4

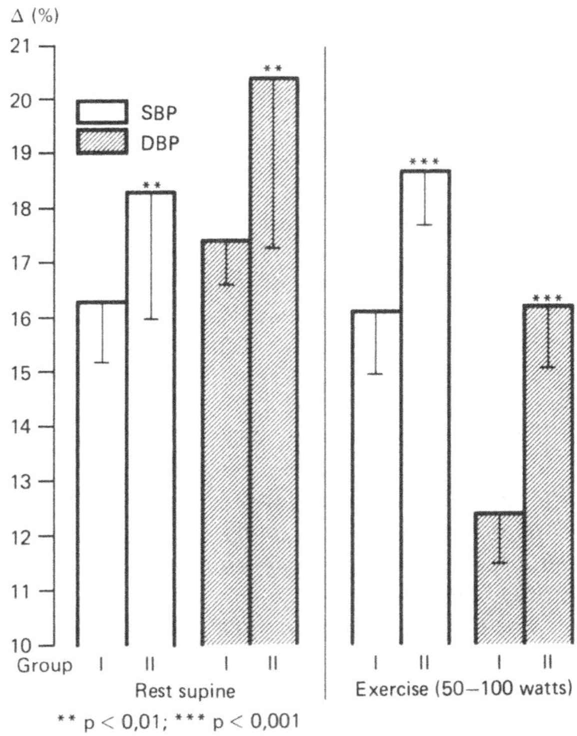

Fig. 58. Percentage reduction of systolic and diastolic blood pressure by 4 weeks' therapy with 400 mg acebutolol (group 1) and a combination of 400 mg acebutolol and 25 mg mefruside (group 2)

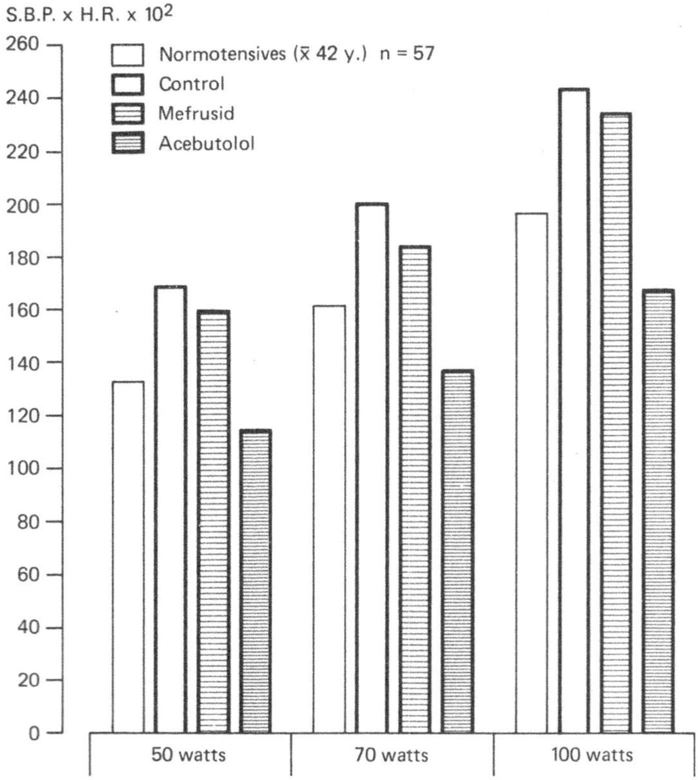

Fig. 59. Effect of 4 weeks' therapy with 25 mg mefruside or 400 mg acebutolol on the rate-pressure product in 15 hypertensives

were lowered into the normotensive range. By the 4th minute after exercise the systolic and diastolic pressures had returned to the high normal range.

When the patients were randomly assigned to groups, it happened that group 2 (height 174 ± 10.3 cm, weight 80 ± 12 kg) had a higher mean blood pressure than group 1 (height 178 ± 7.7 cm, weight 78.5 ± 8.7 kg) at rest and especially during exercise, e.g., 213/118 mm Hg vs. 207/112 mm Hg at 100 watts. Nevertheless, the absolute values of systolic and diastolic blood pressure after the second four-week course of therapy were nearly identical in both groups before, during and after exercise. In other words, the patients in group 2 experienced a virtually identical normalization of blood pressure despite their higher initial readings.

The obvious conclusion to be drawn is that the diuretic enhanced the antihypertensive effect of the beta-blocking drug. This is particularly evident when we compare the therapeutic responses in groups 1 and 2 before, during and after ergometry (Table 47, Fig. 58). At all times the percentage reduction of systolic and diastolic blood pressure on concurrent acebutolol and mefruside therapy in group 2 was significantly ($p < 0.001$) greater than that afforded by beta-blockade alone in group 1. This discrepancy of responses cannot be attributed to

Table 48. Blood pressures and heart rates (means ± SD) of 12 hypertensives (group 3) before and during 4 weeks' therapy with the free combination of 400 mg acebutolol and 25 mg mefruside compared with the fixed combination of 400 mg acebutolol and 20 mg mefruside (*p < 0.05; **p < 0.01; ***p < 0.001)

	Group 3	Rest			Ergometric work (watts)			Recovery period		
		Supine	Standing	Before work	60	80	100	1	3	5
SBP (mmHg)	Before therapy	159.2	157.3	167	195.8	208.5	220.5	196.2	171.3	165.8
		11.7	16.7	18.4	19.0	18.0	15.9	19.2	14.1	14.3
	free combination	136.2	130.2	142	162.8	173.5	187.0	163.5	149.8	142
		14.6***	12.8***	14.4***	16.7***	17.7***	11.7***	10.3***	10.6***	13.1***
	fixed combination	130.5	125.8	137.3	164.3	172.2	185.0	161.0	145.5	136.2
		13.6***	13.8***	10.8***	14.1***	13.6***	13.3***	14.3***	10.0***	10.4***
DBP (mmHg)	Before therapy	104.2	106.9	113.0	120.0	121.7	124.2	110.2	110.0	110.5
		7.1	7.7	9.4	12.2	8.1	10.1	8.2	7.9	10.3
	free combination	89.8	89.5	95.3	101.5	103.7	107.7	97.7	93.5	93.8
		9.3***	9.2***	9.5***	10.8***	10.5***	8.1***	10.2***	10.3***	10.1***
	fixed combination	84.7	86.2	93.0	99.0	103.3	106.2	96.5	92.7	91.0
		9.9***	9.6***	8.8***	10.0***	8.4***	9.2***	8.3***	9.0***	8.6***
HR (bts/min)	Before therapy	67.3	72.0	67.4	98.9	110.4	121.0	87.7	76.9	77.3
		10.8	13.8	12.2	12.6	13.3	13.9	19.2	16.7	14.0
	free combination	60.5	64.3	60.3	86.3	93.4	102.1	72.3	66.6	66.2
		11.9	11.4	11.8	10.6*	10.0**	9.1**	10.7	11.5	10.1
	fixed combination	59.0	63.6	57.3	85.3	93.5	101.6	71.7	65.6	63.6
		10.8	11.4	12.3*	10.4*	10.0**	10.6**	12.5*	11.9	12.4

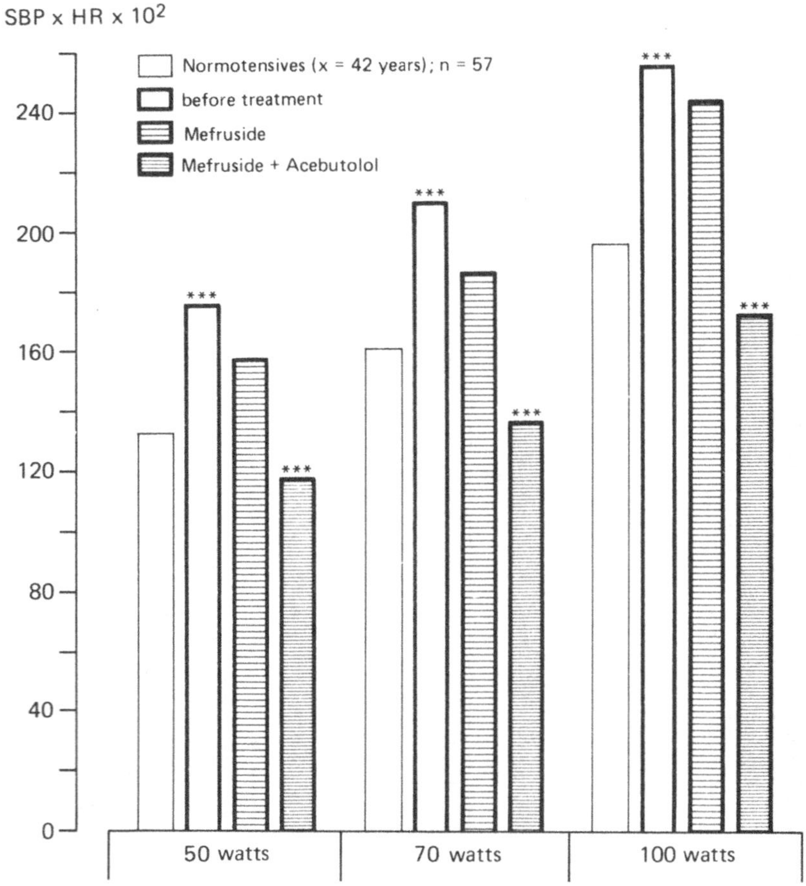

Fig. 60. Effect of 4 weeks' therapy with 25 mg mefruside or 400 mg acebutolol on the rate-pressure product in 15 hypertensives

changes in body weight, as we see from a comparison of the mean body weights of group 1 (78.2 ± 9.3 kg on mefruside, 77.9 ± 9.9 kg on acebutolol) and group 2 (79.3 ± 12.3 kg on mefruside, 79.7 ± 12.2 kg on mefruside and acebutolol). Moreover, no individuals in either group had a weight gain or loss in excess of 1 kg.

In group 3, where we compared the antihypertensive efficacies of the free combination of 400 mg acebutolol and 25 mg mefruside and a fixed combination containing 400 mg acebutolol and 20 mg mefruside (Table 48), we observed no significant differences in blood pressure responses before, during or after ergometry. The systolic and diastolic pressures were significantly lowered ($p < 0.001$) during all phases of the test.

4.2.3. *Effect on Myocardial Oxygen Consumption*

Table 49 and Figs. 59 and 60 show the rate-pressure product as a measure of myocardial oxygen consumption prior to therapy. The results, presented separately for groups 1 and 2, consistently show that the myocardial oxygen consumption, which was markedly elevated before therapy, was not significantly reduced by *diuretic therapy.* On the other hand, both acebutolol and the acebutolol-mefruside combination lowered myocardial oxygen demand at rest (by 30.2 and 30.6%, respectively), during ergometry (32.1 and 33%), and in the first minute of recovery (32.4 and 29.7%) to a highly significant degree ($p<0.001$).

Table 49. Effect of 4 weeks' therapy with 25 mg mefruside or 400 mg acebutolol on the rate-pressure product in 30 hypertensives

Rate-pressure product	Before work	Ergometric work (watts)			Recovery period (min)
		50	70	100	
Group 1 n=15 Before therapy	10192 3106	16930 4881	19935 4867	24305 4914	14564 3764
25 mg Mefruside	9486 2396 **	15920 4337 ***	18447 4532 ***	23362 5498 ***	13167 3600 **
400 mg Acebutolol	7119 1136**	11562 1421***	13703 1665***	16666 2338***	9853 1568***
Group 2 n=15 Before therapy	10307 1792	17616 3158	20952 4061	25528 5508	15139 3659
25 mg Mefruside	9996 1939 ***	15720 2234 ***	18704 2422 ***	24452 3731 ***	14523 2841 ***
25 mg Mefruside and 400 mg acebutolol	7150 1442***	11923 1729***	13686 2017***	17368 2796***	10651 1942***

4.3. Fixed Combination of Timolol and Hydrochlorothiazide/Amiloride Hydrochloride

As we have seen, it is not always possible to normalize the blood pressure with beta-blockers alone (s. Chap. 3.1.1. and 3.2.). Bühler [58] reports that treatment with beta-blockers alone will provide satisfactory control in only about 44% of hypertensives, and that a combination of drugs will usually be required. In these cases a combination product composed of a beta-blocker and diuretic is often the agent of choice, for the need to take only one tablet daily encourages better compliance. In this study we wished not only to investigate the efficacy and tolerance of the fixed combination, but also to learn whether the ergometric testing of antihypertensive effect would permit a meaningful assessment of the dose-response relationship.

4.3.1. Patients and Methods

We tested the antihypertensive efficacy and tolerance of a fixed beta-blocker-diuretic combination containing 10 mg timolol maleate and 25 mg hydrochlorothiazide and 2.5 mg amiloride hydrochloride [121]. Our subjects consisted of 32 patients (29 men, 3 women) ranging in age from 22 to 50 (average age 40.1) with WHO Stage I or II essential arterial hypertension. The patients had a mean blood pressure of 164/107 mm Hg based on multiple determinations at rest. The mean pressure of 231/127 mm Hg at 100 watts of exercise was also markedly elevated.

None of the patients had received antihypertensive therapy prior to the study.

After preliminary exercise testing a total of 21 patients were treated with 1 tablet of the fixed combination per day, and 11 patients were treated with 2 tablets daily. After an average course of 7.5 weeks (4–16 weeks) the patients were retested on the ergometer under identical standardized conditions. All blood pressures were taken by the same examiner using the same calibrated mercury manometer.

All ergometric tests were conducted between 3:30 and 6:00 p.m., always corresponding to the time of preliminary testing. The total daily dose was taken in the morning.

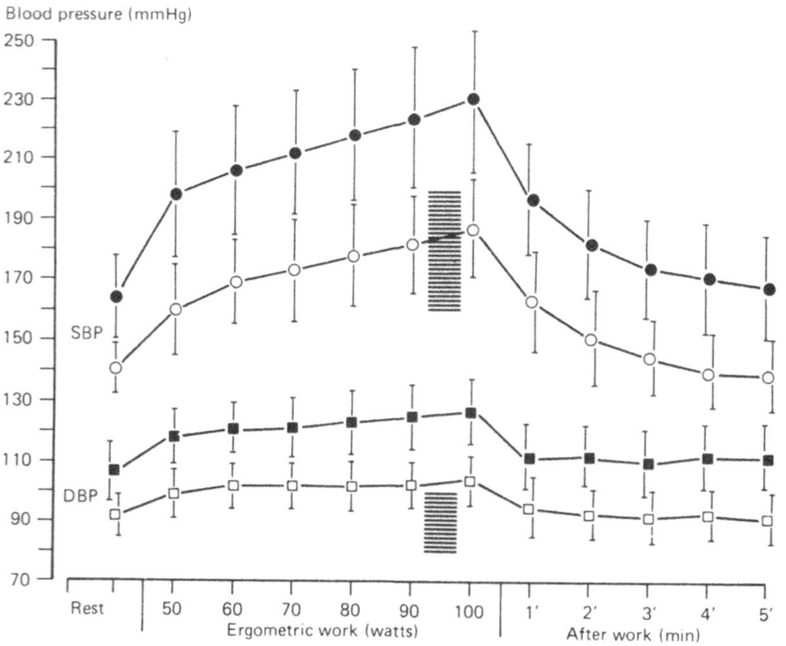

Fig. 61. Blood pressures of 32 younger hypertensives (average age 40.1 years) before (solid symbols) and during (open symbols) several weeks' combined antihypertensive therapy with timolol and hydrochlorothiazide/amiloride. The bars indicate normal blood pressure range at 100 watts

4.3.2. Blood Pressure and Heart Rate Responses

Fig. 61 shows the systolic and diastolic blood pressures of all 32 patients in supine rest and during and after exgometry. Before the start of therapy the patients had a mean blood pressure of 231 ± 26/127 ± 11 mm Hg at 100 watts - well above the normal limit of 200/100 mm Hg.

During therapy the systolic blood pressure was lowered significantly ($p < 0.001$) both at rest and especially during and after exercise, when it entered the normotensive range. The diastolic pressure was also significantly lowered ($p < 0.001$), becoming normotensive before and after exercise. The diastolic pressure remained above the normal range during exercise.

Tables 50 and 51 show the results for patients who responded satisfactorily to 1 tablet (group 1, n = 21; Table 50) and patients who required 2 tablets of the fixed combination to achieve an adequate antihypertensive effect (group 1, n = 11; Table 51).

It is apparent that a single tablet in group 1 was sufficient to produce a normotensive systolic blood pressure under all test conditions and even to lower the markedly elevated diastolic pressure to a highly significant degree ($p < 0.001$), bringing it almost into the normotensive range.

Group 2 had significantly higher systolic and diastolic pressures ($p < 0.01$) before, during and after exercise compared with group 1, e.g., 248.8/135 mm

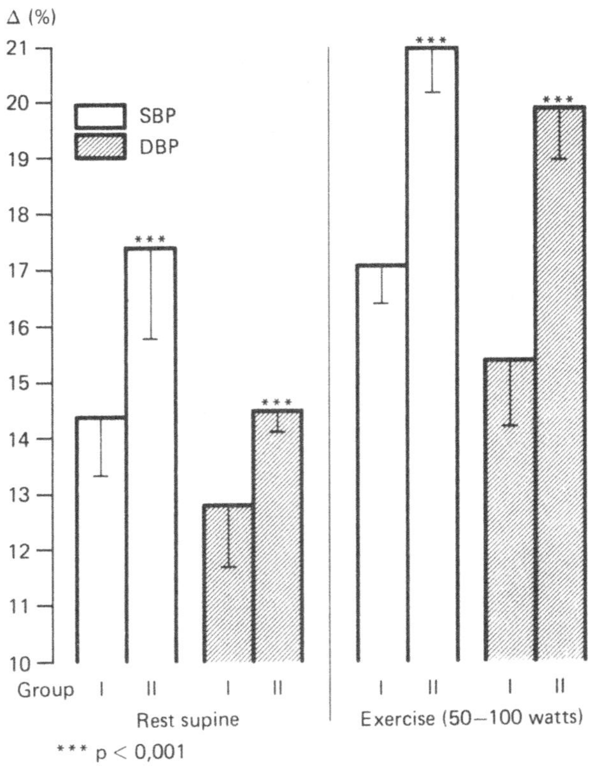

Fig. 62. Percentage reduction of systolic and diastolic blood pressure and of heart rate [sic] by different doses of a fixed beta blocker-diuretic combination (group 1, 1 × 1 tablet; group 2, 2 × 1 tablet)

Table 50. Blood pressures and heart rates (means ± SD) of 21 hypertensives (group 1) before and during therapy with the fixed combination of 10 mg timolol and 25 mg hydrochlorothiazide and 2.5 mg amiloride (***p < 0.001)

	n = 21	Rest		Ergometric work (watts)						Recovery period (min)				
		Supine	Standing	50	60	70	80	90	100	1	2	3	4	5
SBD (mmHg)	Before therapy	160.7	164.1	189.7	198.5	204.9	210.2	215.7	222.5	191.6	177.6	169.2	166.6	163.5
		10.4	20.0	15.4	17.0	17.5	18.3	18.2	21.6	16.0	14.2	10.9	14.8	11.5
	Therapy	148.8	139.4	156.6	166.6	168.6	175.4	178.7	182.7	159.5	149.2	144.5	147.4	146.2
		2.6***	11.6***	12.1***	11.7***	11.5***	13.4***	12.8***	13.7***	15.1***	14.8***	9.4***	7.5***	8.4***
DBP (mmHg)	Before therapy	105.6	109.4	115.3	117.5	117.6	120.0	121.3	123.9	108.8	109.1	107.2	108.8	107.9
		6.9	10.9	8.4	6.7	8.5	9.0	8.7	9.1	10.2	9.2	10.0	10.7	10.4
	Therapy	91.2	96.1	98.1	100.9	100.9	101.2	101.4	102.6	93.3	92.7	91.7	92.2	90.9
		6.9***	9.8***	8.5***	6.8***	7.7***	6.6***	7.3***	7.3***	7.3***	7.8***	7.0***	6.3***	7.5***
HR (bts/min)	Before therapy	91.6	81.5	101.9	106.9	111.4	117.1	122.4	128.1	96.7	89.1	86.1	85.0	84.5
		12.3	14.2	17.5	18.4	19.8	20.9	22.2	22.6	23.0	21.8	19.4	19.7	18.2
	Therapy	57.5	63.0	82.7	86.7	90.0	94.9	98.3	103.7	72.1	69.2	67.4	68.9	68.2
		9.2***	11.2***	12.1***	11.7***	13.2***	14.4***	14.3***	15.7***	14.3***	14.0***	13.7***	14.3***	14.2***

Table 51. Blood pressures and heart rates (means ± SD) of 11 hypertensives (group 2) before and during therapy with 20 mg timolol and 50 mg hydrochlorothiazide and 5 mg amiloride

	n = 11	Rest		Ergometric work (watts)						Recovery period (min)				
		Supine	Standing	50	60	70	80	90	100	1	2	3	4	5
SBP (mmHg)	Before therapy	170.6	175.8	213.2	220.1	224.3	232.5	239.7	247.8	207.5	189.7	183.6	180.5	176.9
		17.2	21.5	22.4	23.9	21.6	22.5	24.9	28.1	20.1	21.3	20.1	22.3	21.5
	Therapy	143.0	143.3	167.5	173.6	180.7	183.5	188.0	195.6	168.2	155.1	147.3	143.6	144.9
		7.3***	6.9***	16.5***	17.5***	22.1***	23.0***	21.1***	19.1***	19.1***	18.9***	16.5***	17.0***	16.8***
DBP (mmHg)	Before therapy	110.0	114.7	124.1	126.5	128.6	130.2	131.6	134.6	117.8	116.4	116.4	117.1	118.4
		10.9	13.9	8.1	8.5	8.2	10.5	10.8	11.7	10.3	9.5	9.3	9.6	9.8
	Therapy	94.3	97.8	100.6	102.4	103.1	103.1	104.9	106.6	97.1	92.6	92.9	93.8	91.1
		6.4***	9.2***	7.0***	9.0***	9.0***	9.3***	9.9***	9.5***	13.1***	9.0***	11.5***	10.6***	11.8***
HR (bts/min)	Before therapy	79.5	89.2	112.0	115.2	120.4	123.9	128.5	133.7	104.5	98.8	95.5	94.1	93.6
		19.5	18.1	16.0	16.1	16.2	16.8	15.9	15.2	28.0	26.3	24.4	22.9	20.9
	Therapy	57.7	63.5	82.0	85.5	88.2	89.7	95.0	99.2	69.6	66.7	67.2	64.5	64.0
		7.5***	9.2***	7.9***	8.8***	7.7***	8.7***	7.6***	8.4***	11.8***	12.4***	12.3***	10.3***	10.8***

Table 52. Percentage reduction of systolic (Δ S.B.P.) and diastolic (Δ D.B.P.) blood pressure by different doses of a fixed betablocker-diuretic combination (group 1, 1 × 1 tablet; group 2, 2 × 1 tablet)

n = 32		Rest	Ergometry	Recovery period
		Supine/standing	50–100 watts	1–5 min
Δ SBP	Group 1 n = 21	14.4 ± 1.1	17.1 ± 0.7	16.4 ± 0.9
	Group 2 n = 11	17.4 ± 1.6	21.0 ± 0.8	19.1 ± 1.0
Δ DBP	Group 1 n = 21	12.8 ± 1.1	15.4 ± 1.2	15.0 ± 0.6
	Group 2 n = 11	14.5 ± 0.3	19.9 ± 0.9	20.2 ± 2.0
Δ HR	Group 1 n = 21	21.2 ± 2.1	19.3 ± 0.7	21.6 ± 2.1
	Group 2 n = 11	28.1 ± 1.0	26.6 ± 0.9	31.7 ± 1.4

Hg vs. 223/124 mm Hg at 100 watts. These higher blood pressure levels under all test conditions explain why these patients required higher-dosage antihypertensive therapy. The benefit of increasing the dosage to 2 tablets in these patients is demonstrated in Table 52 and Fig. 62, which show the mean, therapy-induced percentage reduction of systolic and diastolic blood pressure and heart rate that were achieved in groups 1 and 2. Besides the greater reduction of heart rate in group 2 ($p < 0.01$), which is to be expected, we find significantly greater systolic and diastolic pressure lowering ($p < 0.001$) in all phases of the test.

Despite the overall positive response to this fixed combination, three patients in group 2 additionally required a vasodilator to achieve optimum blood pressure lowering.

Side-effects were mild and infrequent and were characteristic of those caused by beta-blockade. In all patients adverse effects disappeared with continued treatment, aside from occasional instances of acrohypothermy, and there was no case where side-effects required dosage reduction or withdrawal of medication.

4.4. Fixed Combination of Acebutolol and Mefruside in Mild Hypertensives with Coronary Disease

4.4.1. Patients and Methods

A total of 20 mildly hypertensive patients with an average age of 52.9 ± 7 years participated in the study [139]. All had angiographically confirmed coronary heart disease. Two of the patients had single-vessel disease, 5 had 2-vessel disease, and 12 had 3-vessel disease; small-vessel disease was present in 1 patient. All the patients were mildly hypertensive at rest, and none had received prior

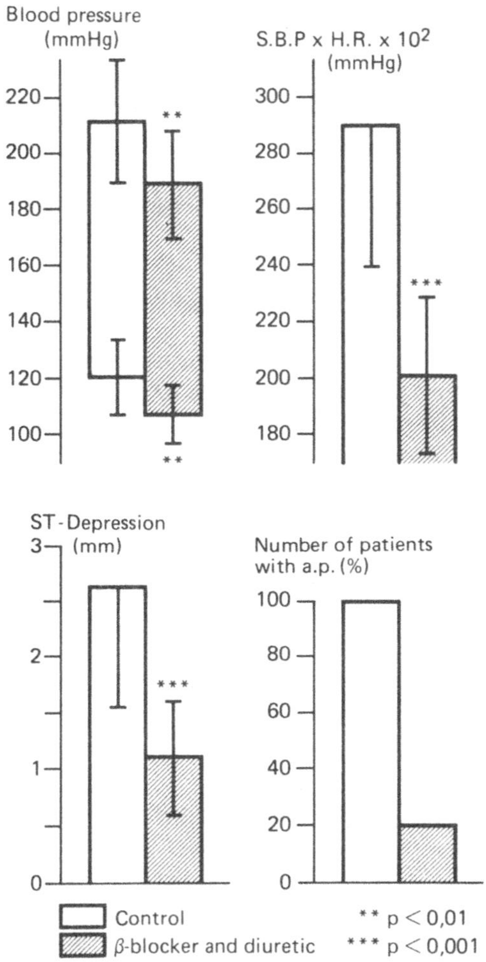

Fig. 63. Blood pressure, rate-pressure product, ST-depression and number of patients with angina pectoris before and after therapy with acebutolol and mefruside in hypertensives with coronary heart disease

antihypertensive drug therapy. All patients were experiencing angina pectoris during ordinary effort despite treatment with long-term nitrates. Our goal in these patients was to learn whether appropriate antihypertensive treatment with a beta-blocker-diuretic combination (400 mg acebutolol + 20 mg mefruside) could improve exercise tolerance in addition to normalizing the blood pressure.

Preliminary testing indicated that the patients had a mean exercise tolerance of 92 ± 25 watts. Ergometry had to be terminated in all patients because of anginal symptoms accompanied by significant ST-segment depression in the ECG. After preliminary testing the patients were treated for 4 weeks with the fixed beta-blocker-diuretic combination, composed of 400 mg acebutolol and 20 mg mefruside, and then retested both at rest and during exercise.

4.4.2. Blood Pressure and Heart Rate Responses

The mildly elevated resting blood pressure of 154 ± 16 mm Hg systolic, 97 ± 9 diastolic was normalized by therapy to 139 ± 14/86 ± 9 mm Hg. The mean blood pressure at the highest workload attained before treatment was 211 ± 22/120 ± 13 mm Hg (Fig. 63). This value was significantly lowered by therapy ($p < 0.001$) to 189 ± 19/107 ± 10 mm Hg. The exercise heart rate also was significantly decreased.

4.4.3. Effect on Myocardial Oxygen Consumption and ST-Segment Depression

The fall in blood pressure and heart rate resulted in a lowering of the rate-pressure product from 28.835 ± 4.900 mm Hg/min to 203012 mm Hg/min ± 2.800 mm Hg/min, representing a highly significant decline ($p < 0.001$). Accordingly, the ST-segment depression decreased from a mean value of 0.263 ± 0.11 mV to 0.113 ± 0.05 mV ($p < 0.001$). The clinical result was that 80% of the patients no longer suffered anginal pain at that level of exercise. The patients also had a much lower frequency of anginal complaints during ordinary exertion and had a reduced need for nitrate therapy.

5. Antihypertensive Effect of Vasodilators Compared with Beta-Blockers and their Combinations

5.1. Comparison of Prazosin and Acebutolol

5.1.1. Patients and Methods

We tested 24 patients (20 men, 4 women) ranging in age from 29 to 55 (average 43.3) who had WHO Stage I–II essential hypertension [134]. Average height was 174.8 ± 7 cm and average weight 66.8 ± 8.7 kg. We investigated and compared the antihypertensive efficacies of the beta-blocker acebutolol (400 mg/day taken once in the morning) and the α_1-blocker prazosin (4 mg/day divided between one morning and one noon dose) at rest and during ergometry. The patients were randomly assigned to 2 groups, with 12 patients started on the beta blocker and 12 on the vasodilator. After 4 weeks the patients were retested under identical conditions. Then the drugs were switched between groups, and this therapy was continued for an additional 4 weeks, whereupon testing was repeated.

5.1.2. Comparison of Monotherapies

Table 53 and Fig. 64 show that both the α_1-blocking drug prazosin and the beta-blocking drug acebutolol lowered the resting blood pressure significantly and to an approximately equal degree ($p < 0.05$–$p < 0.001$) in all pre-exercise resting

Table 53. Blood pressures and heart rates (means ± SD) of 24 hypertensives before and during 4 weeks' therapy with 400 mg acebutolol or 4 mg prazosin (*p < 0.05; **p < 0.01; ***p < 0.001).

	n = 24	Rest			Ergometric work (watts)			Recovery period (min)		
		Supine	Standing	Before work	60	80	100	1.	3.	5.
SBP (mmHg)	Before therapy	166.8 21.8	157.2 24.9	168.5 18.3	192.9 20.8	204.1 24.4	215.3 23.3	188 21.6	170.3 17.1	163.8 15.4
	4 mg Prazosin	150.3 17.3 **	139.2 15.5 **	155.4 17.4 *	182.8 20.9	196.9 22.9	208.3 19.6	181 20.1	161.1 16.4	152.8 15.3 *
	400 mg Acebutolol	145.6 23.4 **	139.7 24.3 *	152.1 25.1 *	167.0 21 ***	173.3 22 ***	182.9 21.9 ***	168.1 23.5 **	151.3 21.1 **	146.2 17.3 ***
DBP (mmHg)	Before therapy	107.7 10	108.2 11.3	110.6 10.3	116.9 10.9	119.8 12.8	122.5 11.7	109.8 10.8	110.3 9.1	109.7 10
	4 mg Prazosin	96.5 11.2 ***	92.6 10.4 ***	102.2 10.3 **	105.0 13 **	106.1 13.8 ***	107.7 14.1 ***	99.7 12.4 **	99.9 12.4 **	99.6 11.1 **
	400 mg Acebutolol	94.1 9.2 ***	94.8 10.2 ***	99.9 11 **	104.9 13.5 **	106.3 13.9 **	106.7 13.5 ***	100.6 12.5 **	97.9 11.4 ***	97.8 10.8 ***
HR (bts/min)	Before therapy	68.3 12.4	71.5 11	69.1 12.9	103.2 13.3	114.7 15.3	126.1 19.7	92 22.6	82 17.5	80 15.6
	4 mg Prazosin	71.8 11.9	82 17.6 *	71.7 13.1	108.5 16.2	117.7 19.5	128.4 21.5	96.2 23.8	85.9 19.8	84 17.9
	400 mg Acebutolol	57.0 5.4 ***	60.2 6.6 ***	59.3 6.7 **	87.1 8.7 ***	94 11.7 ***	102 12.7 ***	73.3 13 ***	67.1 10.5 ***	64.8 8.3 ***

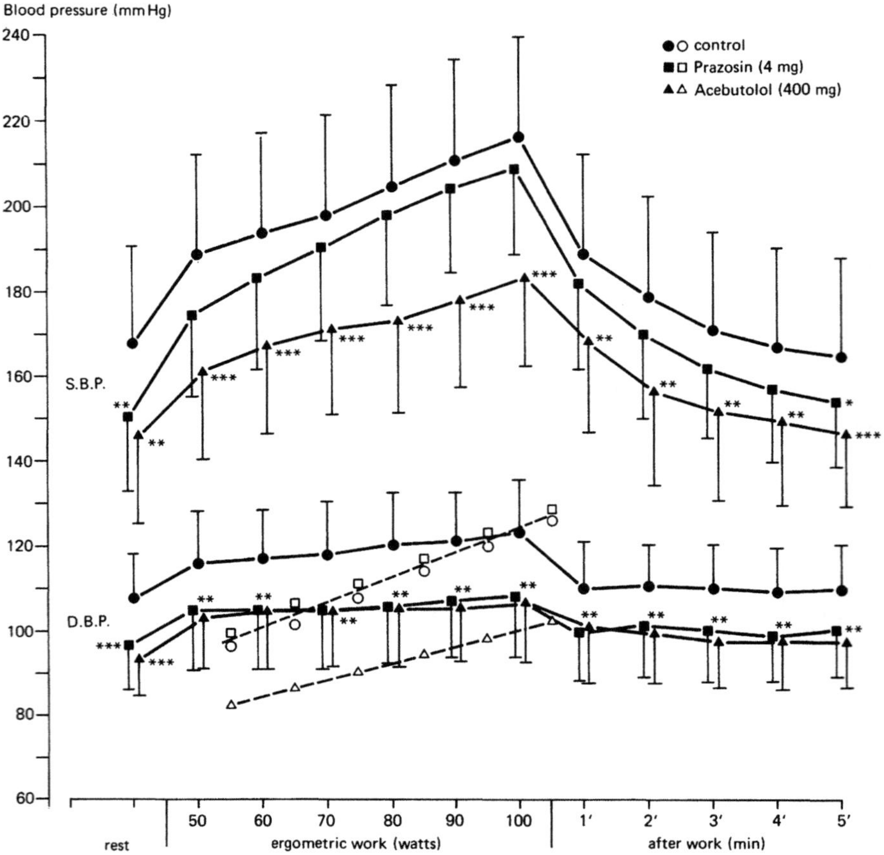

Fig. 64. Systolic (S. B. P.) and diastolic (D. B. P.) blood pressure at rest and during and after exercise in hypertensives before and after therapy with prazosin and acebutolol

states. Both drugs also produced significant diastolic lowering ($p<0.01$–$p<0.001$) during exercise and recovery. The drugs differed markedly in their effect on systolic pressure, however. Thus, prazosin did not produce significant systolic reduction during exercise, and the reduction in the 5th minute of recovery was barely significant ($p<0.05$).

By contrast, the beta blocker acebutolol produced highly significant ($p<0.001$) systolic lowering during and after exercise. Fig. 65 shows that the different effects of prazosin and acebutolol on the blood pressure at 100 watts were not based on the random grouping of the patients, nor were they the result of a carry-over effect. All 12 patients who were started on acebutolol had higher systolic pressures at 100 watts after they switched to prazosin. The reverse pattern was seen in patients who were started on prazosin, i. e., a lowering of the systolic pressure at 100 watts following treatment with the beta blocker. The diastolic reduction at 100 watts did not vary with the type of drug administered.

The greater antihypertensive effect of acebutolol on the systolic blood pressure cannot be attributed to body weight changes, as we realize when we com-

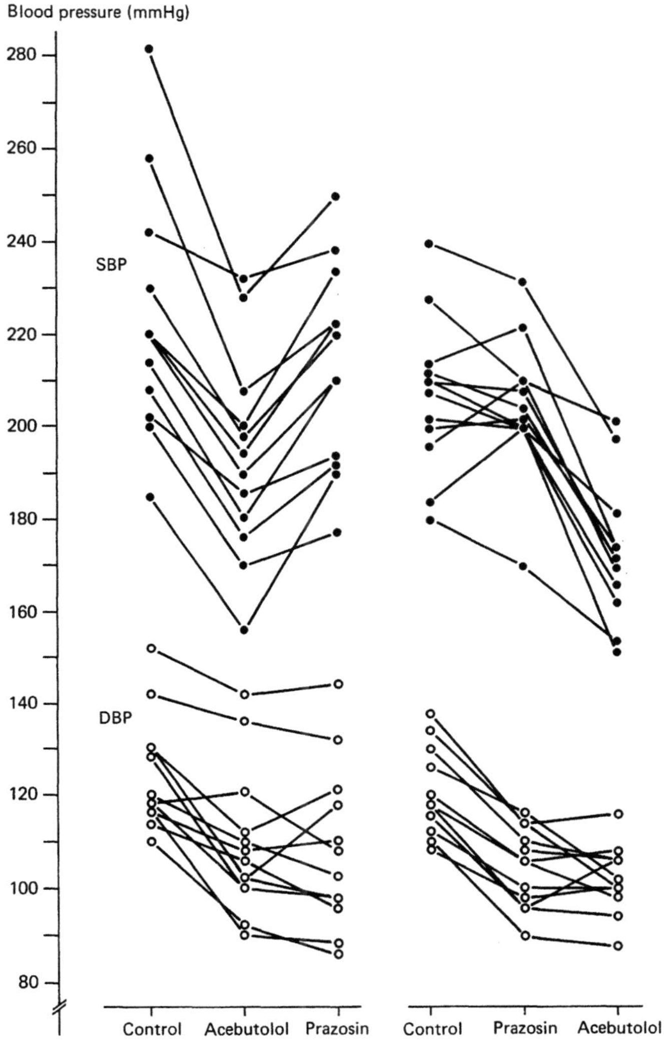

Fig. 65. Systolic (S. B. P.) and diastolic (D. B. P.) at a work load of 100 watts before and during treatment with acebutolol and prazosin. Left side: patients (n = 12) starting with acebutolol; Right side: patients (n = 12) starting with prazosin

pare the mean body weight before treatment, 76.8 ± 8.7 kg, with the body weight on prazosin, 77.9 ± 9 kg, and on acebutolol, 77.2 ± 8.5 kg. None of the patients showed more than a 1-kg gain or loss of weight during either course of therapy.

5.1.3. Efficacy of the Free Combination

Fig. 66 shows the pre-exercise, exercise and postexercise blood pressures of the eight patients who did not respond adequately to prazosin or acebutolol alone. While the monotherapy was unable to produce significant systolic or diastolic

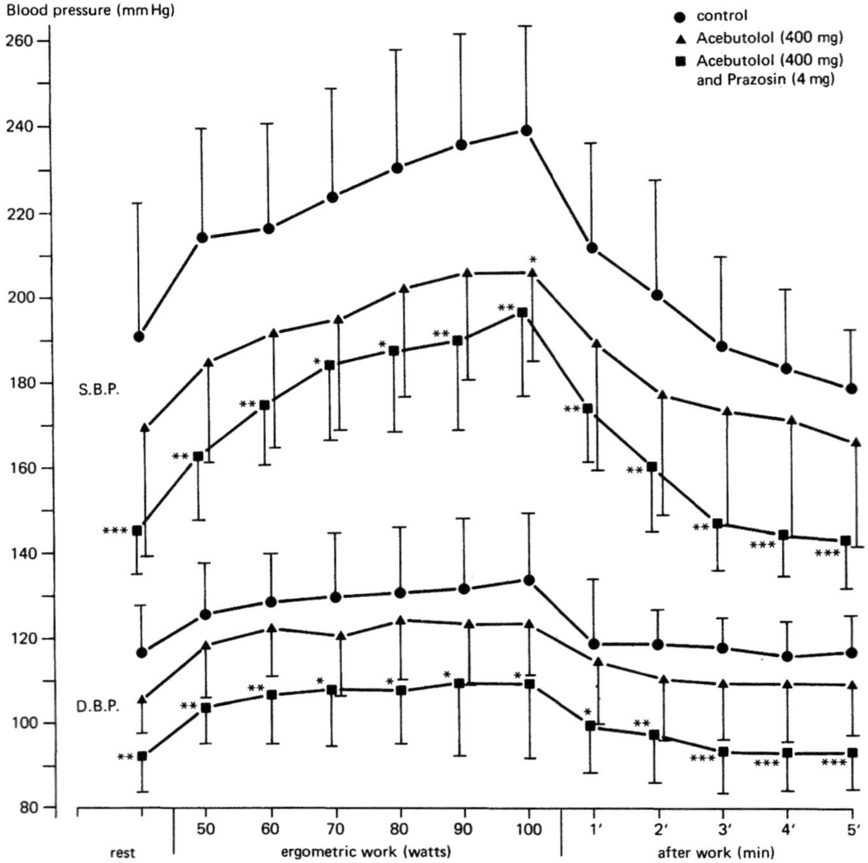

Fig. 66. Systolic (S. B. P.), diastolic (D. B. P.) blood pressure before and during treatment with monotherapy of acebutolol and in combination with prazosin

lowering before, during or after ergometry (except for the standing pressure), the concomitant administration of prazosin and acebutolol lowered the blood pressure significantly ($p<0.05$–$p<0.001$). The effect of this combination on both the systolic and diastolic pressure was not just additive but potentiated, creating a hypotensive effect which was greater than the sum of the individual drug actions under all test conditions.

5.1.4. Effect on Myocardial Oxygen Consumption

Fig. 67 show the effect of antihypertensive therapy with prazosin and acebutolol on the rate-pressure product, which reflects the level of myocardial oxygen uptake. Because prazosin has little influence on systolic blood pressure and none on the heart rate, there is no appreciable lowering of the rate-pressure product with this drug. This contrasts with the highly significant reduction ($p<0.001$) of the rate-pressure product that was obtained with acebutolol.

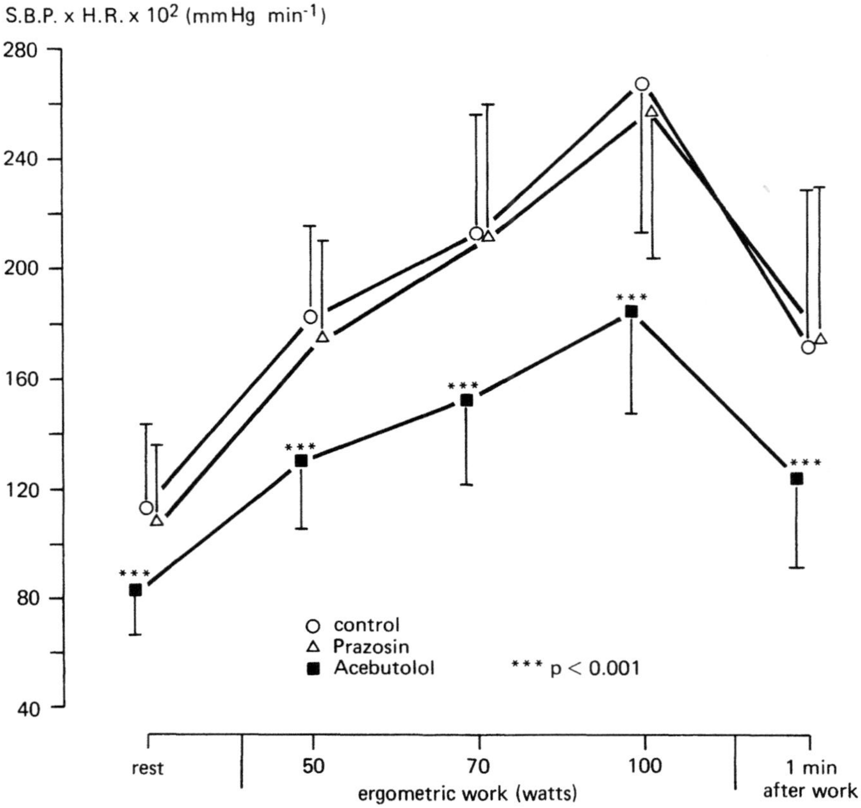

Fig. 67. Rate-pressure product at rest and during and after ergometry before (control) and after therapy with prazosin and acebutolol

5.2. Comparison of Nifedipine, Nitrendipine and Acebutolol

5.2.1. Patients and Methods

We first tested 35 patients (30 men, 5 women) with WHO Stage I-II essential arterial hypertension [135, 142]. The patients ranged in age from 19 to 58 (average age 43.3) and had an average height of 176.3 ± 7 cm and average weight of 80.4 ± 11.4 kg.

Before treatment was initiated the patients were tested twice at 14-day intervals both at rest and during ergometric exercise. The patients were then randomly assigned to 2 groups, and 18 were started on the calcium antagonist nitrendipine (20 mg) and 17 on the calcium antagonist nifedipine (40 mg in delayed release form). After four weeks the patients were retested at rest and during exercise, whereupon the drugs were switched and maintained for an additional four weeks, and testing was repeated. This was followed by a 14-day wash-out period without medication, after which the patients were examined for residual effects of the calcium antagonists, if any. Then the patients were started on a

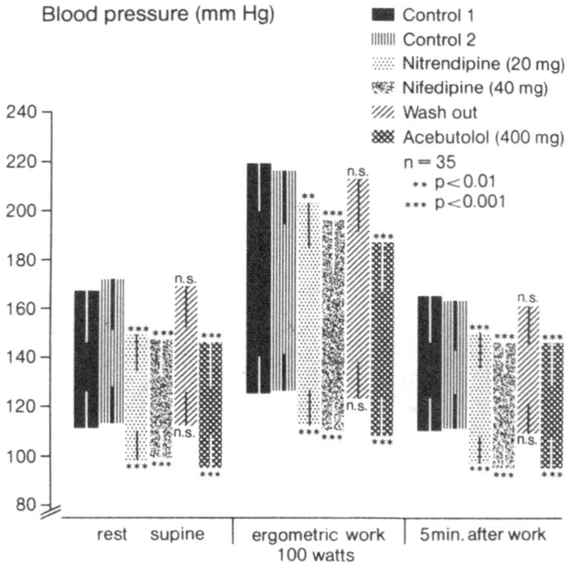

Fig. 68. Blood pressure (mean ± S.D.) at rest and during and after exercise before therapy (control 1 and 2) and under the action of nitrendipine, nifedipine and acebutolol and after a wash out period of 14 days

4-week course of therapy with the β_1-blocking drug acebutolol and retested after that time. Twenty patients whose blood pressures were not normalized by the monotherapy were treated concurrently with 400 mg acebutolol and 40 mg nifedipine for another 4 weeks.

We performed another ergometric study in 10 male subjects age 20–49 (average age 40.8) with WHO Stage I essential hypertension (height 176.8 ± 6.2 cm, weight 84.9 ± 9.5 kg). The men were randomly assigned to 2 groups, and 5 were started on a 4-week course of nifedipine, 40 mg taken once in the morning, and 5 on the beta blocker acebutolol taken in a single 400-mg dose. After four weeks the drugs were switched, followed by another four weeks of therapy. Resting and exercise blood pressures were determined before and during the two treatment periods. The effect of the drugs on the blood pressure response to isometric exercise was also evaluated in these patients.

5.2.2. Comparison of Monotherapies

As Table 54 and Fig. 68 indicate, the subjects showed no differences in their systolic and diastolic blood pressures during the initial 14-day control period without therapy, either at rest or at 100 watts of exercise.

During therapy both calcium antagonists significantly lowered the systolic and diastolic pressure at rest ($p < 0.001$) and the diastolic pressure during exercise ($p < 0.001$), producing an effect equivalent to that of the beta-blocker. The systolic pressure was also lowered significantly by nitrendepine ($p < 0.01$) and nifedipine ($p < 0.001$), although systolic lowering at 100 watts was more pronounced with acebutolol.

Testing after the 14-day wash-out period showed that both the resting and exercise blood pressures had returned to initial pretreatment levels, indicating

Table 54. Blood pressures and heart rates (means ± SD) of 36 hypertensives before treatment (twice at 14-day intervals) and during 4 weeks' therapy with 40 mg nifedipine, 20 mg nitrendipine, after a 14-day wash-out period and during a 4-week treatment period with acebutolol

	Rest						Ergometric work			Recovery period (min) 5 min		
	Supine			Standing								
	SBP	DBP	HR	SBP	DBP	HR	SBP	DBP	HR	SBP	DBP	HR
1st Examination	166,9	110,9	75,2	159,2	111,2	82,4	218,6	124,7	129,3	164,9	110,1	83,8
before therapy	20,9	14,7	12,4	17,2	13,3	11,6	19,7	14,5	20,3	18,8	12,7	18,9
2nd Examination	173,4	112,8	73,2	163,2	111,5	81,8	217,5	125,9	127,8	163,4	110,9	82,1
before therapy	21,0	15,0	14,6	18,4	14,0	15,3	21,0	14,9	22,6	19,6	13,5	18,2
40 mg	146,7	99,3	78,8	138,3	95,4	88,7	203,4	111,9	128,3	149,7	97,1	87,2
Nifedipine	15,0***	11,5**	11,2	12,9***	***	14,0	18,3**	15,3***	23,1	14,5***	11,2***	18,1
20 mg	149,1	97,8	75,9	142,0	96,3	86,0	196,2	109,7	127,2	145,6	95,3	83,9
Nitrendipine	16,1***	12,1***	12,0	15,2***	11,5***	13,9	22,1***	11,4***	21,5	13,4***	9,7***	15,5
Wash-out	168,5	111,9	71,3	159,2	109,9	79,9	212,7	123,1	123,4	160,5	109,0	77,3
	17,5	13,1	12,0	15,5	12,9	13,7	20,6	15,0	21,4	15,6	12,3	17,6
400 mg	145,8	95,4	62,5	139,8	93,4	68,7	186,9	108,1	100,4	145,7	95,2	66,5
Acebutolol	17,5***	12,5**	10,8***	17,3***	11,3***	11,4***	20,4***	14,5***	11,9	16,5***	11,6***	10,3***

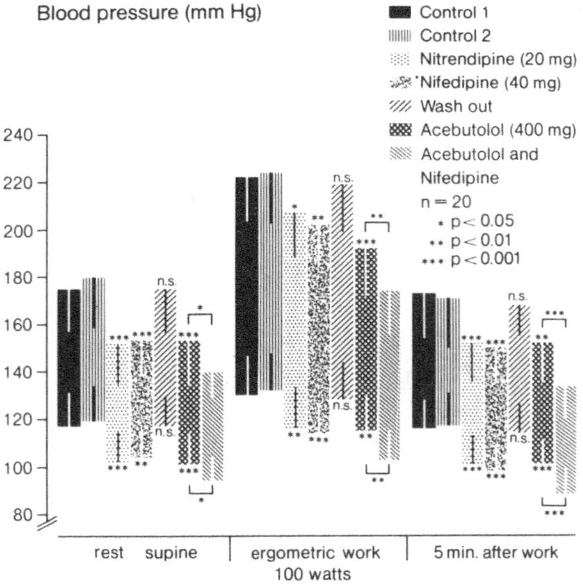

Fig. 69. Blood pressure (mean ± S.D.) at rest and during and after exercise before therapy (control 1 and 2) and under the action of nifedipine, acebutolol and their combination

that the effect of the calcium antagonists had subsided completely by that time. The systolic and diastolic pressures during the recovery period corresponded to readings obtained at rest prior to ergometry.

5.2.3. Efficacy of the Free Combination

Table 55 and Fig. 69 show the results for 20 hypertensive patients who were treated concomitantly with 400 mg acebutol and 40 mg nifedipine for an additional 4 weeks. The systolic and diastolic pressures at rest were lowered to a significantly greater degree ($p < 0.05$) with the combination than with beta blockade alone. This effect is more pronounced during ergometric exercise ($p < 0.01$) and is most conspicuous during postexercise recovery ($p < 0.001$).

5.2.4. Efficacy during Bicycle Ergometry and during Isometric Exercise

Table 56 and Fig. 70 show blood pressure variations before, during and after a 4-week course of acebutolol, 400 mg/day, and nifedipine, 40 mg/day, 2, 8 and 24 hours after the last tablet was taken [137]. At rest we find that the diastolic pressure was significantly ($p < 0.05$) lowered by both the beta blocker and the calcium antagonists even 24 hours after the last dose, whereas the systolic pressure, while 10 mm Hg lower, was not significantly decreased. Two hours after the last dose both classes of drugs lowered the diastolic pressure significantly ($p < 0.01$) and to an approximately equal degree. The systolic pressure was also significantly lowered by acebutolol ($p < 0.01$) and nifedipine ($p < 0.05$). Testing 8 hours after the last dose continued to demonstrate significant systolic and diastolic pressure control with both drugs; the therapeutic results at 2 and 8 hours

Table 55. Blood pressures and heart rates (means ± SD) of 20 hypertensives before treatment (twice at 14-day intervals) and during 4 weeks' therapy with 40 mg nifedipine, after a 14-day wash-out period, during 4 weeks' therapy with 400 mg acebutolol and the combination of acebutolol and nifedipine

	Rest						Ergometric work (100 watts)			Recovery period 5 min		
	Supine			Standing								
	SBP	DBP	HR	SBP	DBP	HR	SBP	DBP	HR	SBP	DBP	HR
1st examination before therapy	175,4 17,7	116,7 13,6	75,7 11,4	164,8 15,6	116,7 10,8	85,0 13,3	222,4 18,6	130,2 15,6	125,9 18,2	173,3 19,1	116,3 12,0	81,5 17,4
2nd examination before therapy	179,9 22,3	119,3 14,8	73,4 13,0	170,1 19,8	117,3 13,8	81,0 13,3	223,5 21,8	131,5 15,8	125,2 18,5	170,5 21,3	117,3 13,5	82,4 16,0
40 mg Nifedipine	153,2 14,7***	103,6 11,5**	80,2 11,2	142,2 13,3	99,2 12,5	90,9 14,1	202,1 17,6**	113,5 12,3***	128,5 21,4	150,1 14,8***	98,8 10,0***	89,6 16,7
Wash-out	174,5 18,6	116,8 12,8	70,6 12,1	162,7 17,3	114,7 12,6	80,2 14,0	218,9 19,9	128,3 15,8	121,7 17,3	167,6 14,9	114,4 12,1	76,2 15,2
400 mg Acebutolol	152,9 18,6***	100,8 13,1***	64,0 11,2	144,8 17,4	98,0 11,6	70,3 12,5	192,4 19,9***	114,8 **	99,9 10,5	152,1 17,1**	101,0 10,3***	66,9 10,5
40 mg Nifedipine and 400 mg Acebutolol	139,5 12,5*	91,9 9,5*	64,8 9,6	131,7 13,3	89,6 10,5	70,7 12,1	174,1 18,1**	102,3 12,0**	98,3 11,3	133,8 12,9***	88 10,2***	69,3 11,6

Table 56. Blood pressures (means ± SD) of 10 hypertensives before and during 4 weeks' therapy with 400 mg acebutolol and 40 mg nifedipine, 2, 8, and 24 hours after the last tablet was taken

mm Hg		Rest supine			Ergometric work 100 watts			Recovery period 5 min		
		Before therapy	Acebutolol	Nifedipine	Before therapy	Acebutolol	Nifedipine	Before therapy	Acebutolol	Nifedipine
8.00 and 10.00	SBP	149,9	140,6	140,0	191,4	173,8	183,6	152,8	137,8	145
a.m.		17,3	14,6	17,7	16,5	14,7*	17,5	18,0	10,4*	18,6
24 h after	DBP	108,6	96,9	97,1	116,2	101,2	108,2	106,4	93,4	100,6
drug intake		11,8	11,5*	10,9*	9,1	5,8***	11,5	11,5	8,5*	11,3
10.00 and	SBP	148	129,2	131,9	191,0	160,4	175,3	149	134,2	134,6
12.00 a.m.		16	12,2**	15,7*	15,7	12,9***	15,8*	13,3	9,7*	12,4*
2 h after	DBP	106,5	93,5	91,3	114,2	100,4	100,8	105,4	91,2	89,2
drug intake		11,5	8,4**	7,7**	9,1	6,7**	11,4**	9,4	7,8**	11,4**
4.00 and	SBP	146,1	132,1	133,7	195,8	168,4	188,6	153,4	133,4	141,4
6.00 p.m.		12,1	10,8*	10,6*	15,6	12,4***	18,7	12,2	9,6***	12,5*
8 h after	DBP	104,8	91,5	94	113,6	94,0	101,0	105,4	87,6	93,6
drug intake		8,3	7,6**	6,7**	6,9	4,7***	9,4	6,9	8,5**	8,8**

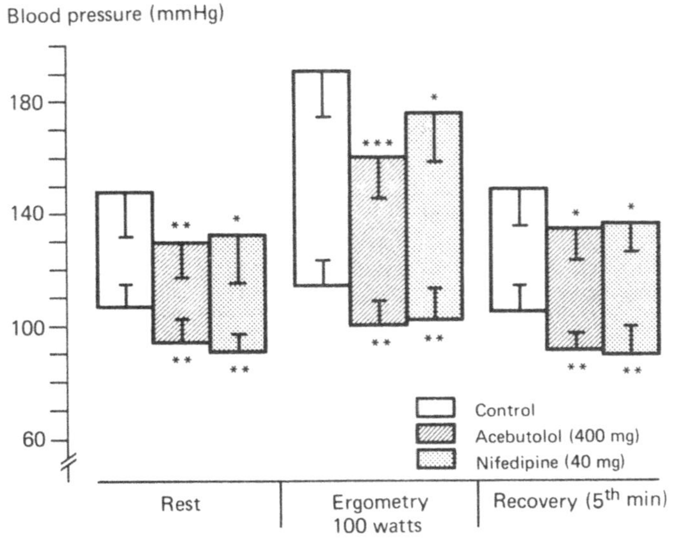

Fig. 70. Blood pressure (mean ± S. D.) at rest and during and after exercise before (control) and after therapy with acebutolol and nifedipine

after dosing were indistinguishable. It is interesting to note that the standing blood pressure at 8 hours after dosing was lowered more effectively by acebutolol than by nifedipine.

The systolic and especially the diastolic blood pressure at 100 watts of exercise were still at a significantly reduced level 24 hours after the last dose of acebutolol. Nifedipine had no such effect on either systolic or diastolic pressure. Two hours after medication both drugs lowered the diastolic pressure significantly ($p < 0.01$) and to an equivalent degree, as shown in Fig. 70. However, acebutolol produced a significantly greater systolic reduction ($p < 0.01$) than nifedipine ($p < 0.05$). At 8 hours, during exercise, nifedipine maintained the same diastolic reduction but could not check systolic elevation. Acebutolol, on the other hand, continued to maintain a systolic and diastolic reduction which was equivalent to its effect at two hours after dosing ($p < 0.001$). The results following ergometry corresponded roughly to the results in recumbency prior to exercise. Thus, the study confirms the results of our investigations comparing atenolol, nadolol and metoprolol. Acebutolol also maintained its full antihypertensive effect at 2 and 8 hours after the last dose; even at 24 hours the diastolic reduction was virtually unchanged, and systolic control was still effective and significant. The calcium antagonist nifedipine maintained roughly the same systolic and diastolic reductions during rest at 2 and 8 hours after last dosing. Nifedipine could not control the systolic elevation during exercise 8 hours after dosing. It produced roughly equal diastolic reductions during exercise at 2 and 8 hours, but the reduction at 24 hours with nifedipine was not significant.

Table 57 and Fig. 71 show the effect of acebutolol and nifedipine on the blood pressure response to isometric exercise, which involved holding a 2.4-kg

Table 57. Blood pressures (means ± SD) of 10 hypertensives at rest (standing) and after 1 min holding a 1.2 or 2.4 kg weight in the left hand with the arm extended horizontally before therapy and after 4 weeks' therapy with 400 mg acebutolol and 40 mg nifedipine, 2 and 8 hours after the last tablet was taken

$\bar{x} \pm s$		Before therapy		Acebutolol		Nifedipine	
		Rest	1.2 kg	Rest	1.2 kg	Rest	1.2 kg
8.00 and	SBP	137,3	151,4	120,5	128,3	127,8	135,4
10.00 a.m.		16,3	18,5	9,9*	16,9**	14,9	14,6*
2 h after	DBP	105,6	115,0	92,2	102,6	91,7	100,6
drug intake		11,4	11,8	7,3**	9,7*	8,3**	10,9*
		Rest	2.4 kg	Rest	2.4 kg	Rest	2.4 kg
4.00 and 6.00 p.m.	SBP	139**	161,2	123	138,6	127,5	143,6
8 h after		12,4	19,4	8,9**	8,9**	10,2*	14,7*
drug intake	DBP	104,5***	118,2	88,8	106,4	94,7	107,6
		6,2	8,4	6,2***	6,0**	7,1**	8,9*

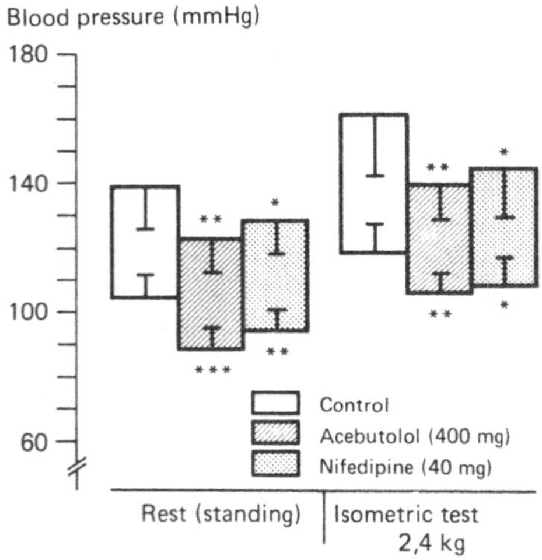

Fig. 71. Blood pressure (mean ± S.D.) at rest during isometric exercise before (control) and after therapy with acebutolol and nifedipine

weight in the left hand with the arm extended horizontally. Both acebutolol and nifedipine significantly lowered the systolic and diastolic pressure elevation after 1 minute of weight holding, with the beta blocker producing a greater systolic reduction. The holding of a 2.4-kg weight caused a significant rise in systolic and diastolic pressure prior to therapy. This elevation was still significantly depressed ($p<0.05$–$p<0.01$) 8 hours after the last dose of acebutolol and nifedipine. As before, the beta-blocker had a more pronounced effect on systolic pressure.

With chronic treatment, then, it is apparent that the beta-blocker can maintain effective blood pressure control during isometric exercise even 2 and 8 hours after the last dose is given. The calcium antagonist nifedipine was found to have an almost equal efficacy.

6. Summary and Conclusions Regarding Beta-Blockers, Diuretics and Vasodilators

6.1. Efficacy and Side-Effects of Beta-Blocking Drugs

Regardless of their *pharmacologic properties* with respect to cardioselectivity, the presence of a sympathomimetic or membranestabilizing action, and plasma half-life, all the beta-blocking drugs investigated here showed equal antihypertensive efficacies both at rest and during exercise when administered in equivalent doses. This was also true during submaximal exercise of longer duration. The results presented here agree closely with the results of Harry et al. [174], who found that four different beta blockers had equivalent effects during exercise.

The therapy-induced reductions of systolic and diastolic pressure demonstrated here by auscultatory blood pressure determinations have been confirmed by other authors using invasive techniques (Reybrouck et al. 351, Lund-Johansen 283, Atterhög et al. 18).

The results presented here on the *duration of the antihypertensive effect* of a single morning dose of a beta blocker during chronic therapy are of major relevance to the practical management of hypertension. Despite differences in their half-lives and plasma levels, all three beta blockers lowered the blood pressure and heart rate significantly and to an equal degree two and eight hours after the last dose was taken. This was true both at rest and during ergometry. Even after 24 hours the diastolic pressure was still virtually unchanged. As for the systolic pressure and heart rate, metoprolol maintained a 49.3% reduction during exercise 24 hours after the last dose compared with its effect at 2 and 8 hours, while atenolol maintained a 58.9% reduction, and nadolol showed no diminution of effect. Corresponding results were obtained for acebutolol.

Rowlands showed that beta-blockers not only lower the blood pressure significantly during submaximal exercise but also lower the mean 24-hour intra-arterial blood pressure profile, resulting in a significant reduction of the left ventricular muscle mass as established by echocardiography [363]. The favorable effect of beta-blockers on the daily blood pressure profile has also been confirmed by Mann et al. [289] and Floras et al. [100] by intra-arterial monitoring.

We see, then, that beta-blocking drugs lower the blood pressure throughout the day without *subsidence of effect,* regardless of their pharmacologic properties, even when given in a single morning dose. This is true at rest and, more importantly, during physical and emotional stress. It should be pointed out that exertional blood pressure increases associated with everyday activities may be caused both by dynamic exercise, as exemplified by bicycle ergometry, and by isometric exercise in which a large force component is involved in muscular contractions. While ergometric blood pressure testing provides a basis for assessing the pressor response to isometric exercise and emotional stress, the therapeutic effects demonstrated during ergometry cannot be applied directly to other forms of stress.

Follow-up studies after one year of beta-blockade have shown no *development of tolerance*. That is, the same doses produced the same antihypertensive effect before, during and after exercise following one year of therapy [118, 143].

The efficacy of antihypertensive therapy also depends in large part on the *frequency of side-effects*. Numerous reports in the literature point to only about a 10% incidence of side-effects with beta-blocking drugs [58, 161, 228]. Other *sympatholytic drugs* cause side-effects in up to 30–50% of patients treated [161, 340]. Diuretics also have been associated with a significantly higher rate of side-effects, such as impotence, than beta-blocking drugs, as indicated by a major English study published in 1981. The most frequently reported side-effect with beta-blockers is increased intestinal motility [165], but this often disappears with continued treatment. A more serious problems relates to the exacerbation of bronchial obstruction in asthmatic individuals. Possible bradycardiac complications and negative inotropic effects are discussed in Chap. IV.6.2.

Beta-blocking drugs also differ from other antihypertensive agents in that they are free of familiar side-effects such as orthostatic or postexertional hypotension. It is particularly noteworthy that beta-blockers do not hamper *driving ability* and can even significantly enhance mental alertness [311]. In addition,

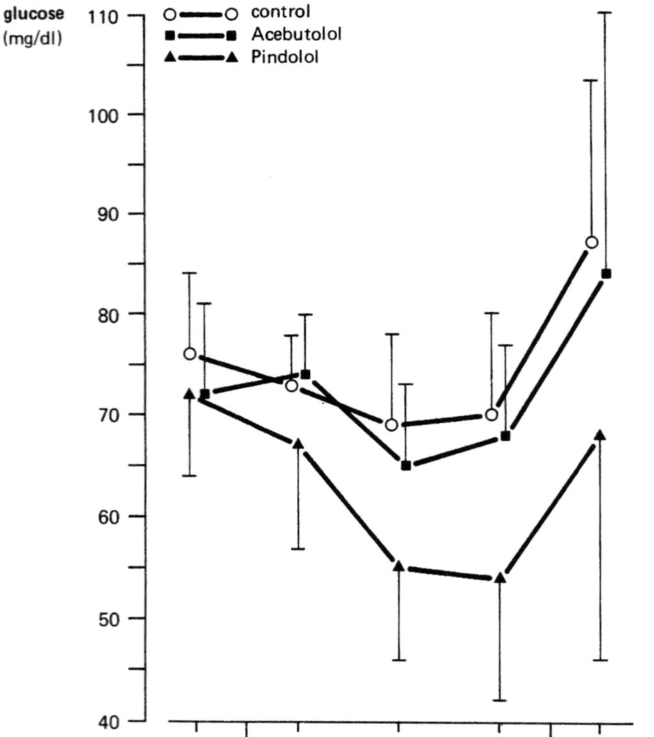

Fig. 72. Blood glucose before and during 4 weeks' therapy with 500 mg acebutolol or 15 mg pindolol at rest and during and after ergometry

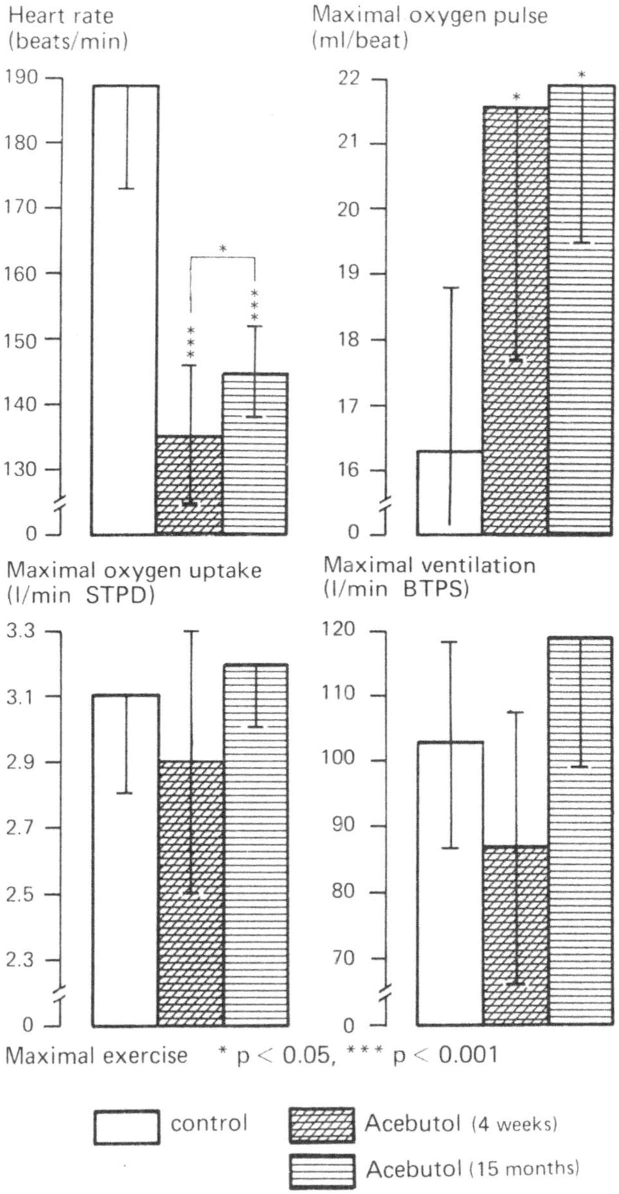

Fig. 73. Heart rate, maximal oxygen uptake, maximal oxygen pulse and maximal ventilation before (control) and after 4 weeks and 15 months of treatment with 500 mg acebutolol in 9 hypertensive patients

the *cardioselective beta-blockers* do not affect *physical performance* owing to the maintenance of an adequate *oxygen uptake* and unaltered *energy metabolism* [15, 111, 115, 126, 143].

As Fig. 72 shows, however, the β_1–β_2 blocker pindolol, unlike the cardioselective β_1-blocker acebutolol, causes a precipitous fall of the *blood glucose* during sustained submaximal exertion [111, 120], because *carbohydrate release* in the skeletal muscles is mediated predominantly by β_2-receptors [11]. The elevated *plasma epinephrine concentration* demonstrated in this study [126] and the marked rise of *adrenocorticotropic hormone* [120] which occurred with *pindolol* alone are viewed as an attempt to compensate for the restriction of *glycogenolysis,* which is more pronounced than with the β_1-selective blocker acebutolol, and thus to forestall *hypoglycemia.* This disturbance of *carbohydrate metabolism* by β_1-β_2 blockers also leads to a restriction of physical performance and accounts for the *muscle pains* reported by some patients. This is reasonable when one considers that oxygen uptake in the submaximal range is not affected by either class of beta blocker [111, 126], but that *maximal oxygen uptake* is reduced by 14% after 4 weeks on the nonselective beta blocker pindolol, compared to only 5% with the β_1-selective acebutolol [126]. After 16 months (Fig. 73), acebutolol no longer has any demonstrable effect on maximal oxygen uptake in WHO Stage I hypertensives [143].

Several reports have been published dealing with the effect of beta blockers on *lipid metabolism* [38, 140, 267]. However, it appears unlikely that this effect is of clinical importance as a cardiovascular risk factor, and long-term studies are needed to resolve the issue. For the present, it appears prudent to check for lipid metabolism disturbances routinely when beta-blockers are used on a long-term basis [140].

The comparative studies presented here on the effect of diuretics and beta-blockers on the pressor response to exercise clearly show that diuretics and the vasodilator prazosin, like many other antihypertensive agents (see Chap. III.2.), are unable to control systolic elevations satisfactorily during exercise and are obviously inferior to beta-blocking drugs. The poor control of exercise blood pressures by diuretics was confirmed by Midekke et al. [305] and Lorimer et al. [275]. Their studies showed that only beta-blocking drugs could significantly lower the rate-pressure product in during exercise and thus reduce the level of myocardial oxygen consumption. It is noteworthy that under conditions of rest, the diuretics, prazosin and the beta-blockers lowered blood pressure significantly and to an approximately equal degree. This is consistent with the findings of Silvertson et al. [393], who compared the effects of 25 mg/day mefruside with 100–400 mg/day atenolol. Lowering of the resting blood pressure by these drugs was found to be equivalent following 6 weeks and 6 months of therapy. Treatment with the diuretic mefruside lowered the resting blood pressure from 172/103 mm Hg to 147/93 mm Hg, while the beta-blocker atenolol lowered pressure from 179/104 to 145/88 mm Hg in a comparable group.

Numerous other studies in many countries have shown that beta-blocking drugs and diuretics are roughly equally effective in lowering mildly to moderately elevated blood pressures at rest [14, 57, 72, 75, 116, 134, 145, 222, 242, 301, 337]. Hence, both classes of drugs are considered to be of equal value in the monotherapy of mild to moderate arterial hypertension.

6.2. Cardioprotective Effect of Beta-Blocking Drugs

An important consideration in hypertensive patients is the fact that the principal risk to these patients is posed not by the level of the resting blood pressure, but by the frequency, magnitude and persistence of blood pressure elevations caused by everyday stresses. This is obvious with regard to the danger of acute events in hypertensives with coronary disease, but it applies equally to the progression of vascular complications (s. Chap. III.1.). The failure of diuretics, prazosin, alpha methyldopa, reserpine and clonidine to control blood pressure during stress is of major clinical relevance not only to all hypertensives who are physically active on the job and in their leisure time, but most especially to patients who have coexisting coronary heart disease and who have embarked upon a rehabilitative training program or other form of exercise therapy. For these patients, an inordinate rise in blood pressure during exercise is considered to be associated with a heightened *cardiovascular risk,* despite treatment with drugs which lower only the resting blood pressure, due to the increased *myocardial oxygen demand* which accompanies the high exercise pressures. Considering the fact that latent or symptomatic coronary artery stenoses are present in a sizable percentage of hypertensive patients [334], we can see that these persons are particularly threatened by an excessive rise in blood pressure during stress.

With regard to myocardial oxygen demand, the significant lowering of the systolic and diastolic blood pressure and of the *rate-pressure product* during and after exercise by *beta-blocking drugs* assumes particular significance. This has been demonstrated convincingly by our own studies in coronary patients with mild hypertension (s. Chap. III.4.4.).

It is interesting to speculate as to why, in recent studies involving treatment mainly with *beta-blockers,* it was possible to decrease morbidity and mortality from myocardial infarction in hypertensives [32, 263, 405, 412]. Earlier studies based chiefly on the use of diuretics revealed the surprising fact that, despite a significant decline in total mortality, antihypertensive treatment was unable to reduce the *incidence of myocardial infarctions* among hypertensive patients [26, 191, 430–433]. This fact has also been confirmed by a more recent clinical study using thiazide diuretics [309].

One possible explanation relates to the electrophysiologic properties of beta-adrenergic blocking drugs [276, 385] and their favorable effect on *free fatty acids* [322] and the *plasma potassium level.* A number of studies have shown that *diuretic-induced hypokalemia* can increase the likelihood of severe *cardiac arrhythmias* [194, 419]. Holland et al. [194] reported that of 21 patients without coronary heart disease who were taking 50 mg hydrochlorothiazide twice daily for their hypertension, 7 developed complex, high Lown-grade ventricular ectopic beats, which responded well to subsequent treatment with spironolactone.

Because earlier studies were based mainly on treatment with diuretics, Glück et al. [155] believed that the failure of the therapy with respect to coronary heart disease could be attributed to the adverse effect of diuretics on the *lipoprotein fractions* [5, 309].

This explanation is called into question by studies showing that *beta-blockers* likewise have a negative effect on the lipoprotein fractions [38, 140, 267]. Yet, as recent studies attest, the total infarction rate and the rate of fatal myocardial infarctions are significantly reduced in hypertensives treated with beta-blocking drugs [263]. The Goteborg study [32] showed that antihypertensive therapy with beta-blockers was effective in preventing serious cardiovascular complications over a 4.3-year follow-up period in patients 47 to 54 years of age. It was also shown that the mortality after myocardial infarction was significantly reduced by beta-blockers, regardless of whether arterial hypertension was present [6, 8].

It is quite possible that the different effects of beta-blockers and diuretics on the progression of coronary heart disease relate to their different effects on the *blood pressure response to stress.* Indeed, this appears to be the most probable explanation when one considers that the risk in coronary patients is determined in part by the severity of the myocardial hypoxia, which in turn depends on the value of the rate-pressure product. As we have seen, the rate-pressure product is significantly lowered by beta-blocking drugs, while it is unaffected by diuretics, prazosin, reserpine, etc. Thus, a patient on diuretic therapy alone is more apt to exceed the tolerance limit for hypoxia, thereby increasing his proneness to myocardial infarction or a fatal hypoxia-induced arrhythmia.

In a prospective study of 169 hypertensives with no recognizable coronary disease, Stewart [405] found that the 121 patients treated with beta-blockers had a 5-year first infarction rate of 7.5%, which was significantly below the 31% rate among 48 patients who had received conventional antihypertensive agents.

The significant risk of *fatal cardiac arrhythmias* in *coronary patients* has been well documented [36]. Studies by Baroldi et al. [25] have shown that this risk is by no means lessened in persons whose coronary disease is asymptomatic. They reported on 208 persons who died suddenly and unexpectedly before witnesses. All were engaged in their usual activities at the time of death; none had a history of coronary disease, and so none were under medical supervision. Of the 208 patients who died suddenly, 157 were found to have severe degrees of coronary stenosis (single-vessel disease in 53, 2-vessel disease in 60, 3-vessel disease in 44), 23 had moderate degrees of stenosis, and 28 showed no evidence of coronary disease. Acute infarction was the presumed cause of death in only 35 patients. These results not only serve to underscore the danger of sudden death from hypoxia-induced arrhythmias, but also remind us that there may be no premonitory symptoms which alert the patient to the danger - one that is present in a large percentage of hypertensives in the form of coronary heart disease [334]. The pronounced reduction of stress blood pressures and thus of hypoxia-related complications may well account for the *cardioprotective effect* of *beta-blocking drugs* in the treatment of hypertension (s. Chap. III.6.3.).

6.3. Importance of Combined Beta Blocker-Diuretic Therapy

In an article published in the *American Journal of Cardiology* in 1974, Gross [163] presented a list of requirements which should be met by the ideal antihypertensive drug. The "ideal" drug should:

1. Produce a decrease in blood pressure that is reliable, of gradual onset, and similar in the supine and standing positions.

2. Have a duration of action between 12 and 24 hours.
3. Be active when taken orally.
4. Cause no negative inotropic cardiac effects and no tachycardia.
5. Cause no tolerance.
6. Cause no or only mild side-effects and no impairment of physical or mental capacity.
7. Be suitable for long-term use.

If one evalutes the beta-blocking drugs in the light of these criteria, one must conclude that they satisfy almost all requirements. This is not to say the "ideal" antihypertensive agent has been found, however. Treatment with *beta-blockers alone* will provide adequate blood pressure control in only about 40% of patients [58]. Prichard [338] states that poor individual responses to beta-blockers are the result of *water retention.*

Of particular interest in this regard are studies done by Rasmussen et al. [343] in 1979 on extracellular fluid volumes in hypertensives treated with beta blockers. In the beta-blocker responders the extracellular fluid volume was increased insignificantly by 205 ml, while the *nonresponders* showed a highly significant, 6% increase of 1025 ml. It is significant that the nonresponders in this study were 20 years older on average than the responders. By combining the beta-blocker with a diuretic in the nonresponding group, it was possible to normalize both the blood pressure and the extracellular fluid volume. It appears, then, that a large percentage of patients, and especially the elderly, will require a combination of beta-blockade and diuretic therapy to achieve an optimum result.

Thus, the special importance of diuretics in antihypertensive therapy is their excellent combinability with beta-blocking drugs [107, 116, 121, 122, 127, 189, 312, 321, 341, 436, 446]. As the studies presented here have shown, diuretics definitely enhance the antihypertensive effect of beta-blockers not only at rest but most especially during stress, as evidenced by the significantly greater degree of diastolic pressure lowering achieved during and after exercise stress testing. This has been demonstrated for the free combination of the beta-blocker acebutolol with hydrochlorothiazide/amiloride or with mefruside.

To explain the enhanced antihypertensive activity of beta-blockers and diuretics administered concurrently, we may invoke the fundamentally different *mechanisms of action* of the two classes of drugs. Hemodynamic studies have shown that beta-blockers cause little or no decrease in the elevated peripheral vascular resistance which is characteristic of arterial hypertension, even with long-term use [277, 280, 281, 283, 368, 415]. It has also been shown that some beta-blockers can raise the *norepinephrine concentration* in the plasma during physical exertion [115, 118, 162, 171, 207, 327]. This could cause an alpha-receptor-mediated constriction of the arterioles, which in turn would raise the total peripheral resistance. On the other hand diuretics can reduce vascular resistance [279], possibly by reducing the effect of noradrenaline on smooth muscles [329]. Moreover β-receptor blockers counterbalance the increase of renin during diuretic therapy [56, 114] and the decrease in potassium [194, 419]. β-receptor blockers also decrease the platelet aggregation [55].

In addition, the study on the fixed combination of timolol and hydrochlorothiazide/amiloride clearly showed that a combination can have good antihypertensive efficacy even when given in relatively small individual doses [107, 121]. The small doses, in turn, result in milder side-effects.

Fig. 64 shows that 4 weeks' treatment with 4 mg prazosin provides a significant ($p<0.01$–$p<0.001$) and satisfactory reduction of the resting blood pressure, comparable to that of a 4-week course of 400 mg acebutolol. However, the systolic pressure during exercise is not significantly influenced compared with beta-blockade. Prazosin does produce a highly significant ($p<0.001$) diastolic pressure reduction of 15 mm Hg, which corresponds to a 12.2% decrease and is substantially greater than the mean 5% reduction obtained with diuretics.

Based on the studies of Lund-Johansen [277], Äarynen et al. [1] and our own results, the main role of prazosin appears to be as an adjunct to beta-blocker therapy. Prazosin has been shown to enhance significantly the antihypertensive effect of beta-blockers on systolic and diastolic pressures during dynamic exercise (Fig. 66), producing a reduction greater than that obtained with a combination of diuretics and beta-blockade.

Monotherapeutic trials with calcium antagonists demonstrated a significant lowering of the systolic and diastolic blood pressure at rest. Calcium antagonists also lowered the systolic pressure significantly during exercise, as confirmed by Ekelund et al. [92], Buchanan et al. [54] and Gould et al. [159], but not to the degree observed with beta-blockers.

Nifedipine and nitrendipine significantly lowered the diastolic blood pressure by 16 and 17 mm Hg, respectively, at 100 watts and thus slightly exceeded the 12.2% reduction obtained with prazosin. It appears, then, that calcium antagonists may offer an alternative antihypertensive monotherapy in cases where beta blockers are contraindicated. In addition, the concomitant use of beta-blockers and nifedipine has proved to be a highly effective (Fig. 69) and well tolerated regimen which has shown greater antihypertensive activity than the combined use of beta-blockers and diuretics. This seems to apply particularly to the more severe forms of hypertension with higher diastolic elevations, which is consistent with the findings of Harris et al. [173].

6.4. Evaluation of Monotherapy and Combined Therapy

Our results clearly indicate that the ergometric monitoring of antihypertensive therapy is capable of answering two questions which have great relevance to daily practice:

1. Is it necessary or beneficial to increase the dosage of a drug already being taken?
2. Is it necessary to add a second antihypertensive drug, and does that drug improve response?

It is not surprising that *ergometry* is so useful in this kind of decision making, because, as stated earlier, the resting blood pressure is subject to emotional influences even in patients who are on *antihypertensive medication,* since the patient may experience some degree of anxiety as awaits the result of treatment.

6.5. Conclusions

1. Hypertensives are jeopardized not only by their elevated resting blood pressure but most especially by the excessive blood pressure increases that may be elicited by everyday stresses. It must be remembered that the level of the resting blood pressure is a poor predictor of the blood pressure response to stress and thus of the vascular risk that is present.
2. If ergometric stress testing shows excessive blood pressure rises in the range from 50 to 100 watts, appropriate antihypertensive therapy should be initiated, particularly if coronary disease is also detected.
3. It is important to realize that a satisfactory antihypertensive effect in the resting state does not mean that the blood pressure will be adequately controlled in exercise. This explains the need for ergometric stress testing to evaluate the antihypertensive efficacy of a particular therapy. The results will aid the physician in adjusting the dosage of a single drug or deciding whether a combination of drugs is needed.
4. Diuretics, reserpine, alpha methyldopa, clonidine and prazosin have no significant effect on the systolic elevation during exercise. The alpha-blocking drug prazosin produces a marked fall of diastolic pressure during exercise, which is more pronounced than that obtained with diuretics.
5. The calcium antagonist nifedipine substantially lowers the diastolic pressure during exercise with an effect similar to that of prazosin. Nifedipine also produces significant systolic lowering during exercise, but less than that obtained with the beta-blockers.
6. Beta-blockers produce the greatest degree of systolic and diastolic blood pressure lowering during dynamic exercise. With chronic use beta-blockers also lower the systolic and diastolic pressure during *isometric exercise* and in situations of *emotional stress* [93].
7. With chronic use beta-blockers produce a reduction of blood pressure and heart rate which is equivalent 2 and 8 hours after the last oral dose, regardless of differences in the pharmacologic characteristics of the drugs. This means that there is no diminution of effect during the course of the day.
8. The antihypertensive effect of beta blockers during exercise is significantly enhanced by diuretics. This effect is even more pronounced when beta-blockers are combined with nifedipine or prazosin.
9. Beta-blockers alone are capable of controlling blood pressure and reducing myocardial oxygen consumption during both dynamic and isometric exercise as well as during emotional stress.
10. Because the cardiovascular risk of arterial hypertension is determined not only by the blood pressure elevation at rest but also by the magnitude of the pressor response to stress, the beta-blocker should be considered an agent of first choice for the mono- or combined therapy of hypertension. If contraindications to beta-blockers exist, calcium antagonists may become increasingly attractive as an alternative.

7. Beta-Blocking Drugs and Diuretics for the Treatment of Hypertension in the Elderly

As the results in Chap. II.3.2., 6.1. and 7.1. indicate, late middle-aged and elderly hypertensives are apt to experience the most *severe blood pressure elevations during stress,* accompanied by a marked rise in myocardial oxygen consumption. Because sequelae of arterial hypertension may already be presumed to exist in older hypertensives, an exaggerated pressor response to exercise is associated with a serious risk of *myocardial hypoxia* and *cerebrovascular complications* in this group. Nowadays it is customary to start antihypertensive treatment in older patients with an oral diuretic. However, because diuretics cannot significantly lower stress-induced blood pressure elevations (s. Chap. IV.4.), we tested a total of 43 hypertensive patients ranging in age from 51 to 74 to determine whether the excellent results of combined beta-blocker and diuretic therapy in younger patients could be reproduced in older subjects. Besides the effects of treatment on blood pressure response and myocardial oxygen consumption (and thus on ST-segment depressions caused by ischemia), particular attention was given to the possible occurrence of ECG changes indicative of bradycardiac rhythm abnormalities.

7.1. Fixed Combination of Metipranolol and Butizide

7.1.1. Patients and Methods

We first tested 13 patients (12 men and 1 women) between 51 and 65 years of age (average age 56.1) with WHO Stage I-II essential hypertension [108].

Following preliminary testing without antihypertensive medication, 11 of the patients were given one tablet daily of a combination product containing 20 mg of the beta-blocker metipranolol and 2.5 mg of the diuretic butizide. The remaining two patients were given the same product but were instructed to take two tablets daily.

The patients were retested twice during therapy, once after 6 weeks and again after 6 months, under the same standardized conditions.

7.1.2. Blood Pressure and Heart Rate Responses

After only 6 weeks of therapy we observed a highly significant ($p < 0.001$) reduction of the systolic and diastolic blood pressure before, during and after ergometry (Table 58, Fig. 74). The resting heart rate before and after exercise was also significantly lowered ($p < 0.05$–$p < 0.01$). Taking a value of 215/105 mm Hg as the upper limit of normal for the older patients at 100 watts of exercise (s. Chap. II.2.5.), we find that the therapy lowered the patients' blood pressures into the normotensive range both at rest and during exercise. Testing after 6 months of therapy demonstrated a lowering of blood pressure and heart rate virtually identical to that shown in Table 58.

Table 58. Blood pressures and heart rates (means ± SD) of 13 hypertensives before and during combined metipranolol (20 mg) and butizide (2.5 mg) therapy

		Rest	Ergometric work (watts)						Recovery period				
		supine	50	60	70	80	90	100	1.	2.	3.	4.	5.
SBP (mmHg)	Before therapy	174,2 16,5	193,4 18,0	207,9 19,4	212,8 20,4	222,5 19,5	230,0 16,9	238,9 17,8	217,0 21,8	200,7 15,5	190,4 18,3	184,5 16,5	177,7 16,0
	Metipranolol and Butizide	142,4 11,8***	156,8 17,3***	165,8 17,1***	172,9 20,3***	182,5 22,1***	191,5 21,7***	199,2 22,0***	171,0 21,8***	157,5 18,5***	149,9 16,8***	147,2 15,0***	140,0 14,2***
DBP (mmHg)	Before therapy	109,4 7,6	115,8 9,0	116,1 8,6	117,7 7,1	120,5 7,8	122,1 7,1	125,4 7,2	108,1 10,1	106,9 11,0	105,1 10,9	106,3 9,8	107,2 8,9
		90,3 5,6***	95,4 8,7***	98,9 8,2***	99,5 7,3***	102,5 9,4***	103,3 8,5***	104,5 8,3***	92,5 6,0***	91,0 7,6***	90,6 8,4***	88,8 7,3***	88,8 7,3***
HR (bts/min)	Before therapy	71,8 10,5	98,2 10,8	104,0 10,6	111,7 9,3	115,2 12,2	123,4 10,5	129,8 12,9	100,5 11,5	96,3 12,4	89,6 14,6	86,5 9,2	84,5 9,5
		61,7 9,8*	89,9 8,7***	90,9 9,5***	95,7 6,4***	99,0 8,2***	104,2 8,4***	112,9 10,8**	84,2 11,6**	79,2 10,8**	77,2 10,9**	75,3 10,3*	75,2 11,4*

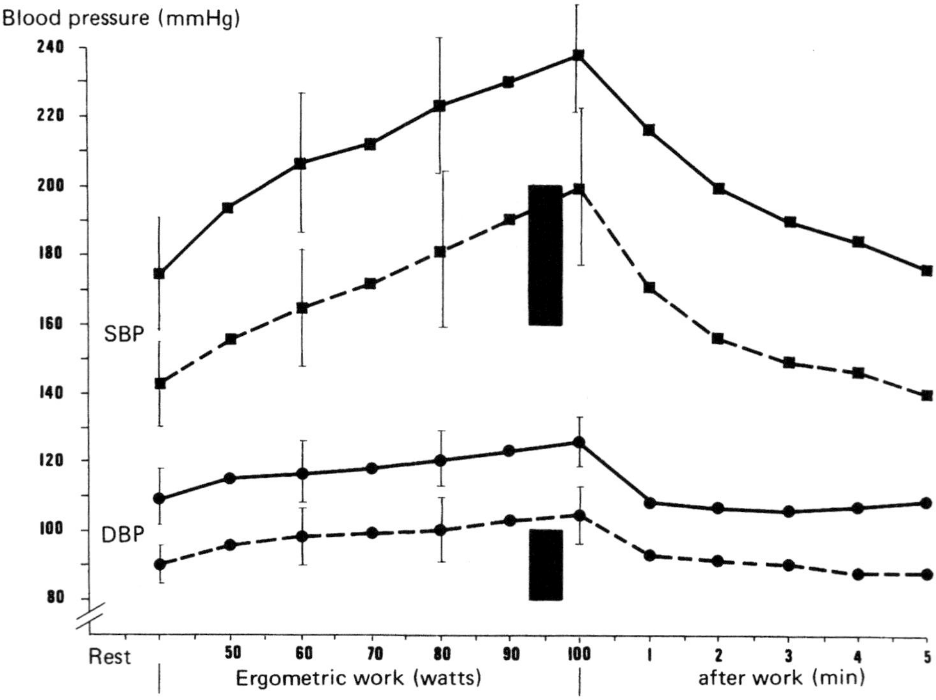

Fig. 74. Systolic (■—■—■) and diastolic (●- -●- -●) blood pressures of 13 hypertensives before (solid lines) and during (dashed lines) combined metipranolol and butizide therapy. The black bars indicate normal blood pressure ranges at 100 watts

Two of the patients complained of fatigue shortly after therapy was initiated, and two others complained of decreased exercise tolerance during their physical training. In all four cases these complaints disappeared with continued therapy, and there was no need to decrease or discontinue the medication.

7.2. Fixed Combination of Timolol and Hydrochlorothiazide/Amiloride Hydrochloride

Based on the encouraging response of these patients to therapy and the minimal side-effects that were experienced, we ran a similar study in a larger group of older hypertensive patients. The goal of the study was to test the antihypertensive efficacy of a fixed beta-blocker-diuretic combination, as before, and also to evaluate the patients for ECG changes in the form of bradycardiac rhythm abnormalities [122].

7.2.1. Patients

A total of 30 hypertensives (8 women and 22 men) with WHO Stage I-III essential hypertension were examined [122]. Only patients who were older than 50 years of age took part in the study. The patients ranged in age from 51 to

74 years (average age 60.3) and were distributed as follows: 10 age 50–55, 7 age 56–60, 6 age 61–65, 4 age 66–70, and 3 over 70. Mean body weight at entry was 77.6 ± 11.3 kg (77.5 ± 11.5 kg after therapy), and mean height was 170.2 ± 7.5 cm.

After preliminary testing the patients were started on a 4-week course of therapy with a fixed diuretic-beta-blocker combination containing 25 mg hydrochlorothiazide or 2.5 mg amiloride hydrochloride and 10 mg timolol. In all cases the total daily dose was taken once in the morning, with 4 patients taking ½ tablet, 20 taking 1 tablet, 2 taking 1½ tablets, and 4 taking 2 tablets.

All ergometric follow-up tests were done at the same time as the preliminary tests, between the hours of 3:00 p.m. and 6:00 p.m. All blood pressures were taken by the same examiner using the same calibrated mercury manometer.

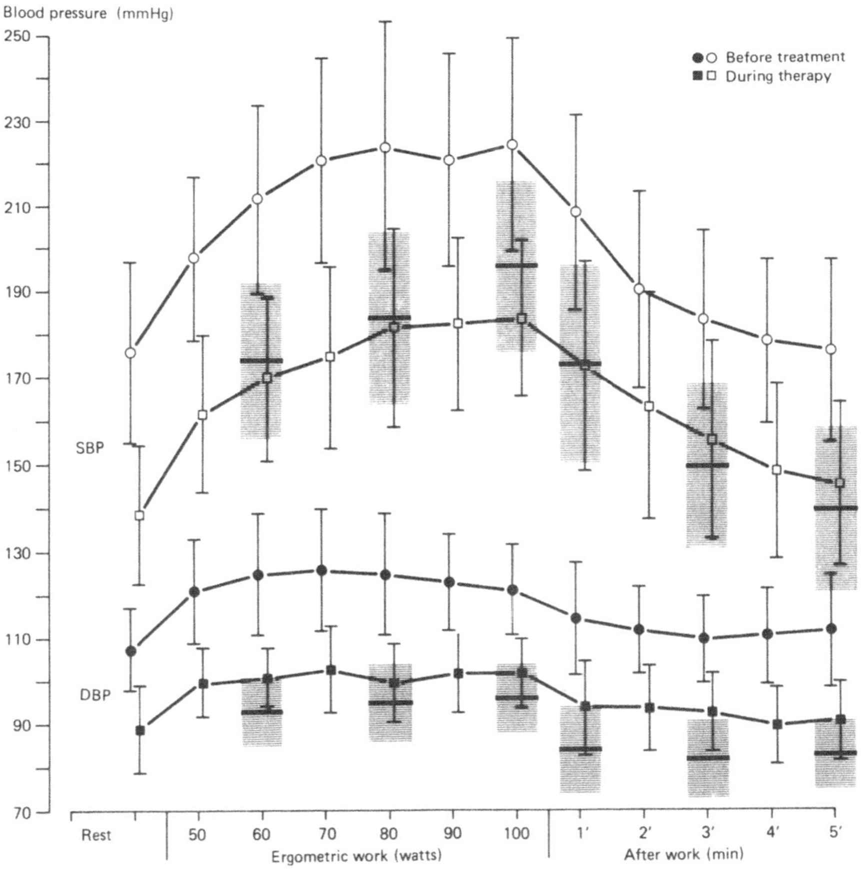

Fig. 75. Systolic and diastolic blood pressures of 30 older hypertensives (average age 60.3 years) before and during several weeks' treatment with a fixed combination of timilol, hydrochlorothiazide and amiloride. The bars indicate the blood pressure range of age-matched normals

Table 59. Blood pressures and heart rates (means ± SD) of 30 older hypertensives (average age 60.3 years) before and during several weeks treatment with a fixed combination of timolol (10 mg), hydrochlorothiazide (25 mg) and amiloride (2.5 mg)

n = 30	Rest		Ergometric work (watts)						Recovery period (min)				
	supine	before work	50	60	70	80	90	100	1	2	3	4	5
SBP (mmHg)													
Before therapy	176,4 22,4	176,9 24,7	197,5 19,0	212,3 22,4	221,3 24	223,7 29,2 n = 27	221,3 24,8 n = 20	224,9 25,3 n = 17	208,9 23,3	190,7 23,2	184,0 20,5	178,5 19,8	177,3 20,6
Therapy	139,3 15,8***	147,0 19,9***	162,1 18,4***	170 19,0***	175,3 21,3***	181,9 23,4***	183,2 19,7***	184,0 18,2***	173,2 24,3***	164,3 25,6***	155,5 23,4***	149,3 20,1***	146,1 18,5***
DBP (mmHg)													
Before therapy	108,3 9,4	112,6 10,5	120,9 11,9	124,6 13,5	125,9 13,5	125,4 14,4	122,5 10,7	121,4 10,7	115,0 12,7	111,7 10,3	110,4 10,5	110,7 11,4	111,9 12,6
Therapy	88,8 9,9***	93,2 9,8***	99,6 8,0***	101,3 8,2***	102,8 9,5***	99,5 9,2***	102,1 8,9***	102,4 8,2***	94,3 10,5***	93,8 9,7***	93,0 9,4***	90,3 9,1***	90,7 8,9***
HR (bts/min)													
Before therapy	70,4 11,1	69,0 10,6	97,9 12,8	104 13,0	109,9 15,1	113,2 17,1	113,0 14,1	117,0 16,1	89,6 13,4	83,7 11,1	81,5 12,6	78,7 11,2	78,4 11,2
Therapy	56,1 8,4***	54,9 8,5***	76,7 10,8***	83,5 12,0***	87,2 12,6***	90,2 11,3***	92,5 11,6***	95,6 10,9***	73,6 10,8***	65,0 8,8***	63,0 9,4***	63,1 8,9***	61,2 10,4***

7.2.2. Blood Pressure Responses

Table 59 and Fig. 75 show the blood pressure changes that occurred during the course of testing. As in the younger patients, the *older hypertensives* experienced excessive blood pressure elevations during exercise. At only 50 watts of exercise the older hypertensives raised their mean blood pressure 32 mm Hg systolic and 30 mm Hg diastolic higher than that of age-matched normotensive controls ($p < 0.001$). The systolic pressure at 50 watts, 196 mm Hg, was attained by the normals only at 100 watts of exercise. The failure of the blood pressure to maintain a continuous rise at 90 and 100 watts is due to the fact that all patients could not be exercised to the highest stages (Table 59).

Blood pressures during the recovery period were also significantly elevated ($p < 0.001$) relative to the normals. Antihypertensive therapy with the fixed beta-blocker-diuretic combination lowered both the systolic and diastolic pressures to a highly significant degree ($p < 0.001$), returning values to the normotensive range before, during and after exercise. This also applied to the standing pressure, which was lowered from an initial value of 169 ± 20/109 ± 10 mm Hg to 136 ± 18/89 ± 12 mm Hg. Comparing this value with the supine blood pressure after therapy, 139/89 mm Hg, we find that the medication caused no significant orthostatic hypotension.

7.2.3. ECG Findings

The heart rate at rest and during exercise was lowered significantly ($p < 0.001$) by the medication (Table 54). It is noteworthy that the heart rate reduction produced by the *beta-blocker,* which amounted to 20.3% at rest and 19.8 ± 1.4% in exercise, was no greater than that observed in earlier studies using considerably younger subjects [107, 111, 116, 120, 127]. The resting heart rate was 40-50/min in 6 patients, 51-60/min in 19 patients, and 61-70/min in 5 patients.

Table 60 shows the variations in the *P-Q interval* at rest and during exercise and how that interval was affected by the beta-blocker-diuretic combination. Before treatment all subjects had a normal P-Q interval which became slightly shorter during exercise. Four weeks' treatment with *beta-blockers* did not significantly prolong the P-Q interval either at rest or during exercise, despite a significant reduction of the heart rate to less than 50/min in some cases. The beta-blockers did not cause a *first- or second-degree AV heart block* in any of the patients tested. One 55-year-old man had a first-degree AV block of 0.24 msec at

Table 60. P-Q-intervals (means ± SD) of 30 older hypertensives before and during therapy with the fixed combination of timolol, hydrochlorothiazide and amiloride at rest and during exercise

	PQ-interval (msec)		
	Rest	Ergometry (watts)	
		50	70
Before therapy	0,156 ± 0,027	0,153 ± 0,019	0,147 ± 0,018
Beta-blocker-diuretic consideration	0,16 ± 0,028	0,154 ± 0,019	0,153 ± 0,018

Table 61. Rate-pressure product of 30 older hypertensives before and during therapy with the fixed combination of timolol, hydrochlorothiazide and amiloride at rest and during exercise

Rate-pressure product	Before work	Ergometric work (watts)			Recovery period 1 min
		50	70	100	
Before therapy	12426 2929	19356 3245	24382 4725	27450 n=17 5239	19133 4200
Therapy	7817 1517***	12881 2839***	15468 3277***	16949 n=17 1785***	12591 3062***

rest prior to treatment, which decreased to 0.2 at 70 watts. Therapy in this patient caused an accentuation of the AV block, which again decreased with exercise. Another 51-year-old man had a P-Q interval of 0.16 msec at rest which decreased to 0.14 at 70 watts. With treatment, the P-Q interval increased to 0.18 at rest and did not change with exercise. The heart rate, however, decreased from 121/min before therapy to 90/min during therapy.

7.2.4. Myocardial Oxygen Consumption and Ergometric Stress Tolerance

Table 61 and Fig. 76 show the rate-pressure product as a measure of *myocardial oxygen consumption* before, during and after exercise. It was found that the older hypertensives also had a significantly ($p<0.001$) increased rate-pressure product, reflecting their higher myocardial oxygen demand [122]. During *therapy* with the fixed combination, the myocardial oxygen consumption showed a highly significant reduction ($p<0.001$) during all phases of the test, i.e., a 37.1% reduction at rest, 36.2% during exercise and 34.2% during recovery, placing the rate-pressure product well within normal limits.

Before treatment was initated, *coronary heart disease* was diagnosed in 14 of the older hypertensives. In 13 cases this was done on the basis of significant *ST-segment depressions* in the ECG (at least 0.1 mV in 2 precordial leads). In the remaining patient, who had a left bundle branch block, coronary disease was diagnosed from reproducible angina pectoris of effort. In 6 of the 14 patients with coronary disease the therapy-related decrease in the *rate-pressure product* proved to be clinically relevant. Before treatment these patients showed pronounced ST-segment depression and had characteristic complaints during ergometry. With *treatment* the ST depression decreased significantly from 0.27 ± 0.08 mV to 0.12 ± 0.01 mV, and 5 of the 6 patients no longer had anginal pain even at 100 watts, even though 2 of them had to stop exercising at 80 watts and one at 90 watts prior to treatment on account of pain. Only one patient, who experienced severe chest discomfort at only 70 watts accompanied by an ST-segment depression of 0.3 mV in V3 to V6, showed virtually no change in his clinical symptoms. Coronary angiography in this patient revealed severe three-vessel disease with diffuse changes.

Eight patients had an asymptomatic ST-segment depression averaging $0.12 + 0.01$ mV at 100 watts prior to therapy. This feature could no longer be demonstrated after therapy was initiated.

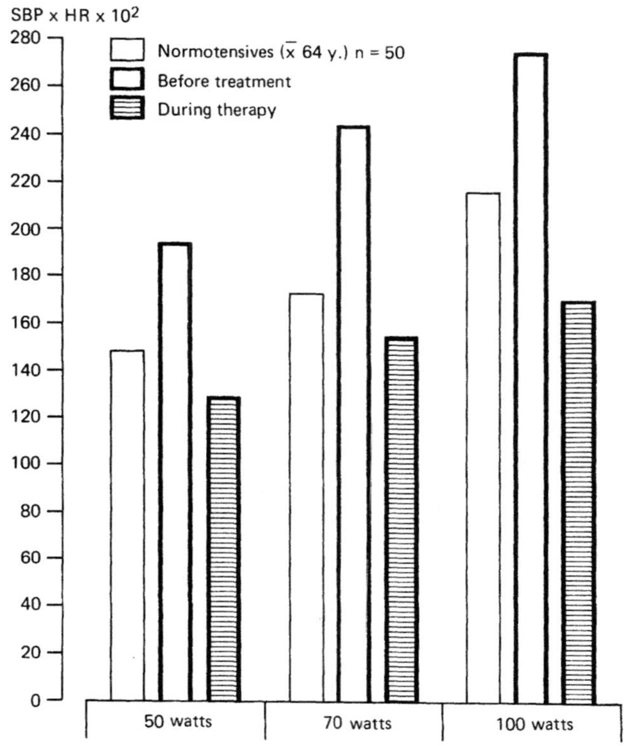

Fig. 76. Effect of combined treatment with timolol, hydrochlorothiazide and amiloride on the rate-pressure product of 30 older hypertensives (average age 60.3 years)

When we compare the *exercise tolerances* of all 30 patients based on the highest stage of exercise that was attained before and during therapy, we find the following: Before treatment all the patients attained 70 watts, 27 attained 80 watts, 20 attained 90 watts, and only 17 could exercise to 100 watts. Of the 13 patients who did not reach the final 100-watt stage because of angina, severe dyspnea or excessive blood pressure elevation, none became worse during therapy. Four exercised to the same stage, while 3 progressed 10 watts higher and 6 progressed 20 watts higher.

7.2.5. Side-Effects

Complaints of adverse effects were considerably more frequent among the older hypertensives than in younger patients. The reported severity of side-effects was also greater, especially with regard to fatigue, depression and in some cases dizziness. However, these complaints either disappeared or became milder with continued therapy, and no patient required dosage reduction or discontinuation.

7.3. Summary and Conclusions

We must require that antihypertensive medications not only normalize the blood pressure in the resting state but also control the excessive blood pressure increases elicited by physical and emotional stress. As pointed out in Chap. IV.2. and 4., however, this is not the case with all antihypertensive agents which have efficacy at rest.

The failure of antihypertensive agents, such as diuretics, to control stress-induced blood pressure elevations is linked to an increased risk of myocardial hypoxia and cerebrovascular complications, especially in the elderly [407, 416]. The *older hypertensives* in our studies showed the highest absolute *blood pressure increases* even at the lowest levels of exercise (50 watts) and at heart rates under 100 beats/min. They also showed a significantly higher myocardial oxygen consumption than younger hypertensives (s. Chap. III.6.). In addition, as Fig. 23 so clearly demonstrates, blood pressure readings obtained at rest are a poor predictor of how the blood pressure will respond to stress.

Given these facts, we are particularly impressed by the significant lowering of the systolic and diastolic blood pressure and of the rate-pressure product that was obtained with the fixed *beta blocker-diuretic combination* during and after exercise stress testing. This seems even more significant when one considers the frequency with which coronary heart disease coexists with hypertension in the elderly, and consequently that these individuals are at particular risk for myocardial ischemia when their blood pressures are raised excessively by stress.

We have demonstrated this fact, as well as the positive effect of therapy on myocardial oxygen consumption, in hypertensive patients with coexisting coronary heart disease. We observed a significant reduction of ST-segment depression and a reduced frequency of anginal episodes without the need for concomitant antianginal therapy. This objective and subjective improvement in clinical symptoms was the result of a significant decrease in the rate-pressure product, which is considered a reliable measure of myocardial oxygen consumption [22, 235, 314, 369]. Numerous studies in patients with coronary disease have documented the positive effect of *beta-blocking drugs* on stress tolerance [418, 425] based upon a significant decrease in the *rate-pressure product* [53, 418] and a resulting improvement in the relationship of oxygen supply to oxygen demand [336].

The fact that *diuretics* cannot lower the rate-pressure product and do not affect myocardial oxygen consumption may account for the surprising result of earlier epidemiologic studies done predominantly with diuretic agents (s. Chap. III.5.2.). Specifically, these studies showed that while the overall mortality was significantly reduced in hypertensives receiving treatment, the incidence of myocardial infarction was not decreased. In addition, a more recent clinical study showed that elderly hypertensives with mild arterial hypertension treated with thiazide diuretics [309] had a significantly higher mortality from myocardial infarction than the group treated with beta-blockers and a control group. This is consistent with the findings of recent Swedish studies demonstrating a decline of mortality and morbidity from coronary heart disease in hypertensives treated with beta-blocking drugs.

When one considers the growing risk of *myocardial complications* with age in hypertensive persons, as well as the increasing risk of stroke, which is three times higher between the ages of 55 and 64 than between 45 and 54 [172, 290], one can appreciate the urgent need for appropriate *antihypertensive therapy* with beta-blocking drugs in older hypertensives. This particularly applies to patients who show excessive pressor responses to stress.

It has also been found that the response of *elderly hypertensives* to treatment can be improved and side-effects minimized by employing an effective combination of antihypertensive agents in relatively small individual doses. For this reason, and because of the tendency of beta-blocking drugs to increase the extracellular fluid volume in older patients [343], a diuretic should always be given concurrently with a beta-blocker when treating hypertension in the elderly. The additive effect is also of benefit to patients with severe coronary atherosclerosis, who are likely to experience marked diastolic blood pressure elevations during ergometry [389] and will not respond adequately to beta-blockers alone.

It need hardly be stated that the physician must exercise special care and diligence when establishing an optimum treatment regimen with beta-blocking drugs in older hypertensive patients. Beta-blockers exert negative chronotropic, dromotropic and inotropic effects on the heart [276]. On the one hand, these drugs inhibit sinus node function, causing a mean 17% reduction in heart rate and prolonging sinus node recovery by 35.3% [385]. In addition, beta-blockers may influence conduction at the AV junction, prolonging the P–Q interval and shortening the A–H interval in the His bundle electrocardiogram [33, 385, 395]. Because of these effects, beta-blocking drugs are generally considered to be contraindicated in the presence of sinus node disease or a second- or third-degree AV block [165, 276, 385, 408]. While a few authors have reported that a lowering of the sinus rate has been able to restore 1:1 conduction in some patients with second-degree AV block [76], it is still wise to observe the contraindications stated above, especially in older hypertensives. At the same time, it should be acknowledged that the danger of a bradycardiac complication tends to be overestimated in patients who have no sinus node disease or heart block. This is clearly indicated by the studies presented here, in which there was no instance of first-degree AV block developing in any of the subjects treated, and the catecholamine-induced shortening of the P–Q interval during ergometry was preserved during beta blockade. This agrees with the report of the Boston Collaborative Drug Surveillance Program [161], which showed only one case of a complete AV block developing in a series of 268 patients treated.

The *resting bradycardia* produced by *beta-blockade* should also be mentioned in this context. It has been recommended [40] that the dosage for the treatment of angina pectoris be stopped when the resting heart rate falls to 50 beats/min. No explanation for this arbitrary limit is given, and presumably it would be most difficult to offer one. A sinus bradycardia is not considered pathologic as long as the heart rate rises adequately during exercise, which was the case in all hypertensives treated here, and the P–Q interval shows no further pathologic changes.

This is evidenced first by the fact that intensive endurance training can lower the heart rate to 40/min or less without adverse clinical effects, even in the elderly. Second, a 10-year follow-up study of 381 patients by Shaw et al. [387] published in the *British Medical Journal* in 1980 showed that patients with isolated *sinus node dysfunction* did not have a higher mortality than the population at large, leading the authors to conclude that sinus bradycardia is a benign condition.

Based on studies conducted to date, the risk of *negative inotropism* from beta-blockers seems to have been greatly overestimated, at least in the treatment of hypertension. Ergometric studies in hypertensives on beta-blockers [59, 71, 148, 277] have shown that the *stroke volume,* which depends strongly on myocardial contractility, was actually increased by the drugs, while the heart rate was reduced. No patient required digitalization.

Even in acute myocardial infarction [284, 448] no decrease in *stroke volume* or rise in *mean pulmonary wedge pressure* was detected – not even in patients with initially marked increases in their left ventricular filling pressures of over 20 mm Hg.

Based on their studies of cardiac valve patients treated with propranolol, Conway et al. [73] concluded that cardiac failure can occur during beta-blockade only if the stroke volume is so low that an elevated heart rate is necessary to maintain an adequate cardiac output. But studies by Waagstein et al. [437] raise some doubt as to the accuracy of this statement, for, even in *congestive cardiomyopathy,* long-term treatment with *beta-blockers* has resulted in a marked improvement of hemodynamic findings.

In practical situations, however, a glycoside or diuretic should always be prescribed concurrently with a beta-blocker whenever frank cardiac failure is present.

Regardless of the type of antihypertensive agent used, side-effects tend to be considerably more frequent in older patients, as the results of our study confirm. Under no circumstances should a patient's subjective complaints on initiation of therapy be considered grounds for discontinuing treatment on the rationale that the hypertension is innocent or "necessary". The initially high rate of side-effect requires first that the physician prepares the patient for any problems that may be experienced and give reassurance that they are only temporary. Second, the side-effects should not mislead the therapist into believing that a beta-blocker-diuretic combination is inappropriate for treating high blood pressure in the elderly. Lower initial doses may be tried if necessary.

In contrast to the sympathicolytic agents ordinarily used in older hypertensives (30–50% rate of side-effects [161, 340]), the beta-blocking drugs cause no orthostatic hypotension. This, in addition to the low frequency of adverse effects (about 10% [58, 161, 228]), represents a significant advantage inasmuch as orthostatic hypotension is one of the most serious complications of antihypertensive therapy in older patients.

Thus, when one weighs the potential risks of treatment against the therapeutic benefits that are to be gained, one must conclude that beta-blocking drugs, combined with a diuretic, represent a first-line medical therapy for hypertension in the elderly. This regimen can provide satisfactory blood pressure control throughout the day following a single morning dose, which is highly advantageous in terms of patient compliance. This is illustrated by the studies of Weber et al. [443], who were able to show that compliance in pill taking was directly proportional to the complexity of the dosing schedule. Thus, 86% patients showed good compliance on a regimen of 1 × 1 tablet/day, as opposed to 60% on a 2 × 1 schedule, 54% on a 3 × 1 schedule, and only 20% on a 4 × 1 schedule.

8. Antihypertensive Effect of Weight Reduction and Endurance Training

The effective control of high blood pressure is essential from the standpoint of preventive medicine and public health. It must be asked, however, whether the *drug therapy of hypertension* will continue to play the dominant role in hypertension management given the large financial burden that is imposed by the use of antihypertensive drugs on a broad scale. It also must be considered that high blood pressure often is only one of several coexisting cardiovascular risk factors [378], which are not eliminated by antihypertensive drug therapy.

In an effort to evaluate the role of nonpharmacologic treatment in hypertension management, we conducted a comparative study to explore the benefits of weight-reduction training, dietary counseling and behavioral modification in overweight persons with arterial hypertension.

8.1. Patients and Methods

We conducted ergometric stress tests in 15 overweight persons with essential hypertension (WHO Stage I–II) age 36.7 + 6.2 years (31–42) who had presented for weight-reduction training. The weight-reduction training consisted of 90-minute periods of endurance training three times weekly, the goal being to exercise the patient to a target heart rate of 170 minus his age. It was extremely difficult to control training intensity exactly, especially in the initial phase, because the patients were poorly conditioned and raised their heart rates sharply even at very low levels of exertion. As training progressed and cardiocorporeal performance improved, the recovery periods were gradually shortened in favor of longer exercise periods. An important part of the weight-reduction program was *behavioral modification* as recommended by Hautzinger, in addition to dietary counseling.

At the conclusion of the three-month program we retested the patients on the ergometer under identical conditions. At the start of the study the patients (10 women, 5 men) had a mean body weight of 94.5 + 12.6 kg with a mean height of 169.7 + 9.5 cm. By the end of the weight-reduction program the mean body weight had decreased by 11.8 kg to 82.7 + 13.1 kg ($p < 0.05$).

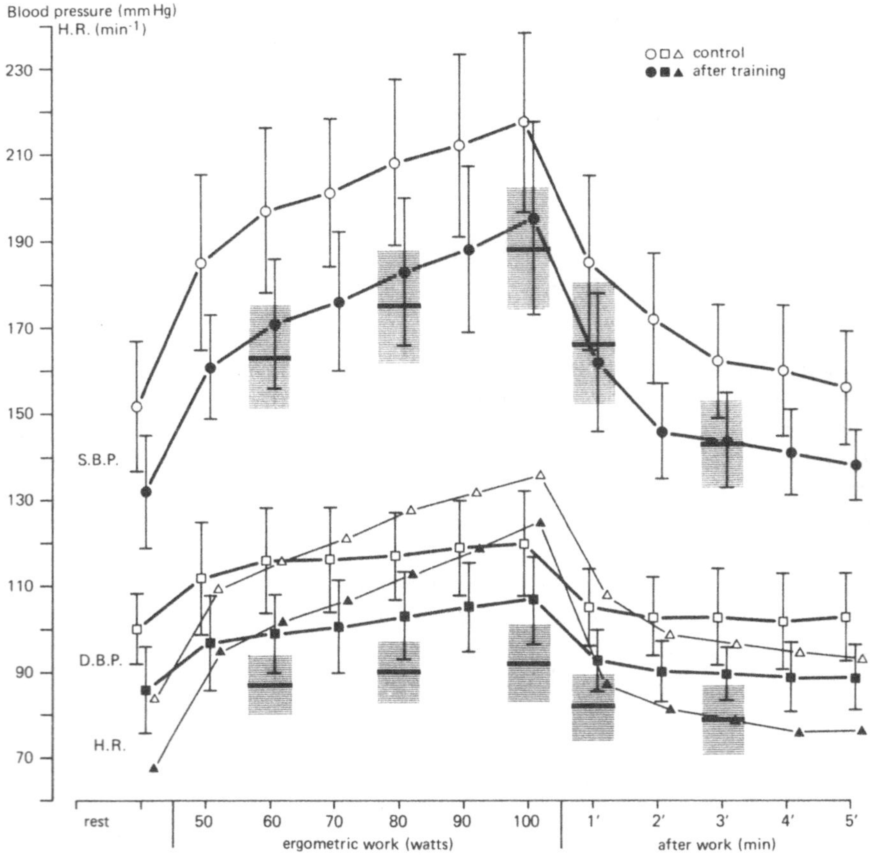

Fig. 77. Blood pressures and heart rates of 15 overweight hypertensives before and after weight reduction combined with 3 months' endurance training. The bars indicate normal blood pressure ranges

8.2. Blood Pressure and Heart Rate Responses

The patients' blood pressures were markedly elevated both at rest and at 100 watts of exercise, with values of 152/100 and 217/120 mm Hg, respectively. The postexercise blood pressure was also typical, maintaining an elevation of 156/103 mm Hg after 5 minutes of recovery (Table 62, Fig. 77).

Weight reduction in the hypertensives normalized the resting, supine blood pressure to 132/86 mm Hg. A significant reduction of systolic and diastolic pressure was also apparent during ergometry ($p<0.05$–$p<0.001$). At that time the systolic pressure was lowered into the normotensive range, while the diastolic pressure, though significantly reduced, was still slightly above normal. During the recovery period both the systolic and diastolic pressures showed a highly significant reduction ($p<0.001$) to normal levels.

When we compare the heart rates before and after endurance training, we find a marked fall in heart rates before, during and after ergometry. On the

Table 62. Blood pressures and heart rates (means ± SD) of 15 overweight hypertensives before and after weight reduction combined with 3 months' endurance training

	Rest		Ergometric work (watts)						Recovery period (min)				
	Supine	Before work	50	60	70	80	90	100	1	2	3	4	5
SBP (mmHg) Before therapy	151,9 15,2	156,1 19,8	185,1 20,0	196,9 19,3	201,4 16,5	207,9 18,6	211,5 20,5	216,8 21,2	185,3 19,7	171,8 14,7	161,5 13,2	159,6 14,8	156,1 13,4
After weight reduction and endurance training	131,9 13,2***	140 12,5*	160,7 11,5***	171,2 15,0***	176,1 15,5***	182,7 16,5***	187,7 18,5**	195,3 22,4*	161,7 15,5**	146 10,6***	144,1 11,1***	141,3 10,4***	138,0 8,3***
DBP (mmHg) Before therapy	100,4 8,3	104,9 10,3	112,0 12,6	116,4 11,9	116,4 11,7	117,1 10,0	119,3 11,1	120,1 11,7	105,1 8,8	102,9 8,8	103,1 10,5	102,1 10,3	103,0 9,9
After weight reduction and endurance training	86,1 10,4***	90,7 7,8***	96,7 11,2**	98,5 9,2***	100,7 10,9***	102,5 10,4***	105,1 10,1**	106,5 9,9**	93,3 6,9***	89,9 7,2***	90,0 6,3***	89,3 7,5***	89,1 8,2***
HR (bts/min)	83,8 20,2	86,1 17,0	109,9 18,4	115,9 20,3	120,6 22	128,1 23	131,6 24,3	136,2 24,2	107,8 24,9	98,6 25,0	96,6 21,6	95,0 22,3	92,9 22,7
	67,7 13,1*	69,3 10,3**	96,4 16,1*	102,2 16,5	106,7 18,6	113,0 18,4	118,5 20,1	124,9 19,8	87,2 20,3*	80,9 19,2*	78,8 17,1*	76,1 16,7*	75,9 15,8*

whole, then, the response of the blood pressure and heart rate to the weight-reduction program was remarkably similar to that achieved with beta-blocking drugs.

8.3. Effect on Myocardial Oxygen Consumption

As Table 63 and Fig. 78 indicate, myocardial oxygen consumption in the hypertensive patients was markedly elevated prior to the weight-reduction program. After three months of *endurance training* and stringent weight control, we found a significant fall in myocardial oxygen consumption at rest (29.6%), during ergometry (18.3%) and after ergometry (26.4%). Two factors were responsible for this effect: the resting and exercise bradycardia produced by the physical training, and the antihypertensive effect of the weight reduction.

8.4. Summary and Conclusions

8.4.1. Importance of Weight Reduction and Endurance Training

Our results clearly demonstrate the beneficial effect of weight reduction and endurance training on the risk factor, arterial hypertension. This is particularly important in view of the prevalence of overweight in hypertensive persons [249, 303, 378]. Besides lowering the resting blood pressure, the program was effective in moderatling the blood pressure response to exercise. This is illustrated by the case of a 31-year-old woman whose heart rate was significantly lowered by training, and who had normal systolic and diastolic blood pressures during ergometry (Fig. 22).

One question raised by our results is whether the blood pressure fall was attributable to the weight reduction itself or to the *endurance training*. As Maill et al. [303] demonstrated in 2051 persons over a 10-year follow-up period, a close correlation exists between a rise of blood pressure and a concomitant gain in body weight. At the same time, it has been shown that weight reduction is of definite value in bringing down the blood pressure even without concurrent salt restriction [346]. Stammler et al. [400] also described a correlation between

Table 63. Rate-pressure product (mean ± SD) of 15 overweight hypertensives before and after weight reduction combined with 3 months' endurance training

Rate-pressure product	Before work	Ergometric work (watts)			Recovery period 1. min
		50	70	100	
Before therapy	12767 3146	20126 4599	23972 4939	29432 6460	20054 5545
After weight reduction and endurance training	8985 2207***	15895 3204**	19450 4449*	24984 5816 n.s.	14764 4214**

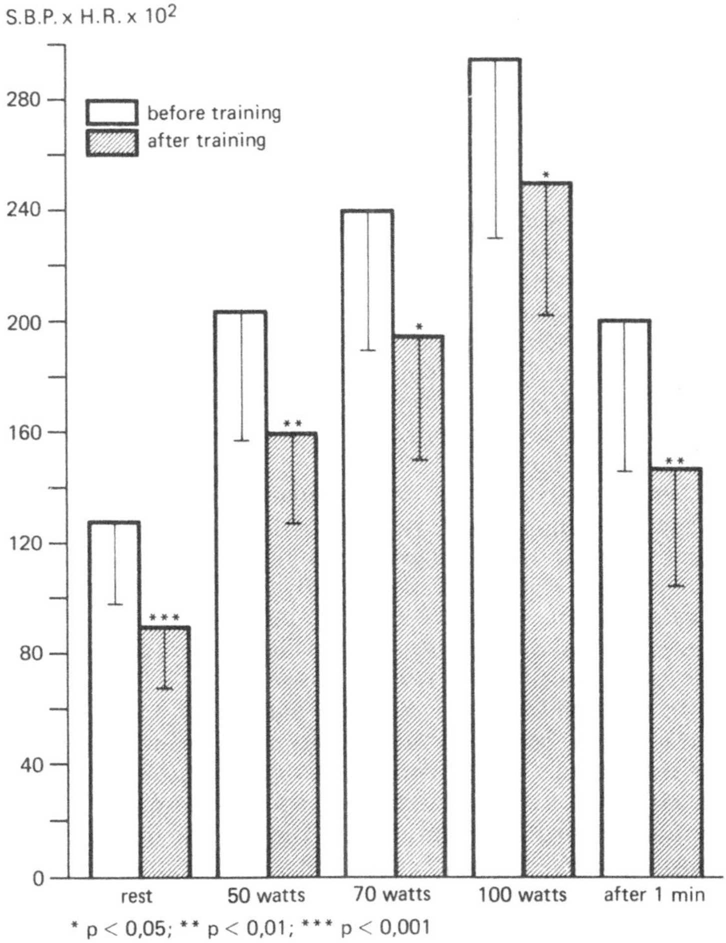

Fig. 78. The rate-pressure product in 15 overweight hypertensives before and after weight reduction combined with 3 months' endurance training

weight reduction and a lowering of the blood pressure, emphasizing that positive long-term effects were a product of better dietary habits and improved physical activity.

It was stated previously that the reduction of blood pressure by physical training depends on the group that is selected for study (s. Chap. III.7.3.). However, a change can definitely be ascribed to the direct effect of endurance training. Our study clearly showed not only a significant fall of systolic and diastolic blood pressure but also a marked reduction of the heart rate, and thus of myocardial oxygen consumption, during exercise stress testing.

8.4.2. Comparison of Weight Reduction and Drug Therapy

Thus, the effect of weight reduction combined with endurance training was similar to that of pharmacologic treatment with beta-blocking drugs. This implies that the combination of weight reduction and endurance training has a value equal to beta blockade in lowering the blood pressure and relieving the load on the heart. However, when we consider that weight loss and physical conditioning also have a salutary effect on other coronary risk factors [121] while stimulating various positive metabolic and hormonal adaptations, we can appreciate the substantial value of this type of therapy. Besides a normalization of blood pressure, the patients on the diet-and-exercise program showed a significant fall in their serum triglyceride levels and a marked improvement in their LDL/HDL ratio over the 3-month period. There is evidence to suggest that the latter quantity may be adversely affected both by beta blockers [38, 140, 267] and by diuretics [155, 360].

When comparing the antihypertensive effects of endurance training and weight reduction with those of drug therapy, one naturally must not disregard the cost factor. To cite an example, a total of 279 million DM was spent on antihypertensive drugs in West Germany in 1979. This figure does not include diuretics and takes into account only the 100 most commonly sold products, so the actual cost may be substantially higher. The costs of weight-reduction training are extremely small by comparison.

In addition to objective clinical parameters and calculable costs, one must not forget the beneficial effect of physical training and behavioral therapy [417] on the patient's subjective sense of well-being. Obesity frequently is damaging to the patient's sense of well-being and, like coronary heart disease, has the effect of lowering the quality of life. There is also the shortness of breath and excessive perspiration that occur when obese persons perform even the most ordinary physical exertion, like stair climbing. From this standpoint preventive training offers not only a longer life expectancy, but also the pleasing prospect of a daily life that is more worth living.

IV. References

1. Äärynen M, Mäkelä M, Hämeenaho P, Mattila MJ (1981) Prazosin enhances the antihypertensive effects of betablockers during isometric and dynamic exercise. Ann Clin Res 13: 71
2. Al-Eshaiker MH, Mellerowicz H (1967) Untersuchungen zur Beurteilung des arteriellen Druckes bei ansteigender ergometrischer Leistung. In: Mellerowicz H, Hansen G (Hrsg) 2. Internationales Seminar für Ergometrie Ergon, Berlin
3. Ammecke E, Rost, R (1984) Prognostic significance of an overshooting exercise blood pressure as an indicator for subsequent manifestation of hypertension. In: Löllgen L, Mellerowicz H (eds) Progress in Ergometry. Springer, Berlin Heidelberg, New York, p 272
4. Amery A, Julius S, Whitlock LS, Conway J (1967) Influence of hypertension on the hemodynamic response to exercise. Circulation 36: 231
5. Ames RP, Hill P (1976) Increase in serum lipids during treatment of hypertension with chlortalidone. Lancet 1: 721
6. A multicentre international study: Improvement in prognosis of myocardial infarction by long term beta-adrenorezeptor blockade using practolol (1975) Br Med J 3: 735
7. Anavekar SN, Louis WJ, Morgan TQ, Doyle AE, Johnston CI (1975) The relationship of plasma levels of pindolol in hypertensive patients to effects on blood pressure, plasma renin and plasma noradrenaline levels. Clin Exp Pharmacol Physiol 2: 203
8. Andersen M, Bechsgaard P, Fredriksen J, Hansen D, Jessen-Jürgensen H, Nielsen P, Pedersen F, Pedersen-Bjergaard O, Lind-Rasmussen S (1975) The effect of alprenolol on mortality among patients with definitive or suspected acute myocardial infarction. Lancet 2: 865
9. Anlauf MG, Schley G, Bock KD (1976) Simultane Messungen des Blutdrucks intraarteriell, mit der Standardmethode und mit dem Ultraschall-Doppelverfahren. Therapiewoche 26: 7582
10. Anschütz F (1970) Über die Zuverlässigkeit der auskultatorisch ermittelten Blutdruckwerte unter körperlicher Belastung. Fortschr Med 88: 1391
11. Arnold A, McAuliff JP, Colella DF, O'Connor WV, Brown TG (1968) β_2-receptor mediated glycogenolytic responses to catecholamines in the dog. Arch Int Pharmacodyn 176: 451
12. Ärztliche Mitteilungen (1980) Ein Drittel für den Bereich der Gesundheit. Dtsch Ärztebl 31: 1887
13. Aschoff J, Wever R (1980) Über Reproduzierbarkeit circadianer Rhythmen beim Menschen. Klin Wochenschr 58: 323
14. Ashton WI (1976) An open, multicentre study of acebutolol in hypertension. Curr Med Res Opin 4: 442
15. Åstrand I (1960) Aerobic work capacity in men and women with special reference to age. Acta Physiol Scand 49: 45
16. Åstrand J (1965) Blood pressure during physical work in a group of 221 women and men 48-63 years old. Acta Med Scand 178: 41
17. Åstrand PO, Rodahl K (1977) Textbook of work physiology. McGraw-Hill, New York
18. Atterhög IH, Duner H, Pernow B (1977) Haemodynamic effects of pindolol in hypertensive patients. Acta Med Scand [Suppl] 606: 55
19. Bachmann K, Thebis J (1967) Die drahtlose Übertragung kontinuierlicher direkter Blutdruckmessungen. Z Kreislaufforsch 56: 188
20. Bachmann K (1969) Arbeitsbelastung und Hypertonie. In: Sasse H (Hrsg) Hypertonie, Pathogenese, Klinik und Therapie. Schattauer, Stuttgart New York
21. Bachmann K, Zerzawy R, Riess PJ, Zölch KA (1970) Blutdrucktelemetrie - kontinuierliche, direkte Blutdruckmessung im Alltag und beim Sport. Dtsch Med Wochenschr 95: 741

22. Baller D, Schenk H, Zipfel J, Hellige G (1979) Möglichkeiten und Grenzen von klinischen O_2-Verbrauchsparametern. Z Kardiol 68: 656
23. Barath E (1927) Blutdruckstudien an alternden Menschen. Ein Beitrag für Pathogenese der arteriellen Hypertension. Z Ges Exp Med 54: 58
24. Barath E (1928) Arterial hypertension and physical work. Arch Intern Med 42: 296
25. Baroldi G, Falzi G, Meriani F (1979) Sudden coronary death. A postmortem study in 208 selected cases compared to 97 "control" subjects. Am Heart J 98: 20
26. Beevers DG, Fairman MJ, Hamilton M, Harpur JE (1973) Antihypertensive treatment and the course of etablished cerebral vascular disease. Lancet 1: 1407
27. Behrenbeck DW, Tauchert M, Meurer KA, Nieheres B, Jansen W, Hötzel J, Hilger H (1977) Der myokardiale Sauerstoffverbrauch bei Patienten mit arterieller Hypertonie vor und nach Drucksenkung. Verh Dtsch Ges Kreislaufforsch 43: 111
28. Bello LT, Sevy RW, Harakal C (1965) Varying hemodynamic patterns in essential hypertension. Am J Med Sci 250: 58
29. Ben Ari E, Kellermann JJ, Lapitod C, Drory Y, Fisman E, Hayat M (1978) Effect of prolonged intensive training on cardiorespiratory response in patients with angina pectoris. Br Heart J 40: 1143
30. Bengtsson E (1956) The working capacity in normal children evaluated by submaximal exercise on the bicycle ergometer compared with adults. Acta Med Scand 154: 91
31. Berger M, Berchtold P (1979) Beta-Rezeptorenblocker. Dtsch Med Wochenschr 24: 888
32. Berglund G, Wilhelmsen L, Sannerstedt R, Hansson L, Anderson O, Sivertsson R, Wikstrand J (1978) Decrease of CHD morbidity by treatment of hypertension. Lancet 1: 1
33. Berkowitz WD, Wit AL, Lan SH, Steiner C, Damato AN (1969) The effects of propranolol on cardial conduction. Circulation 21: 855
34. Berne RM, Levy MN (1972) The cardial pump. In: Berne RM, Levy MN (eds) Cardiovascular physiology. CV Mosby, Saint Louis, p 61
35. Berry CL (1978) Hypertension and arterial development - Longterm considerations. Br Heart J 40: 709
36. Bethge K-P, Klein H, Lichtlen PR (1979) Koronare Herzerkrankung, Rhythmusstörungen und plötzlicher Herztod. Internistische Welt 4: 107
37. Bevegård S, Holmgren A, Jonsson (1960) The effect of body position on the circulation at rest and during exercise, with special reference to the influence on the stroke volume. Acta Physiol Scand 49: 279
38. Bielmann P, Leduc G, Germain M, Davignon J (1980) Betablockers and changes in lipoprotein fractions. N Engl J Med 302: 298
39. Blümchen G, Barthel W, Paparidis C (1981) Häufigkeit der Belastungshypertonie bei Herzinfarkt. Patienten im chronischen Stadium und bei angeblich normalen Patienten. Herz Kreisl 5: 228
40. Bolte HD (1978) Therapie mit Beta-Rezeptorenblockern bei koronarer Herzerkrankung. Internist 19: 520
41. Bowlby JR (1979) The effect of exercise of left ventricular ejection time in patients with hypertension or angina pectoris. Am Heart J 3: 348
42. Boyer J, Kasch F (1970) Exercise therapy in hypertensive men. Am J Med Ass 211: 1668
43. Bock KD, Kreuzenbeck W (1966) Spontaneous blood pressure variations in hypertension: the effect of antihypertensive therapy and correlations with the incidence of complications. In: Gross F (ed) Antihypertensive therapy, principles and practice, an international symposium. Berlin
44. Bock KD (1973) Prophylaxe, Früherkennung und Frühbehandlung der Hypertonie. In: Losse H, Heintz R (Hrsg) Aktuelle Hypertonieprobleme. Stuttgart
45. Bock KD (1977) Pathogenese und Verlauf des essentiellen Hochdrucks. Verh Dtsch Ges Kreislaufforsch 43: 28
46. Bravo L, Tarazi RC, Dustan HP (1975) Beta-adrenergic blockade in diuretic-treated patients with essential hypertension. N Engl J Med 292: 66
47. Brecht HM, Banthien F, Ernst W, Schoeppe WA (1976) Increased plasma noradrenaline concentrations in essential hypertension and their decrease after long-term treatment with a β-receptorblocking agent (Pindolol). Clin Sci Mol Med 51: 485
48. Brest AN (1975) Therapeutic aspects of hypertension. Angiology 26: 584

49. Briedigkeit W, Tittmann F, Honigmann G (1979) Blutdruck im Kindesalter. 4. Mitteilung: Ergometrische Untersuchungen von Kindern und Jugendlichen mit systolischer Grenzwerthypertonie. Z Ärztl Fortbild 73: 378
50. Briedigkeit W (1981) Untersuchungen zur Blutdruckentwicklung bei Jugendlichen. Dtsch Gesundheitswes 36: 1087
51. Brod J, Cachovan M, Bahlmann J, Bauer GE, Celsen B, Sippel R, Hundshagen H, Feldmann U, Rienhoff O (1979) Haemodynamic changes during acute emotional stress in man with special reference to the capacitance vessels. Klin Wochenschr 57: 555
52. Brown ThG (1968) The β_2-receptor mediated glycogenolytic responses to catecholamines in the dog. Arch Int Pharmacoclyn 176: 451
53. Bruce RA, Hossack KF, Kusumi F, Clarke L (1979) Acute effects of oral propranolol on hemodynamic responses to upright exercise. Am J Cardiol 44: 132
54. Buchanan N, Weir RJ (1982) A comparison of nifedipine and mefruside in the treatment of mild/moderate hypertension. Abstract Ninth scientific meeting of the International Society of Hypertension, Mexico City
55. Bucher HW, Stucki P (1969) The effect of various beta-receptor blocking agents on platelet aggregation. Experienta 25: 280
56. Bühler FR, Laragh JH, Baer LB, Vaughan ED, Brunner HR (1972) Propranolol inhibition of renin secretion. N Engl J Med 287: 1209
57. Bühler FR, Bertel O, Kiowski DW (1978) Plasmanoradrenaline and adrenaline and β-adrenoreceptor responsiveness in renin subgroups of essential hypertension. Clin Sci Mol Med 55: 57
58. Bühler FR, Kiowski W, Bolli P, Bertel O (1978) Das Potential der Beta-Blocker in der Hochdruckbehandlung. Internist 19: 510
59. Burkart F, Bühler FR, Pfisterer M, Küng M (1976) Belastungshämodynamik und Renin vor und nach akuter β-Blockade bei Patienten mit essentieller Hypertonie. Schweiz Med Wochenschr 106: 1732
60. Carey RM, Ayers C (1976) Labile hypertension. Precursor of sustained essential hypertension? Am J Med 61: 811
61. Carlson LA, Böttiger LE, Åhfeldt P (1979) Risk factors for myocardial infarction in the Stockholm prospective study. Acta Med Scand 206: 351
62. Carlström S, Westling H (1970) Metabolic, circulatory and respiratory effects of a new sympathomimetic β-receptor-stimulating agent, terbutaline, compared with those of orciprenaline. Acta Med Scand [Suppl] 512: 33
63. Carvalho AC, Colman RW, Lees RS (1974) Platelet function in hyperlipoproteinaemia. N Engl J Med 290: 434
64. Chodakowska J, Nazar K, Wocial B, Jarecki M, Skorka B (1975) Plasma catecholamines and renin activity in response to exercise in patients with essential hypertension. Clin Sci Mol Med 49: 511
65. Choquette E, Ferguson R (1973) Blood pressure reduction in borderline hypertensives following physical training. Can Med Ass J 108: 699
66. Christensen NJ, Brandsborg O (1973) The relationship between plasma catecholamine concentration and pulse rate during exercise and standing. Eur J Clin Invest 3: 199
67. Chrysant SG, Fröhlich ED, Papper S (1976) Why hypertension is so prevalent in the elderly and how to treat it. Geriatrics 32: 101
68. Clausen JP, Trap-Jensen J, Lassen NA (1970) The effect of training on the heart rate during arm and leg exercise. Scand J Clin Lab Invest 26: 295
69. Clausen JP, Trap-Jensen J (1970) Effects of training on the distribution of cardiac output in patients with coronary artery disease. Circulation 42: 611
70. Colandrea MA, Friedmann SD, Nichamann MZ, Lynd CN (1970) Systolic hypertension in the elderly. Circulation 41: 239
71. Colemann AJ, Leary WP (1972) Cardiovascular effects of acebutolol in exercising man: A comparative study with practolol and propranolol. Curr Ther Res 14: 673
72. Conway J, Lauwers P (1960) Hemodynamic and hypotensive effects of long-term therapy with chlorothiazide. Circulation 21
73. Conway N, Seymor J, Gelson A (1968) Cardiac failure in patients with valval heart disease after use of propranolol to control atrial fibrillation. Br Med J 2: 213
74. Corday E, Corday StR (1975) Prevention of heart disease by control of risk factors: The time has come to face the facts. Am J Cardiol 35: 330

75. Cranston WI, Juel-Jensen BE, Semmence AM, Handfied Jones RCP, Forbes JA, Mutch LMM (1963) Effects of oral diuretics in raised arterial pressure. Lancet 2: 966
76. Csapo G, Weisswange A, Roskamm H (1978) Beta-Rezeptorenblocker bei atrioventrikulären Block II. Grades: Intrakardiale elektrographische Untersuchungen an 9 Patienten. Z Kardiol 67: 420
77. Currens JH (1948) A comparison of the blood pressure in the lying and standing position: A study of five hundred men and five hundred women. Am Heart J 35: 646
78. Detry JM, Rousseau M, Vandenbrouche G, Kusumi F, Brasseur LA, Bruce RA (1971) Increased arterio-venous oxygen difference after physical training in coronary heart disease. Circulation 44: 109
79. Deutsche Liga zur Bekämpfung des hohen Blutdruckes: Merkblatt, Normwerte des Blutdruckes und Entstehung der chronischen arteriellen Hypertonie (1976)
80. Deutsche Liga zur Bekämpfung des hohen Blutdruckes: Merkblatt, Empfehlungen zur Blutdruckmessung (1976)
81. Deutsche Liga zur Bekämpfung des hohen Blutdruckes: Merkblatt, Indikationen zur medikamentösen Hochdrucktherapie (1979)
82. Diehls HS (1929) The variability of blood pressure. Morning and evening studies. Arch Intern Med 43: 835
83. Dock DS, Fukushima K (1978) A longitudinal study of blood pressure in the Japanese, 1959-72. J Chron Dis 31: 669
84. Distler A, Philipp Th (1976) Stellenwert der β-Rezeptorenblocker im Vergleich zu Diuretika in der Basistherapie der Hypertonie. Med Welt 26: 1022
85. Dlin RA, Hanne N, Silverberg DS, Bar-Or, O (1983) Follow-up of normotensive men with exaggerated blood pressure response to exercise. Amer Heart J 106: 316
86. Drexler H, Löllgen H, Bodemann H, Just A (1983) Zur Reproduzierbarkeit ergometrischer und hämodynamischer Meßgrößen. In: Mellerowicz H, Franz I-W (Hrsg) Ergometrie: Kalibrierung, Standardisierung, Methodik. Peri-Med, Erlangen p 88
87. Drews A (1967) Bedeutung und Ergebnisse ergometrischer Leistungskontrollen bei aktiver Bewegungstherapie. Arbeitsmed Sozialmed Arbeitshyg 2: 441
88. Dufey K, Krönig B (1974) Kritischer Belastungsdruck bei Hochdruckkranken, Ergebnisse direkter Blutdruckmessung unter alltäglichen und fahrradergometrischen Belastungen, Schlußfolgerungen für die Praxis. Fortschr Med 92: 1339
89. Dunn FG, Melville DJ, Jones JV, Lorimer AR, Lawrie TDV (1978) Standardized stress and hypertension: Comparison of effect of propranolol and methyldopa. Br J Clin Pharmacol 5: 223
90. Dustan HP (1977) Vascular diseases of hypertension: mechanism, recognition, and control. In: Paoletti R, Gotto AM (eds) Atherosclerosis reviews, vol 2. Raven, New York, p 1
91. Eckberg DL (1979) Carotid baroreflex function in young men with borderline blood pressure elevation. Circulation 59: 632
92. Ekelund L-G, Ekelund C, Rössner S (1982) Antihypertensive effects at rest and during exercise of a calcium blocker, nifedipine, alone and in combination with metoprolol. Acta Med Scand 212: 71
93. Eliasson K, Hjemdahl P, Hylander B, Kahan T, Lins L-E (1982) Circulatory and sympathoadrenal responses to stress after long-term beta blockade. Abstract Ninth scientific meeting of the International Society of Hypertension, Mexiko City
94. Epstein SE, Robinson BF, Kahler RL, Braunwald E (1965) Effects of beta-adrenergic blockade on the cardiac response to maximal and submaximal exercise in man. J Clin Invest 44: 1745
95. Epstein FH (1977) Evaluation of epidemiology concerning prevention and therapy of atherosclerosis. In: Hauss WH, Wissler RW, Lehmann R (eds) State of prevention and therapy in human atherosclerosis and in animal models. Wiesbaden
96. Epstein FH, Gutzwiller F, Howald H, Junod B, Schweizer W (1979) Prävention der Arteriosklerose: Grundlagen heute. Schweiz Med Wochenschr 109: 1171
97. Fahrenkamp K (1921) Beitrag zur Kenntnis der Tagesschwankungen des Blutdrucks bei der Hypertonie. Med Klin 17: 776
98. Falkner B, Questi G, Affrime MB, Löwenthal DT (1982) The effect of a centrally acting agent versus diuretics on the cardiovascular response to mental stress in adolescent hypertension. Abstract Ninth scientific meeting of the International Society of Hypertension, Mexico City

99. Fineberg MH (1927) Systolic hypertension: its relationship to atherosclerosis of the aorta and the larger arteries. Am J Med Sci 173: 835
100. Floras JS, Fox P, Hassan MO, Jones JK, Sleight P, Turner KL (1979) Assessment of the antihypertensive effect of atenolol with 24 h ambulatory monitoring of blood pressure. Clin Sci 57: 387
101. Floras JS, Hassan MO, Sever PS, Jonas JV, Osikowska B, Sleight P (1981) Cuff and ambulatory blood pressure in subjects with essential hypertension. Lancet, II: 107
102. Folkow B (1975) Vascular changes in hypertension - review and recent animal studies. In: Berglund G, Hansson L, Werkö L (eds) Pathophysiology and management of arterial hypertension. Mölndal, Schweden
103. Found FM, Tarazi RC, Dustan HP, Bravo EL (1978) Hemodynamics of essential hypertension in young subjects. Am Heart J 96: 646
104. Franke H, Schramm A (1980) Herz- und Kreislaufbefunde im höchsten Lebensalter. Aktuel Gerontol 10: 137
105. Franz I-W, Mellerowicz H (1977) Vergleichende Messungen der PWC_{170} mit Leistungsstufen von unterschiedlicher Größe und Dauer. Z Kardiol 66: 670
106. Franz I-W (1978) Äthiologie, klinische Symptomatik und Diagnostik orthostatischer Kreislaufregulationsstörungen. Ther Ggw 117: 1199
107. Franz I-W, Lohmann FW (1978) Die Bedeutung der ergometischen Untersuchung zur Beurteilung der antihypertensiven Therapie. Dtsch Med Wochenschr 38: 1478
108. Franz I-W, Lohmann FW (1979) Der Einfluß einer Saluretikum-β-Rezeptorenblocker-Kombination auf überhöhte Belastungsblutdrücke. Med Klin 74: 396
109. Franz I-W (1979) Untersuchungen über das Blutdruckverhalten während und nach Ergometrie bei Grenzwerthypertonikern im Vergleich zu Normalpersonen und Patienten mit stabiler Hypertonie. Z Kardiol 68: 107
110. Franz I-W (1979) Das Elektrokardiagramm während ergometrischer Leistung. Med Klin 74: 896
111. Franz I-W, Lohmann FW (1979) Der Einfluß einer chronischen kardioselektiven und nichtselektiven β-Rezeptorenblockade auf den Blutdruck, die O_2-Aufnahme und den Kohlenhydratstoffwechsel. Z Kardiol 68: 503
112. Franz I-W (1979) Welchen Sport dürfen und sollen Hypertoniker betreiben? Med Trib 36: 27
113. Franz I-W (1979) Indikationen, Dosierung und Kontraindikationen präventiven Trainings. In: Mellerowicz H, Franz I-W (Hrsg) Training als Mittel der präventiven Medizin. Perimed, Erlangen S. 27
114. Franz I-W, Lohmann FW, Koch G (1979) Vergleichende Untersuchungen über die Wirkung einer chronischen kardioselektiven und nicht kardioselektiven β-Rezeptorenblockade auf die Plasmareninaktivität und den Blutdruck vor, während und nach Ergometrie bei Hochdruckkranken. Therapiewoche 29: 7753
115. Franz I-W, Lohmann FW, Koch G (1980) Differential effects of long-term cardioselective and nonselective beta-receptor blockade on plasma catecholamines during and after physical exercise in hypertensive patients. J Cardiovasc Pharmacol 2: 35
116. Franz I-W (1980) Differential antihypertensive effect of acebutolol and the fixed combination hydrochlorothiazide/amiloridehydrochloride on elevated exercise blood pressures in hypertensive patients. Am J Cardiol 46: 301
117. Franz I-W, Kothari P (1980) Blood pressure control during ergometric work in mild hypertension. Indian Heart J 32: 8
118. Franz I-W, Lohmann FW, Koch G (1980) Excessive dopamine increase at rest and during exercise after long-term betaadrenoreceptor blockade in hypertensive patients. Br Heart J 44: 25
119. Franz I-W, Mellerowicz H (1980) Vergleichende ergometrische Untersuchungen über den Tension-Time-Index und die körperliche Leistungsbreite bei Patienten mit grenzwertiger und stabiler Hypertonie und Normalpersonen. Z Kardiol 69: 587
120. Franz I-W, Lohmann FW (1980) Unterschiedlicher Einfluß einer chronischen, überwiegend β_1-selektiven und β_1-β_2-Rezeptorenblockade auf den Kohlenhydratstoffwechsel. Ergometrische Untersuchungen bei Hochdruckkranken. Klin Wochenschr 58: 1155
121. Franz I-W (1980) Die antihypertensive Wirksamkeit einer fixen β-Rezeptorenblocker-Diuretikum-Kombination auf Ruhe- und Belastungsblutdruck von essentiellen Hypertonikern. Schweiz Med Wochenschr 110: 1616

122. Franz I-W (1981) Einfluß einer fixen β-Rezeptorenblocker-Diuretika-Kombination auf den hohen Blutdruck im Alter. Herz Kreislauf 4: 187
123. Franz I-W (1981) Ergometrische Untersuchungen zur Beurteilung des hohen Blutdruckes im Alter. Herz Kreislauf 4: 197
124. Franz I-W (1981) Herzschlagfrequenz und arterieller Blutdruck bei Ergometrie - Physiologischer Bereich und pathologische Abweichungen. Kassenarzt 4: 274
125. Franz I-W (1981) Belastungsblutdruck bei Hochdruckkranken. Springer, Berlin Heidelberg New York
126. Franz I-W, Lohmann FW, Koch G (1982) Effects of chronic antihypertensive treatment with acebutolol and pindolol on blood pressure, plasma catecholamines, and oxygen uptake at rest and during submaximal and maximal exercise. J Cardiovasc Pharmacol 4: 180
127. Franz I-W (1982) Vergleichende ergometrische Untersuchungen über die Wirkung von β-Rezeptorenblockern und Diuretika und deren Kombination auf den Blutdruck und das Doppelprodukt bei Hochdruckkranken. Z Kardiol 71: 129
128. Franz I-W, Mellerowicz H (1982) Methodische und leistungsphysiologische Grundlagen der Ergometrie. Herz 7: 29
129. Franz I-W, Bartels F, Müller R: Blood-pressure response to ergometric work in normotensive subjects, aged 20-50 years. Z Kardiol 1982; 71: 458
130. Franz I-W Assessment of blood pressure response during ergometric work in normotensive and hypertensive patients. Acta med Scand 1982; Suppl 670: 35
131. Franz I-W, Lohmann FW Reproducibility of blood pressure measurements in hypertensives during and after ergometry. Dtsch med Wschr 1982; 107: 1379
132. Franz I-W (1982) Ergometrie bei Hochdruckkranken. Springer, Berlin, Heidelberg, New York
133. Franz I-W (1983) Beeinflussung des Belastungsblutdrucks durch antihypertensive Pharmaka. In: Distler A, Philipp T (Hrsg) Neuere Entwicklungen in der Hochdrucktherapie. Thieme, Stuttgart, p 71
134. Franz I-W The effects of prazosin and acebutolol and their combination on blood pressure and pressure-rate product during ergometric work in hypertensive patients. Z Kardiol 1983; 72: 746-754
135. Franz I-W, Wiewel D (1983) Antihypertensive Wirkung von Kalziumantagonisten auf Ruhe- und Belastungsblutdruck im Vergleich zu β-Rezeptorenblockern. 89 Verh Dtsch Ges Innere Med, Bergemann, München, p 1138
136. Franz I-W (1983) Effect of acebutolol on elevated exercise blood pressures in hypertensives. In: Lichtlen P, Maranhão MF (eds) Advances in β-blocker therapy. Schattauer, Stuttgart, New York, p 147
137. Franz I-W (1984) Isometrische und dynamische Belastung als Kriterium für die Therapiebeurteilung. In: Holzgreve H, Rost R (eds) Aktuelles und Kontroverses aus der Hochdruckforschung. MMV, München, p 107
138. Franz I-W (1984) Prognostische Bedeutung des Belastungsblutdruckes. In: Anlauf M, Bock KD (eds) Blutdruck unter körperlicher Belastung, p 79
139. Franz I-W, Paeprer H, Schmutzler H (1984) Zur Behandlungsbedürftigkeit der milden Hypertonie bei Koronarkranken. 90 Verh Dtsch Ges Inn Med Bergmann, München, p 739
140. Franz I-W, Lohmann FW, Röcker L (1984) Differential effects of long term β_1-selective and nonselective β-receptor blockade on lipid metabolism in hypertensive patients. Herz/Kreislauf 3: 116
141. Franz I-W (1985) Ergometry in the assessment of arterial hypertension. Cardiology 72: 147
142. Franz I-W, Wiewel O (1985) Antihypertensive effects of Calciumantagonists, β-receptor blockers and their combination on blood pressures at rest and during exercise in hypertensive patients. J Cardiovasc Pharmacol 6 (Suppl 7): 1037
143. Franz I-W, Lohmann FW, Koch G (1985) Long term effect of β-receptor blockade on maximal oxygen uptake and plasma catecholamines in hypertensive patients. Int J Sports Med
144. Franz I-W, Wiewel D, Ketelhut R (in print) Regression of left ventricular hypertrophy in hypertensive patients during chronic β-receptor blockade. Dtsch med Wschr
145. Freis ED, Wanko A, Wilson IM, Parrish AE (1958) Treatment of essential hypertension with chlorothiazide. JAMA 166: 137-140
146. Frick MH, Katila M (1968) Hemodynamic consequences of physical training after myocardial infarction. Circulation 37: 192

147. Frisch P (1978) Herzgröße, Puls und Blutdruck in Ruhe unter Atenolol. Med Klin 73: 1477
148. Frisk-Holmberg M, Juhlin-Dannfeldt A, Jorfeldt L, Aström H (1976) Effect of long-term antihypertensive β-receptorblocking treatment on hemodynamic and metabolic responses to prolonged exercise in man. Clin Sci Mol Med 51: 489
149. Fry J (1974) Natural history of hypertension. A case of selective non-treatment. Lancet 2: 431
150. Fuchs G (1980) Umgang mit statistischen Zahlenangaben bei der ärztlichen Begutachtungspraxis. Lebensversicherungsmedizin 5: 115
151. Garraway WM, Whisnant JP, Phillips LH, Kurland T, O'Fallon WM (1979) The declining incidence of stroke. N Engl J Med 300: 449
152. Gattenlöhner W, Schneider KW (1966) Das Verhalten des Herzschlagvolumens in Ruhe, während und nach körperlicher Arbeit beim kompensierten Patienten mit Cor pulmonale, Hypertonie und Herzklappenfehler im Vergleich zum Gesunden und Sportler. Verh Dtsch Ges Inn Med 72: 869
153. Geddes LA, Whistler SJ (1978) The error in indirect blood pressure measurement with the incorrect size of cuff. Am Heart J 96: 4
154. Gleichmann M (1984) Diskussionsbeitrag. In: Anlauf M, Bock KD (Hrsg) Blutdruck unter körperlicher Belastung. Steinkopff, Darmstadt, p 64
155. Glück Z, Weidmann P, Mordasini R, Peheim E, Bachmann L, Keusch G, Riesen W (1979) Einfluß einer Diuretikatherapie auf die Serumlipoproteine: ein unerwünschter Effekt. Schweiz Med Wochenschr 109: 104
156. Goldberg LI (1972) Cardiovascular and renal actions of dopamine: Potential clinical applications. Pharmacol Rev 24: 1
157. Goldring D, Hernandez A, Choi S, Lee JL, Londe S, Lindgren FT, Burton RM (1979) Blood pressure in high school population. J Pediatr 95: 298
158. Gollnick PD (1973) Factors controlling glycogenolysis and lipolysis during exercise. In: Keul J (ed) Limiting factors of physical performance. Thieme, Stuttgart, p 81
159. Gould BA, Mann S, Davis AB, Altmann DG, Raftery EB (1981) Does placebo lower blood pressure? Lancet II: 1377
160. Granath A, Jonsson B, Strandell T (1964) Circulation in healthy old men, studied by right heart catheterization at rest and during exercise in supine and sitting position. Acta Med Scand 176: 425
161. Greenblatt DJ, Koch-Weser J (1973) Adverse reaction to propranolol in hospitalized medical patients. A report from the Boston Collaborative Drug Surveillance Program. Am Heart J 86: 478
162. Grobecker H, Planz G, Wiethold G, Simsrock R, Becker HJ, Lutz E, Petersen P (1976) Specific and non-specific effects of β-adreno-receptor blocking drugs in man. Klin Wochenschr 54: 783
163. Groß F (1974) Drug therapy in hypertension. What we have, what we need, what we except. Am J Cardiol 34: 471
164. Groß F (1978) Klinische Pharmakologie der β-Adrenorezeptoren Blocker. Internist 19: 504
165. Gugler R (1978) Therapie mit Beta-Rezeptorenblockern. Nebenwirkungen und Kontraindikationen. Internist 19: 547
166. Gutzwiller F (1976) Öffentliche Hypertonie. Erfassung und Problematik der individuellen Langzeitkontrolle. Schweiz Med Wochenschr 106: 1687
167. Gutzwiller F, Bühler FR (1978) Die Erfassung des unbekannten Hypertonikers. Muench Med Wochenschr 13: 427
168. Halhuber MJ (1966) Längsschnittuntersuchungen an Hochdruckkranken während einer Klima- und Terrainkur in 2000 m Höhe. Sportarzt Sportmed 17: 473
169. Hallock P, Benson JC (1937) Studies in the elastic poperties of human isolated aorta. J Clin Invest 16: 595
170. Hansson B-G, Hökfelt B (1975) Long-term treatment of moderate hypertension with penbutolol. Eur J Clin Pharmacol 9: 9
171. Hansson B-G (1976) Long-term non-selective and cardioelective receptor blockade in hypertensive patients. Acta Med Scand [Suppl] 598: 1
172. Harmsen P, Berglund G, Larsson O, Tibblin G, Wilhelmsen L (1979) Stroke registration in Göteborg, Sweden, 1970–1975. Acta Med Scand 206: 337
173. Harris L, Dargie HJ, Lynch PG, Bulpitt J, Krikler DM (1982) Blood pressure and heart rate in patients with ischaemic heart disease receiving nifedipine and propranolol. Br Med J 284: 1148

174. Harry JD, Knapp MF, Linden RJ, Stoker JB, Newcombe L (1979) Effects of 4 β-adrenoceptor-blocking drugs on blood pressure and exercise heart rate in hypertension. Eur J Cardiol 10: 131
175. Hauss WH (1982) Zur Pathogenese der Arteriosklerose. Med Welt 1: 20
176. Hayduk K (1978) Nebenwirkungen der Antihypertensiva bei Langzeittherapie. Muench Med Wochenschr 120: 459
177. Hayduk K (1979) Ist die Grenzwerthypertonie eine behandlungsbedürftige Erkrankung? Nieren Hochdruckkr 4: 140
178. Hedstrand H, Åberg A (1975) A three-year follow up of middle aged men with borderline blood pressure. Acta Med Scand 198: 389
179. Held B, Scherer B, Weber PC (1979) Grenzwerthypertonie - maximale Diagnostik und Therapie? Pro Maximalprogramm. Internist 20: 102
180. Heidbreder E, Ziegler A, Heidland A (1982) Verhindern sympatholytische Antihypertensiva den Blutdruckanstieg bei mentalem Streß? Herz Kreisl 3: 135
181. Heller RF, Rose G (1977) Current management of hypertension in hospital. Br Med J I: 1441
182. Heller RF, Rose G (1977) Current management of hypertension in general practice. Br Med J I: 1442
183. Henquet JW, Kho TL, Rahn KH (1978) Grenzwerthypertonie. Muench Med Wochenschr 13: 437
184. Henschel AF, de la Vega F, Taylor HL (1954) Simultaneous direct and indirect blood pressure measurements in man at rest and work. J Appl Physiol 6: 506
185. Heyden S, Bartel AG, Hames CG, McDonough JR (1969) Elevated blood pressure levels in adolescents, Evans County, Georgia. JAMA 209: 1683
186. Heyden S (1974) Ergebnisse und Konsequenzen der Post-Framingham-Studie. Risikofaktoren für das Herz. Mannheim
187. Hines EA, Brown GB (1936) The cold pressure test for measuring the reactibility of the blood pressure: Data concerning 571 normal and hypertensive subjects. Am Heart J 11: 1
188. Hines EA (1940) Range of normal blood pressure and subsequent development of hypertension. JAMA 115: 271
189. Hintzen AHJ, Henquet JWM, Chappin JJML, Slagboom G (1978) Concomitant administration of timolol and hydrochlorothiazide/amiloride in hypertensive patients. J Int Med Res 6: 213
190. Hochdruck-Ratgeber: Sport und Bewegung. Bayer AG, Pharma Wiss Abteilung
191. Hodge JV, Smirk FH (1967) The effect of drug treatment of hypertension on the distribution of deaths from various causes. Am Heart J 73
192. Hoffmann K, Kuhlmann E (1983) Meßtechnische Untersuchungen an Fahrrad-Ergometern. - Zur Kalibrierung von Ergometern. In: Mellerowicz H, Franz I-W (Hrsg) Ergometrie: Kalibrierung, Standardisierung, Methodik. Peri-Med, Erlangen p 14
193. Hoher Blutdruck: Antworten auf 10 Fragen. Informationsbroschüre der Deutschen Liga zur Bekämpfung des hohen Blutdruckes
194. Holland OB, Nixon JV, Kuhnert L (1981) Diuretic-induced ventricular ectopic activity. Am J Med 70: 762
195. Hollmann W, Barg W, Weyer G, Heck H (1970) Der Alterseinfluß auf spiroergometrische Meßgrößen im submaximalen Arbeitsbereich. Med Welt 21: 1280
196. Hollmann W (1974) Leistungsphysiologische Grundlagen zur rehabilitativen Kardiologie. In: Mellerowicz H, Weidener J, Jokl E (Hrsg) Rehabilitative Kardiologie. Karger, Basel, S 44
197. Holmgren A (1956) Circulatory changes during muscular work in man. With special reference to arterial and central venous pressures in the systematic circulation. Scand J Clin Lab Invest 8 [Suppl 24]: 1
198. Holmgren A, Mossfeld F, Sjöstrand T, Ström G (1960) Effect of training on work capacity, total hemoglobin, blood volume, heart volume and pulse rate in recumbent and upright position. Acta Physiol Scand 50: 72
199. Holzgreve H (1973) Die Frühbehandlung der leichten Hypertonie. Internist 14: 313
200. Holzgreve H (1978) Hypertonie: Dunkelziffer verringern, Kooperation verbessern. Muench Med Wochenschr 13: 425
201. Holzgreve H, Middecke M (1979) Über die Behandlungsbedürftigkeit der Hypertonie im Alter. Nieren Hochdruck 4: 114

202. Holzgreve H (1980) Die Kooperation des Patienten bei der Hochdrucktherapie. Muench Med Wochenschr 122: 267
203. Hull DH, Wolthius RA, Cortese T, Longo MR, Triebwasser JH (1977) Borderline hypertension versus normotension: Differential response. Am Heart J 34: 414
204. Hultmann EL, Nilsson L (1974) Liver glycogen as a glucosesupplying source during exercise. In: Keul J (ed) Limiting factors of physical performance. Thieme, Stuttgart, p 179
205. Hypertension Detection and Follow-up Program Cooperative Groups. Five-year findings of the Hypertension Detection and Follow-up Program. I. Reduction on mortality of persons with high blood pressure including mild hypertension. JAMA 242: 2562
206. Hypertension Detection and Follow-up Program Cooperative Group. Five-year follow-up Program. II. Mortality by race, sex and age. JAMA 242: 2572
207. Irving MH, Britton BJ, Wood WG, Padgham C, Carruthers M (1974) Effects of adrenergic blockade on plasma catecholamines in exercise. Nature 248: 531
208. Irving GB, Kerr F, Ewing DJ, Kirbi BJ (1974) Value of prolonged recording of blood pressure in assessment of hypertension. Br Heart J 36: 859
209. Irving JB, Bruce R, Deronen T (1977) Variations and significance of systolic blood pressure during maximal exercise testing. Relation to severity of coronary artery disease and cardiac mortality. Am J Cardiol 39: 841
210. Jackson G, Pierscianowski TA, Mahon W, Condon J (1976) Inappropriate antihypertensive therapy in the elderly. Lancet 2: 317
211. Jahnecke J (1974) Risikofaktor Hypertonie. Mannheim
212. Johnson W, Grover J (1967) Hemodynamic and metabolic effects of physical training in four patients with essential hypertension. Can Med Ass J 96: 842
213. Jokl E, Ball M, Frankel L (1967) Ergometry, exercise and hypertension. In: Mellerowicz H, Hansen G (Hrsg) 2. Int Seminar für Ergometrie. Ergon
214. Jörgensen CR, Wang K, Gobel FL (1974) Effect of proprandol on myocardial oxygen consumption during static and dynamic exercise. Circulation 50: 1179
215. Julius S, Pascual AV, Sannerstedt R (1971) Relationship between cardial output and peripheral resistance in borderline hypertension. Circulation 43: 382
216. Julius S, Schork MA (1971) Borderline hypertension - a critical review. J Chron Dis 23: 723
217. Julius S, Esler M (1975) Autonomic nervous cardiovascular regulation in borderline hypertension. Am J Cardiol 36: 685
218. Julius S (1976) Abnormalities of autonomic nervous control in borderline hypertension. Schweiz Med Wochenschr 106: 1698
219. Julius St (1977) Classification of hypertension. Borderline hypertension: Epidemiologie and clinical implications. In: Genest J, Koiw E, Küchel O (eds) Hypertension. McGraw-Hill, New York, pp 9, 613
220. Julius St (1978) Clinical and physiological significance of borderline hypertension at youth. Pediatr Clin North Am 25: 35
221. Kain HK, Hinman AT, Sokolow M (1964) Arterial blood pressure measurements with a portable recorder in hypertensive patients. I. Variability and correlation with casual pressures. Circulation 30: 882
222. Kampffmeyer H, Conway I (1968) The antihypertensive and diuretic effects of amiloride and of its combination with hydrochlorothiazide. Clin Pharmacol Ther 9: 350
223. Kannel WB, Widmer LK, Dawber TR (1965) Gefährdung durch coronare Herzkrankheit. Folgerungen für die Praxis aus 10 Jahren Framigham-Studie. Schweiz Med Wochenschr 95: 18
224. Kannel WB, Gordon T, Schwartz MJ (1971) Systolic versus diastolic blood pressure and risk of coronary disease. Am J Cardiol 27: 335
225. Kannel WB (1975) Role of blood pressure in cardiovascular disease: The Framigham study. Angiology 26: 1
226. Kannel WB, Sorlie P (1975) Hypertension in Framigham. In: Oglesby P (ed) Epidemiology and control of hypertension. Thieme, Stuttgart, p 553
227. Karlefors T, Nilsen R, Westling H (1966) On the accuracy of indirect auscultatory blood pressure measurement during exercise. Acta Med Scand 180: 81
228. Kellaway GSM (1976) Adverse drug reactions during treatment of hypertension, Drugs [Suppl 1] 11: 91

229. Kellermann JI, Ben-Ari E, Chaquet M, Lapidot C, Drory Y, Fisman E (1977) Cardiocirculatory response to different typs of training in patients with angina pectoris. Cardiology 62: 218
230. Kennedy PGE, Hoffbrand BJ (1978) Strokes and hypertension: contribution of poor blood pressure control. Br Med J 2: 1605
231. Kilpatrick JA (1948) The variation of casual, basal and supplemental blood pressure in health and in essential hypertension. Br Heart J 10: 48
232. Kindler J, Schulz V, Sieberth HG, Gross R (1978) Dauerbehandlung der Hypertonie. Dtsch Ärztebl 49: 2971
233. Kirchhoff H-W, Beckmann P (1965) Regulationsstörungen des Herzens und Kreislaufs. München
234. Kirchhoff H-W (1967) Körperliche Aktivität in der Behandlung des Hochdrucks. Ärztl Prax 19: 1733
235. Kitamura K, Jörgensen CR, Göbel F (1972) Hemodynamic correlates of myocardial oxygen consumption during upright exercise. J Appl Physiol 32: 516
236. Klein W (1980) Moderne Hypertoniebehandlung bei älteren Menschen. Aktuel Gerontol 10: 21
237. Kleinhanss G, Jürgel S, Passmann (1971) Zum Aussagewert indirekter Blutdruckbestimmungen in Ruhe und bei Kreislaufbelastungen durch Ergometerarbeit. Z Kreislaufforsch 60: 136
238. Knauf H (1969) Die Wirkung der Betarezeptorenhemmstoffe auf die Durchblutung des arbeitenden Skelettmuskels. Z Kreislaufforsch 58: 749
239. Koch G (1977) Plasma renin activity, epinephrine and norephephrine at rest and during exercise in young adults and boys. Scand J Clin Lab Invest [Suppl] 147: 37, 107
240. Koch G (1978) Plasma catecholamines and plasma renin activity during submaximal and nearmaximal exercise in normotensive adolescents and adults, and in hypertensive patients (Abstr). Fifth Scientific Meeting of the International Society of Hypertension, p 140
241. Koch G, Johansson U, Arvidsson E (1980) Determination of epinephrine, norepinephrine and dopamine in 0,1 ml plasma samples. J Clin Chem Clin Biochem 18: 367
242. Koch-Weser J (1973) Correlation of pathophysiology and pharmacotherapy in primary hypertension. Am J Cardiol 32: 499
243. Koch-Weser J (1978) Arterial hypertension in old age. Herz 3: 235
244. König K, Reindell H, Steim H, Musshoff K (1959) Beitrag zur Hämodynamik hypertoner Regulationsstörungen. Z Kreislaufforsch 48: 923
245. König K, Gebhardt W, Ullmann HW, Reindell H (1968) Veränderungen des Herzvolumens sowie einiger wichtiger spiroergometrischer Parameter nach β-Rezeptoren-Blockade. Z Kreislaufforsch 57: 415
246. König K, Ruck H, Brusis O (1977) Der Effekt körperlichen Trainings im Rahmen der Frührehabilitation nach Herzinfarkt. Herz Kreislauf 4: 192
247. Koerker DJ, Goodner CJ, Toivola PTK, Gale CC, Ensink JW (1974) Adaption to fasting in baboon. I. Influence of feeding schedule. Am J Physiol 227: 520
248. Koerker DJ, Goodner CD, Chideckel EW, Ensink JW (1975) Adaption to fasting in baboon. II. Regulation of lipolysis early and late in fasting. Am J Physiol 229: 350
249. Kornhuber HH, Lison G (1981) Bluthochdruck, Übergewicht und Alter: Zur Frühbehandlung der Hypertonie. Dtsch Med Wochenschr 106: 1692
250. Kooperstein SI, Schifrin A, Leahy TJ (1962) Level of initial blood pressure and subsequent development of essential hypertension. Am J Cardiol 10: 416
251. Korofkov NS (1905) K vopruso o metodakh issledonaniya krovianogo davleniya. Izo Voenno Med Akad 11: 365
252. Kotler MN, Bermann L, Rubenstein AH (1966) Hypoglycaemia precipitaded by Propranolol. Lancet 1: 1389
253. Krönig B, Moergel K, Jakob H, Graulich M, Jahnecke J (1973) Blutdrucktelemetrie-Untersuchungen zum Vergleich von Basis- und Entspannungsblutdruck bei Hochdruckkranken. Verh Dtsch Ges Inn Med 79: 781
254. Krönig B, Dufey K, Moergel K, Michaelis J, Jahnecke J (1974) Telemetrische Untersuchungen zur Wertigkeit eines Basalblutdruckes bei Hochdruckkranken. Klin Wochenschr 52: 809
255. Krönig B, Dufey K, Meuter K, Wolff HP, Knappen F (1976) Ausmaß des Belastungsblutdruckes bei 40–65jährigen Blutdruckgesunden, an behandelten und unbehandelten Hochdruckkranken. Verh Dtsch Ges Inn Med 82: 1278

256. Krönig B (1977) Spezielle Aspekte der Blutdruckvariabilität Hochdruckkranker, Autoreferateband 43. Jahrestagung Dtsch Ges Kreislaufforsch 67
257. Krönig B (1978) Die Beurteilung der Blutdruckmessung zur Diagnose und Therapiekontrolle der Hypertoniker. Muench Med Wochenschr 13: 43
258. Krönig B (1981) Blutdruckvariabilität bei Hochdruckkranken - Ergebnisse telemetrischer Langzeitmessungen. In: Franz I-W (Hrsg) Belastungsblutdruck bei Hochdruckkranken. Springer, Berlin Heidelberg New York, S 23
259. Krönig B (1976) Blutdruckvariabilität bei Hochdruckkranken. Hüthig, Heidelberg
260. Kubicek F (1973) Der Einsatz der Ergometrie in der Beurteilung der kardiovaskulären Arbeitskapazität. Wien Klin Wochenschr 19: 1
261. Kuchel O (1977) Autonomic nervous system in hypertension: Clinical aspects. In: Gevest I, Koiw E, Kuchel O (eds) Hypertension - physiopathology and treatment. McGraw Hill, New York
262. Lake BJ (1982) Arterial pressures and dynamic exercise. Colloquium at the University of New England Armidale, August 1982
263. Lambert D (1974) Hypertension and myocardial infarction. Br Med J 3: 685
264. Lassvik C (1978) Reproducibility of work performance and serial exercises in patients with angina pectoris. Scand J clin Lab Invest 38: 747
265. Laughlin KD, Fisher L, Sherrad DJ (1980) Blood pressure reductions during self-recording of home blood pressure. Am Heart J 98: 629
266. Leary WP (1974) The cardioselectivity of acebutolol in man. Clin Trials J 11: 33
267. Lehtonen A, Viikari J (1979) Longterm effects of soltalol on serum lipids. Clin Sci 57: 405_s
268. Leibel B, Kobrin I, Ben-Ishay D (1982) Exercise testing in assessment of hypertension. Br Med J 285: 1535
269. Lew EA (1967) Blood pressure and mortality. Life insurance experience. In: Stanley J, Stamler R, Pullmann TN (eds) The epidemiology of hypertension. Grune & Stratton, New York, p 392
270. Linss G, Böthig S (1974) Normotonie oder Hypertonie? Dtsch Gesundheitswes 29: 635
271. Linzbach AJ, Boateng EA (1979) Das Herz im Alter. Mat Med Nordm 31: 140
272. Littler WA, Honour AJ, Pugsley DJ, Sleight P (1975) Continuous recording of direct arterial pressure in untreated patients: its role in the diagnosis and management of high blood pressure. Circulation 51: 1101
273. Littler WA, Watson RDS (1978) Circulation variation in blood pressure. Lancet I: 995
274. Löllgen H (1983) Zur Bedeutung der Tretgeschwindigkeit in der Ergometrie. In: Mellerowicz H, Franz I-W (Hrsg) Ergometrie: Kalibrierung, Standardisierung, Methodik. Perimed, Erlangen p 46
275. Lorimer AR, Barbour MP, Comerfeld MB, Lawrie DV (1982) Assessment of blood pressure responses in hypertension to isometric and varying form of dynamic exercise, and their modification by treatment. Abstract Ninth Scientific Meeting of the International Society of Hypertension. Mexico City
276. Lüderitz B (1978) Beta-Rezeptorenblocker bei kardialen Rhythmusstörungen. Internist 19: 532
277. Lund-Johansen P (1981) Hämodynamik bei der essentiellen Hypertonie in Ruhe und während Ergometrie und deren Beeinflussung durch Diuretika, β-Rezeptorenblocker und Vasodilatatoren. In: Franz I-W (Hrsg) Belastungsblutdruck bei Hochdruckkranken. Springer, Berlin Heidelberg New York S 107
278. Lund-Johansen P (1967) Hemodynamics in early essential hypertension. Acta Med Scand [Suppl 482] 183: 1
279. Lund-Johansen P (1970) Hemodynamic changes in long-term diuretic therapy of essential hypertension. Acta Med Scand 187: 509
280. Lund-Johansen P (1974) Hemodynamic changes at rest and during exercise in long-term therapy of essential hypertension. Acta Med Scand 195: 177
281. Lund-Johansen P, Ohm OI (1976) Hemodynamic long-term effects of β-receptor blocking agents in hypertension: Comparison between alprenolol, atenolol and timolol. Clin Sci Mol Med 51: 481
282. Lund-Johansen P (1976) Hemodynamic effects of clonidine in man. In: Onesti G, Fernandes M, Kim KE (eds) Regulation of blood pressure by the central nervous system. Grune & Stratton, New York

283. Lund-Johansen P (1976) Haemodynamic long-term effects of timolol at rest and during exercise in essential hypertension. Acta Med Scand 199: 263
284. Malek I, Waagstein F, Hjalmarson A, Holmberg S (1978) Hemodynamic effects of the cardioselective β-blocking agent metoprolol in acute myocardial infarction. Acta Med Scand 204: 195
285. Mallion JM, Debru JL, Avezon F, Cau G, Mueller JM (1975) Intérêt de l'étude à l'effort chez le normotendu et chez l'hypertendu des chiffres de la pression artérielle. Arch Mal Coeur 68: 1001
286. Management Committee (1980) The Australian therapeutic trial in mild hypertension. Lancet 6: 1261
287. Management Committee of the Australian Therapeutic Trial in Mild Hypertension (1982) Untreated mild hypertension. Lancet II, 185
288. Mancia G, Ferrari A, Bertinieri G, Grassi G, Zanchetti A (1982) Blood pressure rises associated with the cuff measurement procedure in hypertension. Abstract Ninth Scientific Meeting of the International Society of Hypertension, Mexico City
289. Mann S, Millar-Craig MW, Altmann DG, Melville D, Raftery EB (1979) The effects of metoprolol on ambulatory blood pressure. Clin Sci 57: 375
290. Matsumoto N, Whisnant JP, Kurland LT, Okazaki N (1973) Natural history of stroke in Rochester, Minnesota, 1955 through 1969: An extension of previous study, 1945 through 1954. Stroke 4: 20
291. Matthes D, Schütz P, Hüllemann K-D (1978) Unterschiede zwischen indirekt und direkt ermittelten Blutdruckwerten. Med Klin 11: 371
292. Matzdorff F (1975) Herzinfarkt, Prävention und Rehabilitation. Urban & Schwarzenberg, München Berlin Wien
293. Mayer S, Moran NC, Fain J (1961) The effect of adrenergic blocking agents on some metabolic actions of catecholamines. J Pharmacol Exp Ther 134: 8614
294. McAllister RG (1979) Effects of adrenergic receptor blockade on the responses to ergometric handgrip: Studies in normal and hypertensive subjects. J Cardiovasc Pharmacol 1: 253
295. McFate Smith W (1977) Treatment of mild hypertension. Results of a ten-year intervention trial. Circ Res [Suppl 1] 40: 1
296. Meesmann W, Stöveken HJ, Billing CP (1968) Eine einfache Methode zur Bestimmung des Basisblutdrucks und deren Bedeutung für die Praxis. Lebensversicherungsmedizin 20: 118
297. Meesmann W, Stöveken HJ, Billing CP (1970) Die Bestimmung des Basisblutdrucks in der Praxis durch die Ermittlung des sogenannten Entspannungswertes. Dtsch Med Wochenschr 95: 734
298. Mellerowicz H (1956) Vergleichende Untersuchungen über das Ökonomieprinzip in Arbeit und Leistung des trainierten Kreislaufs und seine Bedeutung für die präventive und rehabilitative Medizin. Arch Kreislaufforsch 24: 70
299. Mellerowicz H, Roskamm H, Hettinger Th, Hollmann W, Klaus EJ, König K, Mies H, Reindell H, Stoboy E (1964) Vorschläge zur Standardisierung der ergometrischen Leistungsmessung. 2. Mitteilung. Z Kreislaufforsch 53: 856
300. Mellerowicz H (1979) Ergometrie. Urban & Schwarzenberg, München Wien Baltimore
301. Menard J, Bertagna X, N'Guyen PT, Degoulet P, Corwe P (1976) Rapid identification of patients with essential hypertension sensitive to acebutolol. Am J Med 60: 886
302. Metropolitan Life Insurance Company: Blood pressure: Insurance experience and its implications. New York, 1961
303. Miall WE, Bell RA, Lovell HG (1968) Relation between changes in blood pressure and weight. Br J Prev Soc Med 22: 73
304. Miall WE, Chinn S (1974) Screening for hypertension: Some epidemiological observations. Br Med J 7: 595
305. Middeke M, Burkhart A, Holzgreve H (1982) Blutdruckverhalten während dynamischer und isometrischer Belastungen unter antihypertensiver Langzeittherapie mit Beta-Rezeptorenblockern und Diuretika. Verh Dtsch Ges Inn Med 88: 737
306. Mocellin RJ, Rutenfranz (1970) Methodische Untersuchungen zur Bestimmung der körperlichen Leistungsfähigkeit (PWC_{170}) im Kindesalter. Z Kinderheilkd 108: 61
307. Moeller J, Heyden O (1959) Die labile Blutdrucksteigerung. Z Kreislaufforsch 48: 413

308. Mordasini R, Glück Z, Weichmann P, Keusch G, Meyer A, Riesen W (1980) Zur Pathogenese der Diuretikainduzierten Hyperlipoproteinämie. Klin Wochenschr 58: 359
309. Morgan T, Adam W, Carney S, Gibbard R, Brown S, Wheeler D (1979) Treatment of mild hypertension in elderly males. Clin Sci 57: 355_s
310. Morgenroth J, Maron BJ, Henry WL, Epstein SE (1975) Comparative left ventricular dimensions in trained athlets. Am Intern Med 82: 521
311. Moser L, Schmidt M, Lundt PV (1979) Die Wirkungen eines Beta-Rezeptorenblockers auf die Kraftfahreigenschaft. Med Klin 74: 1134
312. Muiesan G, Magnani B, Agabati-Rosei E, Alicandri C, Ambrosionie E, Miele N (1976) Evaluation of the effect of timolol alone and in combination with hydrochlorothiazide and amiloride in the treatment of mild to moderate arterial hypertension: a doubleblind controlled study. Clin Sci Mol Med 51: 529
313. Nagle FJ, Naughton J, Balke B (1966) Comparison of direct and indirect blood pressure with pressure flow dynamics during exercise. J Appl Physiol 21: 317
314. Nelson RR, Gobel FL, Jorgensen CR (1973) Hemodynamic predictors of myocardial oxygen consumption during static and dynamic exercise. Circulation 50: 1173
315. Nerem RM, Cornhill JF (1980) Hemodynamics and atherogenesis. Atherosclerosis 36: 151
316. Neuendörfer B, Kömof D, Marx P (1979) Risikofaktoren beim Hirninfarkt. Med Welt 49: 1837
317. Neus H, Schulte W, Friedrich G, Rüddel H, Schirmer G, Eiff AW von (1981) Relationship between blood pressure reactions on an ergometric and an emotional stress test. Klin Wochenschr 59: a47
318. Neus H, Eiff AW von, Friedrich G, Heusch G, Schulte W (1981) Das Problem der Adaptation in der klinisch-therapeutischen Hypertonieforschung. Dtsch Med Wochenschr 106: 622
319. Nüssel E (1977) Some new results from the epidemiological research in Heidelberg. World Health Organization meeting on comprehensive cardiovascular community control programs. Geneva
320. Nyberg G (1976) Effect of β-adrenoreceptor blockers on heart rate and blood pressure in dynamic and isometric exercise. Drugs [Suppl 1] 11: 185
321. O'Brien ET, McKinnon J (1972) Propranolol and polythiazide in treatment of hypertension. Br Heart J 34: 1042
322. Oliver MB, Kurien VA, Greenwood TW (1968) Relation between serum-free-fatty-acids and arrhythmias and death after acute myocardial infarction. Lancet 1: 710
323. Patyna WD (1981) Die Beeinflussung des Blutdruckverhaltens Hochdruckkranker während Ergometrie durch eine Reserpin-Diuretikum-Kombination und β-Rezeptorenblockade. In: Franz I-W (Hrsg) Belastungsblutdruck bei Hochdruckkranken. Springer, Berlin Heidelberg New York, S 139
324. Payen DM, Safar ME, Levenson JA, Totomokono JA, Weiss YA (1982) Prospective study of predictive factors determining borderline hypertensive individuals who develop subtained hypertension: Prognostic value of increased diastolic orthostatic blood pressure tilt-test response and subsequent weight gain. Am Heart J 103: 379
325. Peart WS (1976) The problems of morbidity and therapy in borderline hypertension. Schweiz Med Wochenschr 106: 1706
326. Perry HM (1982) Are we overdiagnosing mild hypertension? Abstract Ninth Scientific Meeting of the International Society of Hypertension. Mexico City
327. Philipp Th, Cordes U, Distler A (1977) Sympathetic responsiveness and antihypertensive effect of beta-receptor blockade in essential hypertension. Dtsch Med Wochenschr 102: 569
328. Philipp Th, Distler A, Cordes U (1978) Sympathetic nervous system and blood pressure control in essential hypertension. Lancet 11: 559
329. Philipp Th, Distler A (1979) Gefäßreagibilität unter Diuretika. Med Welt 26: 1015
330. Pickering TG, Harshfield GA, Kleinert HO, Blank S, Laragh JH (1982) Blood pressure during normal daily activities, sleep and exercise. JAMA 247, 992
331. Placheta Z, Novak A (1971) Einige Probleme der Funktionstests bei submaximaler Belastung. Med Sport 5: 153
332. Poliner LR, Dehmer GJ, Lewis SE, Parkey RW, Blomquist CG, Willerson JT (1980) Left ventricular performance in normal subjects: a comparison of the response to exercise in the upright and supine position. Cir 62: 123

333. Ponari O, Civardi E, Poti R (1972) Action of some betablockers on plasma fibrinolysis in vitro and in vivo in man. Arzneim Forsch 22: 629
334. Prachar H, Heller G, Jobst Ch, Kiss E, Nobis H, Spiel R, Enenkel W (1976) Zum koronaren Risiko bei Hypertonikern. Herz Kreisl 8: 174
335. Prachar H, Enenkel W, Nobis H, Ogis E (1979) Zur Wertigkeit verschiedener Untersuchungen bei der arteriellen Hypertonie. Wien Klin Wochenschr 91: 552
336. Prennschütz-Schützenau H, Baller D, Hellige G, Sigmund-Duchanova H, Vennebusch HJ (1977) Wirkungen von Isobiddinnitrat und Pindolol auf Herzdynamik, O_2-Verbrauch des Herzens und Koronarzirkulation bei alleiniger und kombinierter Applikation. Herz Kreisl 9: 217
337. Prichard BNC (1964) Hypotensive action of pronethalol. Br Med J 1: 1227
338. Prichard BNC (1977) Pressor responses to betaadrenergicblocking drugs. Lancet 1: 536
339. Pruett ED, Maehlum S (1973) Muscular exercise and metabolism in male juvenile diabetics. Energy metabolism during exercise. Scand J Clin Lab Invest 32: 139
340. Putzeys MR, Hoobler SW (1972) Comparison of clonidin and methyldopa on blood pressure and side effects in hypertensive patients. Am Heart J 83: 464
341. Pyörälä K, Mattila S, Leirisalo M, Taivonen S (1974) A new beta-adrenergic blocking drug, timolol maleate, in combination with hydrochlorothiazide in the treatment of arterial hypertension. In: Magnani B (ed) Beta-adrenergic blocking agents in the management of hypertension and angina pectoris. Raven, New York, p 59
342. Rabkin SW, Mathewson FAL, Tate RB (1978) Predicting risk of ischemic heart disease and cerebrovascular disease from systolic and diastolic blood pressures. Ann Intern Med 88: 342
343. Rasmussen S, Rasmussen K (1979) Influence of metoprolol, alone and in combination with a thiazid diuretic, on blood pressure, plasma volume, extracellular volume and glomerular filtration rate in essential hypertension. Eur J Clin Pharmacol 15: 305
344. Recklinghausen H von (1901) Über Blutdruckmessung beim Menschen. Arch Exp Pathol Pharmakol 46: 78
345. Reindell H, König K, Roskamm H (1967) Funktionsdiagnostik des gesunden und kranken Herzens. Schattauer, Stuttgart
346. Reisin E, Abel R, Modan M, Silverberg DS, Eliahon HE, Modan B (1978) Effect of weight loss without salt restriction on the reduction of blood pressure in oberweight hypertensive patients. N Engl Med 298: 1
347. Relman AS (1980) Mild hypertension: no more benign neglect. N Engl J Med 302: 293
348. Remington JW (1963) The physiology of the aorta and major arteries. In: Hamilton WF, Dow P (eds) Handbook of physiology, section 2, Circulation, vol II. American Physiological Society, Washington DC, p 799
349. Renner F, Haber P, Rainer P (1981) Ergebnisse elektrokardiographischer und ergometrischer Untersuchungen an 18jährigen männlichen Stellungspflichtigen. Z Kardiol 70: 495
350. Report of Medical Research Council Working Party on Mild to Moderate Hypertension (1981) Adverse reactions to bendrofluazide and propranolol for the treatment of mild hypertension. Lancet 9: 539
351. Reybrouck T, Amery A, Billiet L (1977) Hemodynamic response to graded exercise after chronic beta-adrenergic blockade. J Appl Physiol 42: 133
352. Richardson DW, Honour AJ, Fenton GW, Stoff FH, Pickering GW (1964) Variation in arterial pressure throughout the day and night. Clin Sci 26: 445
353. Ricci DR, Orlick AE, Cipriano PR, Guthaner DF, Harrison DC (1979) Altered adrenergic activity in coronary arterial spasm: Insight into mechanism based on study of coronary hemodynamics and the electrocardiogramm. Am J Cardiol 43: 1073
354. Richter-Heinrich E, Borys M, Sprung H, Läuter J (1971) Psychophysiologische Reaktionsprofile von Hypo- und Hypertonikern. Dtsch Gesundheitswes 26: 1481
355. Ritter G (1973) Neuere Ergebnisse über das Blutdruckverhalten junger Männer. Muench Med Wochenschr 115: 763
356. Riva-Rocci S (1896) Un nuova sigmomanometro. Gaz Med Torino 47: 981
357. Rizza RA, Cryer PE, Gerich JE (1979) Role of glucagon, catecholamines and growth hormone in human glucose counter regulation. J Clin Invest 64: 62, 71
358. Robinson SK (1973) Indentification of mild hypertension and some risk factors that influence prognosis. J Am Geriatr Soc 21: 379

359. Rosenman RH, Scholtz RI, Brand J (1976) A study of comparative blood pressure measures in prediciting risk of coronary heart disease. Circulation 54: 51
360. Rosenthal T, Holtzman E, Segal P (1980) The effect of chlortalidone on serum lipids and lipoproteins. Atherosclerosis 36: 111
361. Rost R, Hollmann W, Liesen H (1976) Körperliches Training mit Hochdruckpatienten, Ziele und Probleme. Herz Kreisl 2: 680
362. Rost R (1979) Kreislaufreaktion und -adaptation unter körperlicher Belastung. Osang, Bonn
363. Rowlands DB, Ireland MA, Stallard TJ, Glover DR, McLeay RAB, Watson RDS, Littler WA (1982) Assessment of left-ventricular mass and its response to antihypertensive treatment. Lancet II: 467
364. Sackett DL (1974) Screening for disease: cardiovascular disease. Lancet 2: 1189
365. Safar ME, Weiss YA, London GM, Frackowiak RF, Milliez PL (1974) Cardiolpulmonary blood volume in borderline hypertension. Clin Sci Mol Med 47: 153
366. Sannerstedt R (1966) Hemodynamic response to exercise in patients with arterial hypertension. Acta Med Scand [Suppl] 180: 458
367. Sannerstedt R (1969) Hemodynamic findings at rest and during exercise in mild arterial hypertension. Am J Med Sci 258: 70
368. Sannerstedt R (1975) Haemodynamic effects of adrenergic beta-receptor-blocking agents in arterial hypertension. In: Berglund G, Hansson L, Werkö L, Lindgren A (eds) Pathophysiology and management of arterial hypertension. Mölndal, p 194
369. Sarnoff S, Case JRB, Stainsky WN, Macruz R (1958) Hemodynamic determinants of oxygen consumption of the heart with special reference to the tension-time-index. Am J Physiol 192: 148
370. Schalch DS, Kipnis DM (1965) Abnormalities in carbohydrate tolerance associated with elevated plasma nonesterified fatty acids. J Clin Invest 44: 2010
371. Scheler F (1977) Warum Hochdrucktherapie? Therapiewoche 27: 7168
372. Schellong F, Heinemeier M (1933) Über die Kreislaufregulation in aufrechter Körperstellung und ihre Störungen. Z Ges Exp Med 89: 49
373. Schettler G (1979) Ist der Kampf gegen die Herz- und Gefäßkrankheiten zu gewinnen? Z Allg Med 55: 667
374. Schimert E (1965) Körperbelastung und Koronarerkrankungen. Muench Med Wochenschr 18: 894
375. Schneider KW (1962) Einfluß einer mäßigen körperlichen Belastung auf die wichtigen hämodynamischen Parameter des Hypertonikers. Verh Dtsch Ges Kreisl Forsch 28: 102
376. Schneider KW (1968) Pathogenese der Herzinsuffizienz bei Hypertonie. In: Reindell H, Keul J, Doll E (Hrsg) Herzinsuffizienz. Schattauer, Stuttgart, S 396
377. Schmidt HD, Hoppe H, Heidenreich L (1979) Direct effects of dopamine, orciprenaline and norepinephrine on the right and left ventricle of isolated canine hearts. Cardiology 64: 133
378. Schoknecht G, Thefeld W, Hoffmeister H (1980) Bluthochdruck, Übergewicht und Hypercholesterinämie - unabhängige Faktoren? Med Welt 31: 588
379. Schulte W (1981) Blutdruckreaktivität unter emotionalem Streß bei essentieller Hypertonie - pathophysiologische und diagnostische Aspekte. In: Franz I-W (Hrsg) Belastungsblutdruck bei Hochdruckkranken. Springer, Berlin Heidelberg New York, S 59
380. Schulte W, Neus H, Noffke HK, Eiff AW von (1978) Zur Problematik der Einteilung in Blutdruckgruppen aufgrund von Ruhemessungen. Verh Dtsch Ges Inn Med 84: 789
381. Schulte W, Neus H, Noffke H-K, Malsch B (1978) Zur Problematik der Hypertonieeinteilung nach klinischen Blutdruckwerten. Med Welt 43: 1669
382. Schulte W, Neus H (1979) Bedeutung von Streßreaktionen in der Hypertoniediagnostik. Herz Kreisl 11: 541
383. Schwalb H, Eberl J, Meier G (1970) Sauerstofftransportökonomie und Leistungsbreite des Kreislaufs in Beziehung zum Blutdruck bei Männern mittleren Lebensalters. Arch Kreisl Forsch 63: 78
384. Schwalb H (1974) Training bei Hypertonikern. In: Mellerowicz H, Weidener J, Jokl E (Hrsg) Rehabilitative Kardiologie. Karger, Basel, S 105
385. Seipel L, Breithardt G, Döhring HP (1977) Die Wirkung von Atenolol auf den Sinusknoten und die intrakardiale Erregungsleitung beim Menschen im Vergleich zu Propranolol. Z Kardiol 66: 719

386. Seliger V, Buchberger J, Pachlopnikova I (1968) Zur Untersuchungsmethodik der physischen Arbeitskapazität des Menschen. Teor Praxe Tel Vych 16: 730
387. Shaw DB, Holman RR, Gowers JI (1980) Survival in sinoatrial disorder. Br Med J 1: 139
388. Shekelle RB, Ostfeld AM, Klawans HL (1974) Hypertension and risk of stroke in an elderly population. Stroke 5: 71
389. Sheps DS, Ernst JC, Briese FW, Myerburg RJ (1979) Exercise-induced increase in diastolic pressure: Indicator of severe coronary artery disease. Am J Cardiol 43: 708
390. Simon H (1978) Herzwirksame Pharmaka. Urban & Schwarzenberg, München Wien Baltimore
391. Simon AC, Safar MA, Levenson JA, Kheder AM, Levy BT (1979) Systolic hypertension: hemodynamic mechanism and choice of antihypertensive treatment. Am J Cardiol 44: 505
392. Sinclair RG (1975) Hypertension. In: Hart CR (Hrsg) Screening in general practice. Edinburgh
393. Sivertson R, Andersson O, Hansson L (1979) Blood pressure reduction and vascular adaption. Acta Med Scand 205: 477
394. Smirk FH (1944) Casual and basal blood pressure. IV. Their relationship to the supplemental pressure with a note on statistical implications. Br Heart J 6: 176
395. Smithen CS, Balcon R, Sowton E (1971) Use of his potentials to assess changes in atrioventricular conduction produced by a series of beta-adrenergis blocking agents. Br Heart J 33: 995
396. Snedecor CW (1971) Statistical methods, 6th edn. Towa State University Press, Towa
397. Soltero I (1978) Trends in mortality from cerebrovascular diseases in the United States, 1960 to 1975. Stroke 9: 549
398. Sokolow M, Perloff D, Cowan R (1982) A 10-year prospective study of the incidence of cardiovascular events in hypertensive patients utilizing ambulatory blood pressure measurements. Abstract, Ninth Scientific Meeting of the International Society of Hypertension. Mexico City
399. Stamler J (1973) Epidemiology of coronary heart diseases. Med Clin North Am 57: 5
400. Stamler JSt, Farinario E, Mojounier LM, Haie Y, Moss D, Stamler R (1980) Prevention and control of hypertension by nutritional-hygienic means. JAMA 18: 1819
401. Stegemann J, Kenner T (1974) A theory on heart control by muscular metabolic receptors. Arch Kreislaufforsch 64: 185
402. Stein G (1981) The heart load of several kinds of sports in rehabilitation after heart infarction (Abstr) II. World Congress on Cardial Rehabilitation, Jerusalem
403. Steinmann B (1980) Physiologische Altersveränderungen als Risikofaktoren. Aktuel Gerontol 10: 149
404. Stephan E (1979) Kombination Schirmbild-Blutdruckmessung, Erfahrungen und Ergebnisse im Kanton Bern. Schweiz Med Wochenschr 109: 234
405. Stewart McDG (1976) Compared incidence of first myocardial infarction in hypertensive patients under treatment containing propranolol or excluding β-receptor-blockade. Clin Sci Mol Med 51: 509s
406. Stoker JB, Sreeharan N, Linden RJ, Barbour MP, Lorimer AR, Hillis WS, Lawrie TDV (1979) The effects of exercise in hypertension controlled with metoprolol or methyldopa. Clin Sci 57: 391_s
407. Strauer BE (1979) Das Hochdruckherz. Springer, Berlin Heidelberg New York
408. Strauss HC, Gilbert M, Svenson RH, Miller HC, Wallace AG (1976) Electrophysiological effects of propranolol on sinus node function in patients with sinus node dysfunction. Circulation 54: 452
409. Strong JP, Eggen DA, Oalmann MC (1972) The natural history, geographic, pathology and epidemiology of atherosclerosis. In: Wiss RW, Geer JC (eds) The pathogenesis of atherosclerosis. Williams & Wilkins, Baltimore, p 20
410. Studer A, Baumgärtner R, Siebenschein R, Satz N, Grimm J, Siegenthaler W, Vetter W (1980) Prävalenz der Hypertonie und Grenzwerthypertonie bei Studenten. Schweiz Med Wochenschr 110: 338
411. Sturm A, Schuster P (1977) Rehabilitation bei Hypertonie. Dtsch Med Wochenschr 102: 1732
412. Svärdsudd K, Berglund G, Tibblin G (1976) Morbidity and mortality in treated and untreated hypertension: results from the Göteborg 50-year-old men study. Drugs [Suppl] 1: 34
413. Svärdsudd K, Tibblin G (1979) Mortality and morbidity during 13,5 year's follow-up in relation to blood pressure. Acta Med Scand 205: 483
414. Tammen A-T, Bierck G, Fentrop Th, Blümchen G (1984) Prognostische Bedeutung des Bela-

stungsblutdrucks bei Herzinfarktpatienten. In: Anlauf M, Bock KD (eds) Blutdruck unter körperlicher Belastung. Steinkopff, Darmstadt, p 103
415. Tarazi RC, Dustan HP (1972) Beta adrenergic blockade in hypertension. Practical and theoretical implications of long-term hemodynamic variations. Am J Cardiol 29: 633
416. Taylor SH (1975) The circulation in hypertension. In: Burley DM, Birdwood GFB, Fryer JH, Taylor SH (eds) Hypertension - its nature and treatment. Metropolis, London, p 29
417. Taylor CB, Farguhar JW, Nelson B (1977) Relaxation therapy and high blood pressure. Arch Gen Psychiatr 34: 339
418. Thadani U, Parker JO (1979) Propranolol in angina pectoris. Duration of inproved exercise, tolerance and circulatory effects after acute oral administration. Am J Cardiol 44: 118
419. Thomas RD (1981) Ventricular fibrillation in myocardial infarction and hypokalaemia (Abstr). Symposium: Potassium, the Heart and Hypertension. Rome
420. Thulesius O (1974) Die Diagnose der orthostatischen Hypertonie anhand einfacher Kreislaufparameter. In: Dengler H-J (Hrsg) Das Orthostasesyndrom. Schattauer, Stuttgart New York, S 177
421. Tibblin G, Wilhelmsen L, Werkö L (1975) Risk factors for myocardial infarction and death due to ischemic heart disease and other causes. Am J Cardiol 35: 514
422. Trafford JAP, Horn CR, O'Neal H, McGonigk R, Halford-Maw L, Evans R (1981) Five year follow-up of effects of treatment of mild and moderate hypertension. Br Med J 282: 1111
423. Traub YM, Aygen MM, Rosenfeld JB (1979) Hazards in treatment of systolic hypertension. Am Heart J 2: 174
424. Trieb G, Nüsser E, Aschke HJ (1973) Untersuchungen der Blutdruckregulation bei essentieller Hypertonie unter Orthostasebelastung vor und nach Therapie. Herz Kreisl 5: 202
425. Turner GG, Nelson RR, Nordstrom LA, Diefenthal HC, Gobel FL (1978) Comperative effect of nadolol and propranolol on exercise tolerance in patients with angina pectoris. Br Heart J 12: 1361
426. Undeutsch K, Lang E (1976) Besonderheiten der Hochdruckkrankheit des alternden Menschen. Geriatrie 6: 284
427. United States Public Health Service Hospitals: Morbidity and mortality in mild essential hypertension. Circ Res [Suppl II] 30, 31: 110
428. Varnauskas B, Cramer G, Malmcrona R, Werkö L (1961) Effect of chlorothiazide on blood pressure and blood flow at rest and on exercise in patients with arterial hypertension. Clin Sci 20: 406
429. Vedin A, Wilhelmson C, Werkö L (1975) Chronic alprenolol treatment of patients with acute myocardial infarction after discharge from hospital. Acta Med Scand [Suppl] 575: 7
430. Veterans Administration Cooperative Study Group on Antihypertensive Agents: Effects of treatment on morbidity in hypertension: results in patients with diastolic blood pressure averaging 115 through 129 mm Hg. JAMA 202: 1028 (1967)
431. Veterans Administration Cooperative Study Group on Antihypertensive Agents. Effects of treatment on morbidity in hypertension. II Results in patients with diastolic blood pressure averaging 90 through 114 mm Hg. JAMA 213: 1143 (1970)
432. Veterans Administration Cooperative Study Group on Antihypertensive Agents. Effects of treatment on morbidity in hypertension. III Influence of age, diastolic pressure and priorcardiovascular disease; further analysis of side effects. Circulation 45: 991 (1972)
433. Veterans Administration Cooperative Study Group on Antihypertensive Agents: Effects of treatment on morbidity in hypertension. Circulation 51: 1107 (1975)
434. Von Eiff AW (1967) Essentielle Hypertonie. Klinik, Psychophysiologie und Psychopathologie. Thieme, Stuttgart
435. Von Eiff AW, Neus H, Schulte W (1978) Streßreagibilität als Charakteristikum von Blutdruckgruppen. Verh Dtsch Ges Inn Med 84: 792
436. Vorburger C (1977) Die antihypertensive Wirkung von Timololmaleat (Blocadren) in gestaffelter Kombination mit einem Diuretikum. Schweiz Med Wochenschr 106: 1474
437. Waagstein F, Hjalmarson A, Varnauskas B, Wallentin I (1975) Effects of chronic beta-adrenergic receptor blockade in congestive cardiomyopathie. Br Heart J 37: 1022
438. Waern U, Åberg H (1979) Blood pressure in 60-year-old men. Acta Med Scand 206: 99
439. Wahlund H (1948) Determination of the physical working capacity. Acta Med Scand [Suppl 215] 132: 1

440. Wagner G (1976) Hypertonie. Methodik und Ergebnisse einer Vorsorgeuntersuchung in einem chemischen Großbetrieb. BASF-Studie III. Schattauer, Stuttgart
441. Wald H, Guerney M, Stoff FH (1937) Some effects of alteration of posture on arterial blood pressure. Am Heart J 14: 319
442. Watson RDS, Stallard TJ, Littler WA (1979) Influence once-daily administration of β-adrenoceptor antagonists on arterial pressure and its variability. Lancet 6: 1210
443. Weber E, Gundert-Remy U, Schrey A (1977) Patienten Compliance. Witzstrock, Baden-Baden
444. Weidener J, Mellerowicz H (1970) Dosiertes Training bei hypertonen Kreislaufregulationsstörungen. Internist 11: 287
445. Weidmann P, Glück Z (1979) Grenzwert-Hypertonie. Schweiz Med Wochenschr 109: 417
446. Wessels F, Heinze A, Werth HW (1977) Antihypertensive therapy with a new β-blocking agent timolol. Double blind study and comparison with aprenolol and pindolol. Med Klin 72: 1689
447. Wilson L, Meyer B, Albury J (1979) Early prediction of hypertension using exercise blood pressures. Med Sci Sports 11: 110
448. Wirtzfeld A, Klein G, Delius W, Sack D (1978) Behandlung des akuten Myokardinfarktes mit Metoprolol. Dtsch Med Wochenschr 103: 566
449. Wolff G (1978) Bluthochdruck - die Pest unserer Zeit. Mod Med 2: 87
450. Wollheim E (1975) 50 Jahre Hochdruckforschung, Probleme und Ergebnisse. Vortrag anläßlich der 1. Mitgliederversammlung der Deutschen Liga zur Bekämpfung des hohen Blutdruckes, Bonn
451. World Health Organization (1959) Hypertension and coronary heart disease: classification and criteria for epidemiological studies. Technical Report series No 168
452. World Health Organization: Arterial hypertension and ischaemic heart disease. Technical Report series No 231 (1962)
453. Zerzawy R, Bachmann K, Fleischer H (1976) Telemetrische Untersuchungen der Herz- und Kreislaufbelastung auf einem Trimmpfad. Dtsch Med Wochenschr 17: 664
454. Zerzawy R, Reis A, Bachmann K (1977) Belastungshypertonie bei Hochdruckkranken und Grenzwerthypertonikern. Autoreferateband 43, Jahrestagung. Dtsch Ges Kreislaufforsch 112
455. Zerzawy R (1981) Belastungshypertonie bei stabiler und grenzwertiger Hypertonie - Vergleich geistiger, isometrischer und dynamischer Belastungen. In: Franz I-W (Hrsg) Belastungsblutdruck bei Hochdruckkranken. Springer, Berlin Heidelberg New York, S 49
456. Zerzawy R (1981) Telemetrie von arteriellem Druck und Herzfrequenz unter alltäglichen und sportlichen Belastungen im Vergleich zur Fahrradergometrie. In: Franz I-W (Hrsg) Belastungsblutdruck bei Hochdruckkranken. Springer, Berlin Heidelberg New York, S 161

Subject Index

GPSR Compliance

The European Union's (EU) General Product Safety Regulation (GPSR) is a set of rules that requires consumer products to be safe and our obligations to ensure this.

If you have any concerns about our products, you can contact us on ProductSafety@springernature.com

In case Publisher is established outside the EU, the EU authorized representative is:

Springer Nature Customer Service Center GmbH
Europaplatz 3
69115 Heidelberg, Germany

Batch number: 10620881

Printed by Printforce, the Netherlands